W9-ARF-016

Infant & Toddler Health Sourcebook

Infectious Diseases Sourcebook

Injury & Trauma Sourcebook

Learning Disabilities Sourcebook,
2nd Edition

Leukemia Sourcebook

Liver Disorders Sourcebook

Lung Disorders Sourcebook

Medical Tests Sourcebook, 2nd Edition

Men's Health Concerns Sourcebook,
2nd Edition

Mental Health Disorders Sourcebook,
3rd Edition

Mental Retardation Sourcebook

Movement Disorders Sourcebook

Muscular Dystrophy Sourcebook

Obesity Sourcebook

Osteoporosis Sourcebook

Pain Sourcebook, 2nd Edition

Pediatric Cancer Sourcebook

Physical & Mental Issues in Aging
Sourcebook

Podiatry Sourcebook, 2nd Edition

Pregnancy & Birth Sourcebook,
2nd Edition

Prostate Cancer Sourcebook

Prostate & Urological Disorders
Sourcebook

Public Health Sourcebook

Reconstructive & Cosmetic Surgery
Sourcebook

Rehabilitation Sourcebook

Respiratory Diseases & Disorders
Sourcebook

Sexually Transmitted Diseases
Sourcebook, 3rd Edition

Sleep Disorders Sourcebook,
2nd Edition

Smoking Concerns Sourcebook

Sports Injuries Sourcebook, 2nd Edition

Stress-Related Disorders Sourcebook

Stroke Sourcebook

Substance Abuse Sourcebook

Surgery Sourcebook

Thyroid Disorders Sourcebook

Transplantation Sourcebook

Traveler's Health Sourcebook

Urinary Tract & Kidney Diseases &
Disorders Sourcebook, 2nd Edition

Vegetarian Sourcebook

Women's Health Concerns Sourcebook,
2nd Edition

Workplace Health & Safety Sourcebook

Worldwide Health Sourcebook

Teen Health Series

Alcohol Information for Teens

Allergy Information for Teens

Asthma Information for Teens

Cancer Information for Teens

Complementary & Alternative
Medicine Information for
Teens

Diabetes Information for Teens

Diet Information for Teens,
2nd Edition

Drug Information for Teens,
2nd Edition

Eating Disorders Information
for Teens

Fitness Information for Teens

Learning Disabilities Information
for Teens

Mental Health Information for
Teens, 2nd Edition

Sexual Health Information for
Teens

Skin Health Information for
Teens

Sports Injuries Information
for Teens

Suicide Information for Teens

Tobacco Information for Teens

Congenital Disorders
SOURCEBOOK

Second Edition

Health Reference Series

Second Edition

Congenital Disorders
SOURCEBOOK

*Basic Consumer Health Information about
Nonhereditary Birth Defects and Disorders Related to
Prematurity, Gestational Injuries, Congenital Infections,
and Birth Complications, Including Heart Defects,
Hydrocephalus, Spina Bifida, Cleft Lip and Palate,
Cerebral Palsy, and More*

*Along with Facts about the Prevention of Birth Defects,
Fetal Surgery and Other Treatment Options, Research
Initiatives, a Glossary of Related Terms, and Resources
for Additional Information and Support*

Edited by
Sandra J. Judd

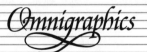

615 Griswold Street • Detroit, MI 48226

Bibliographic Note

Because this page cannot legibly accommodate all the copyright notices, the Bibliographic Note portion of the Preface constitutes an extension of the copyright notice.

Edited by Sandra J. Judd

Health Reference Series

Karen Bellenir, *Managing Editor*
David A. Cooke, M.D., *Medical Consultant*
Elizabeth Collins, *Research and Permissions Coordinator*
Cherry Stockdale, *Permissions Assistant*
Laura Pleva Nielsen, *Index Editor*
EdIndex, Services for Publishers, *Indexers*

* * *

Omnigraphics, Inc.

Matthew P. Barbour, *Senior Vice President*
Kay Gill, *Vice President—Directories*
Kevin Hayes, *Operations Manager*
David P. Bianco, *Marketing Director*

* * *

Peter E. Ruffner, *Publisher*

Frederick G. Ruffner, Jr., *Chairman*

Copyright © 2007 Omnigraphics, Inc.

ISBN 978-0-7808-0945-1

Library of Congress Cataloging-in-Publication Data

Congenital disorders sourcebook : basic consumer health information about nonhereditary birth defects and disorders related to prematurity, gestational injuries, congenital infections, and birth complications, including heart defects, hydrocephalus, spina bifida, cleft lip and palate, cerebral palsy, and more; along with facts about the prevention of birth defects, fetal surgery and other treatment options, research initiatives, a glossary of related terms, and resources for additional information and support / edited by Sandra J. Judd. -- 2nd ed.
    p. cm. -- (Health reference series)
  Summary: "Provides basic consumer health information about nonhereditary birth defects and disorders. Includes index, glossary of related terms, and other resources"--Provided by publisher.
  Includes bibliographical references and index.
  ISBN 978-0-7808-0945-1 (hardcover : alk. paper) 1. Abnormalities, Human--Popular works. 2. Developmental disabilities--Popular works. I. Judd, Sandra J.
  RG626.C597 2007
  618.3'2--dc22

                                                                    2006037186

Table of Contents

Visit www.healthreferenceseries.com to view *A Contents Guide to the Health Reference Series*, a listing of more than 12,000 topics and the volumes in which they are covered.

Preface xiii

Part I: Prenatal Concerns and Preventing Birth Defects

Chapter 1—Birth Defects: An Overview 3

Chapter 2—Prenatal Care and the Prevention of
Birth Defects 11

    Section 2.1—Prenatal Care:
               What to Expect 12

    Section 2.2—Understanding
               Prenatal Tests 17

    Section 2.3—Pregnancy and a
               Healthy Diet 33

    Section 2.4—Folic Acid 39

Chapter 3—Smoking and Pregnancy 45

Chapter 4—Alcohol Use during Pregnancy 51

    Section 4.1—What You Should Know
               about Fetal Alcohol
               Syndrome 52

    Section 4.2—Alcohol in Pregnancy May
               Cause Permanent Fetal
               Nerve Damage 54

Section 4.3—Fetal Alcohol Spectrum
Disorders through the
Lifespan 56

Chapter 5—Illicit Drug Use during Pregnancy 61

Chapter 6—Pregnancy and Medication 67

Section 6.1—Medication Use during
Pregnancy: An Overview 68
Section 6.2—Risk of Birth Defects
with Accutane 72
Section 6.3—Risk of Birth Defects
with Angiotensin Converting
Enzyme (ACE) Inhibitors 77
Section 6.4—Risk of Birth Defects
with Paxil 78
Section 6.5—Risk of Birth Defects
with Thalidomide 80
Section 6.6—Vaccines and Pregnancy 82

Chapter 7—X-Rays, Pregnancy, and You 85

Chapter 8—Chemical and Other Environmental
Risks and Pregnancy 89

Chapter 9—Fetal Risks Associated with
Maternal Conditions 97

Section 9.1—Maternal Asthma...................... 98
Section 9.2—Maternal Cancer 101
Section 9.3—Maternal Diabetes 104
Section 9.4—Maternal High Blood
Pressure 113
Section 9.5—Maternal Obesity 119
Section 9.6—Maternal Phenylketonuria
(PKU) 121

Chapter 10—Fetal Risks Associated with
Infectious Diseases 127

Section 10.1—Chicken Pox and Pregnancy ... 128
Section 10.2—Fifth Disease and Pregnancy... 130
Section 10.3—Congenital Rubella 134
Section 10.4—Sexually Transmitted
Infections in Pregnancy........... 137

Section 10.5—Cytomegalovirus and
        Pregnancy 143
Section 10.6—Listeriosis and Pregnancy:
        What Is Your Risk? 147
Section 10.7—Toxoplasmosis and
        Pregnancy 150

Chapter 11—Rh Incompatibility 155

Chapter 12—Gestational Concerns 159

Section 12.1—Fetal Growth Restriction 160
Section 12.2—Amniotic Fluid
        Abnormalities 163
Section 12.3—Placental Conditions 171
Section 12.4—Umbilical Cord
        Abnormalities 177

Chapter 13—Fetal Surgery and Other Fetal
Treatment Techniques 183

Part II: Prematurity and Other Birth Complications

Chapter 14—Premature Labor and Delivery 191

Section 14.1—Premature Labor 192
Section 14.2—Premature Birth
        Complications 196
Section 14.3—What to Expect in the
        Neonatal Intensive
        Care Unit 200

Chapter 15—Medical Complications of Prematurity 205

Section 15.1—Apnea of Prematurity 206
Section 15.2—Bronchopulmonary
        Dysplasia 210
Section 15.3—Retinopathy of Prematurity 215

Chapter 16—Multiple Births 221

Section 16.1—Preparing for Twins,
        Triplets, and More 222
Section 16.2—Twin Pregnancy
        Complications 228
Section 16.3—Fetal Surgery for Twin-Twin
        Transfusion Syndrome 232

Section 16.4—High Order Multiples:
    Special Concerns 236

Chapter 17—Birth Complications Associated with
Birth Defects 245

    Section 17.1—Cesarean Childbirth:
    Why and How It Is
    Performed 246
    Section 17.2—What to Expect in
    Labor and Delivery
    When Your Baby Has
    a Health Problem 249

Chapter 18—Medical Evaluations for the Newborn 253

    Section 18.1—Apgar Score 254
    Section 18.2—Newborn Screening Tests 256

Chapter 19—Perinatal Infections 259

    Section 19.1—Group B Streptococcal
    Disease and Neonatal Risks ... 260
    Section 19.2—Hepatitis B: Mother to
    Newborn Infection 266

Chapter 20—What to Expect When Your Baby
Has a Birth Defect 269

Part III: Structural Abnormalities and Functional Impairments

Chapter 21—Cardiovascular Defects 275

    Section 21.1—Diagnosing Congenital
    Heart Defects with Fetal
    Echocardiography 276
    Section 21.2—Defects of the Heart and
    Blood Vessels 279
    Section 21.3—Patent Foramen Ovale 290
    Section 21.4—Arteriovenous
    Malformation 294
    Section 21.5—Persistent Pulmonary
    Hypertension of the
    Newborn 305
    Section 21.6—Vascular Rings 311

Chapter 22—Congenital Brain Defects 315

    Section 22.1—Hydrocephalus 316
    Section 22.2—Other Cephalic Disorders 322
    Section 22.3—Agenesis of the Corpus
                       Callosum 333
    Section 22.4—Chiari Malformation 334
    Section 22.5—Craniosynostosis 336
    Section 22.6—Dandy-Walker Syndrome........ 337

Chapter 23—Craniofacial Defects 339

    Section 23.1—Cleft Lip and Palate 340
    Section 23.2—Facial Palsy 347
    Section 23.3—Goldenhar Syndrome.............. 351
    Section 23.4—Hemifacial Microsomia 353
    Section 23.5—Microtia 355
    Section 23.6—Pierre Robin Sequence 357

Chapter 24—Cerebral Palsy 359

    Section 24.1—What You Should Know
                       about Cerebral Palsy............... 360
    Section 24.2—Botox in the Management
                       of Children with Cerebral
                       Palsy 384
    Section 24.3—Hyperbaric Oxygen
                       Therapy for Cerebral
                       Palsy 386
    Section 24.4—Hypothermia in the
                       Prevention of Cerebral
                       Palsy among Newborn
                       Infants 391

Chapter 25—Spina Bifida 395

    Section 25.1—What You Should Know
                       about Spina Bifida 396
    Section 25.2—Urinary Tract Concerns in
                       Spina Bifida 403
    Section 25.3—Latex Allergy in
                       Spina Bifida 405
    Section 25.4—Fetal Surgery for
                       Spina Bifida 407
    Section 25.5—Tethering Spinal Cord............ 409

Chapter 26—Congenital Lung Lesions 415

Chapter 27—Defects of the Liver and Pancreas 421

    Section 27.1—Annular Pancreas 422
    Section 27.2—Pancreas Divisum 424
    Section 27.3—Biliary Atresia 425

Chapter 28—Defects of the Upper Gastrointestinal Tract 429

    Section 28.1—Esophageal Atresia and
                Tracheoesophageal Fistula 430
    Section 28.2—Congenital Diaphragmatic
                Hernia....................................... 432
    Section 28.3—Fetal Surgery for
                Congenital Diaphragmatic
                Hernia....................................... 435
    Section 28.4—Gastroschisis 437
    Section 28.5—Omphalocele 441

Chapter 29—Defects of the Lower Gastrointestinal Tract 447

    Section 29.1—Bowel Obstruction 448
    Section 29.2—Intestinal Malrotation 450
    Section 29.3—Hirschsprung Disease 454
    Section 29.4—Imperforate Anus.................... 462

Chapter 30—Kidney Defects 465

    Section 30.1—Ectopic Kidneys 466
    Section 30.2—Hydronephrosis 468
    Section 30.3—Multicystic Dysplastic
                Kidney...................................... 470
    Section 30.4—Renal Fusion (Horseshoe
                Kidney) 471
    Section 30.5—Detecting Kidney and
                Urinary Tract Abnormalities
                before Birth 473

Chapter 31—Defects of the Urinary Tract 477

    Section 31.1—Urinary Tract Obstruction 478
    Section 31.2—Fetal Surgery for
                Obstructive Uropathy.............. 480
    Section 31.3—Bladder Exstrophy.................... 484
    Section 31.4—Epispadias 487
    Section 31.5—Ectopic Ureter 489
    Section 31.6—Megaureter 494
    Section 31.7—Ureterocele 498

Section 31.8—Vesicoureteral Reflux 502
Section 31.9—Urachal Anomalies 504

Chapter 32—Defects of the Reproductive Organs 509

Section 32.1—Undescended Testes 510
Section 32.2—Hypospadias 512
Section 32.3—Hydroceles and Inguinal
                    Hernias 514
Section 32.4—Urogenital Sinus 517
Section 32.5—Vaginal Agenesis 519
Section 32.6—Cloacal Exstrophy 523
Section 32.7—Ambiguous Genitalia 525

Chapter 33—Musculoskeletal Defects 531

Section 33.1—Arthrogryposis 532
Section 33.2—Clubfoot 534
Section 33.3—Congenital Amputation 542
Section 33.4—Congenital Torticollis 544
Section 33.5—Fibrous Dysplasia 546

Chapter 34—Fetal Tumors 549

Section 34.1—Cervical Teratoma 550
Section 34.2—Sacrococcygeal Teratoma 553
Section 34.3—Fetal Surgery for
                    Sacrococcygeal Teratoma 556

Chapter 35—Birthmarks 559

Part IV: Additional Help and Information

Chapter 36—Glossary of Terms Related to Congenital
                    Disorders 567

Chapter 37—Congenital Disorders: Resources for
                    Information and Support..................................... 579

Index **591**

Preface

About This Book

According to the March of Dimes, 150,000 U.S. babies—one in twenty-eight—are born each year with a birth defect. In fact, birth defects are the leading cause of death in the first year of life. Yet the future is brightening. Recent medical advances have allowed doctors to diagnose and treat some birth defects before birth, allowing affected children a much greater chance at survival. Additionally, advances in our understanding of the causes of birth defects allow prospective parents to take steps to minimize the chance that an infant will be born with these types of disorder.

Congenital Disorders Sourcebook, Second Edition, describes the most common types of nonhereditary birth defects and disorders related to prematurity, gestational injuries, congenital infections, and birth complications, including disorders of the heart, brain, gastrointestinal tract, musculoskeletal system, urinary tract, and reproductive organs. Cerebral palsy, spina bifida, and fetal alcohol syndrome and their related complications are also discussed in detail. Causes, diagnostic tests, and innovative treatment strategies, including fetal surgery, are explained, and current research initiatives are described. The book concludes with a glossary of related terms and a directory of resources for further help and information.

Readers seeking information about related topics may wish to consult other books in the *Health Reference Series*:

- *Breastfeeding Sourcebook* provides information about the benefits of breastfeeding, including in such special situations as multiple births and with infants who have special needs.

- *Infant and Toddler Health Sourcebook* describes the physical and mental development of newborns, infants, and toddlers.

- *Genetic Disorders Sourcebook, Third Edition* offers facts about chromosome abnormalities and disorders linked to mutations in specific genes.

- *Mental Retardation Sourcebook* includes detailed information about disorders that cause mental retardation, prevention strategies, and parenting issues.

- *Muscular Dystrophy Sourcebook* explains the causes, diagnosis, treatment, and management of congenital and other forms of muscular dystrophy.

- *Pregnancy and Birth Sourcebook, Second Edition* provides detailed information about prenatal care, physical changes during pregnancy, fetal development, labor, delivery, and the postpartum period.

How to Use This Book

This book is divided into parts and chapters. Parts focus on broad areas of interest. Chapters are devoted to single topics within a part.

Part I: Prenatal Concerns and Preventing Birth Defects begins with a look at prenatal care. It discusses the importance of a nutritious diet and explains the vital role folic acid plays in the prevention of neural tube defects. Exposure to substances in the environment that can be harmful to the developing fetus are also discussed. These include cigarette smoke, alcohol, medications, chemicals, and infectious diseases. Maternal conditions that can have adverse affects on the unborn baby and amniotic fluid, placental, and umbilical cord abnormalities are also described. The part concludes with a discussion of fetal surgery and other fetal treatment techniques.

Part II: Prematurity and Other Birth Complications provides a detailed look at the complexities associated with premature and multiple births.

It also describes labor and delivery complications commonly associated with the presence of birth defects. Apgar scoring and newborn screening tests are explained, and risks associated with perinatal infections are discussed.

Part III: Structural Abnormalities and Functional Impairments describes the causes, symptoms, diagnostic tests, treatment techniques, and research advances for different types of birth defects. These include spina bifida, cerebral palsy, fetal tumors, cardiovascular and brain defects, craniofacial defects, and malformations of the urinary tract, reproductive organs, gastrointestinal tract, liver, pancreas, and musculoskeletal system.

Part IV: Additional Help and Information provides a glossary of terms related to congenital disorders and a directory of organizations able to provide additional help and support.

Bibliographic Note

This volume contains documents and excerpts from publications issued by the following U.S. government agencies: Agency for Healthcare Research and Quality (AHRQ); Center for the Evaluation of Risks to Human Reproduction (CERHR); Centers for Disease Control and Prevention (CDC); National Eye Institute (NEI); National Heart, Lung, and Blood Institute (NHLBI); National Institute of Child Health and Human Development (NICHD); National Institute of Dental and Craniofacial Research (NIDCR); National Institute of Diabetes and Digestive and Kidney Diseases (NIDDK); National Institute of Environmental Health Sciences (NIEHS); National Institute of Neurological Disorders and Stroke (NINDS); National Women's Health Information Center (NWHIC); U.S. Department of Agriculture (USDA); and U.S. Food and Drug Administration (FDA).

In addition, this volume contains copyrighted documents from the following organizations: A.D.A.M., Inc.; American College of Surgeons; American Academy of Orthopaedic Surgeons; American Heart Association; American Lung Association; American Pregnancy Association; American Society of Clinical Oncology; American Urological Association; Children's Craniofacial Association; Children's Hospital Boston; Children's Hospital of Philadelphia; Cincinnati Children's Hospital Medical Center; Cleveland Clinic; Donna D'Alessandro, M.D.; Fetal Treatment Center, University of California San Francisco; Fetal Treatment Program, Brown University; Gale Group; Hepatitis C Support Project; Institute for Fetal Health at Children's Memorial Hospital, Chicago; March of Dimes; Massachusetts Department of Public Health; Massachusetts Medical Society; National Craniofacial Association (FACES); National Infertility Association (RESOLVE); National Kidney Foundation; National Organization on Fetal Alcohol Syndrome; Nemours Foundation; Organization of Teratology Information Specialists; Shriners Hospitals for Children-Spokane; Shriners International Headquarters; Spina Bifida Association; Texas Pediatric Surgical Associates; United Cerebral Palsy; University of Missouri Children's Hospital; and Washington University in St. Louis-Program in Pediatric and Adolescent Gynecology.

Full citation information is provided on the first page of each chapter or section. Every effort has been made to secure all necessary rights to reprint the copyrighted material. If any omissions have been made, please contact Omnigraphics to make corrections for future editions.

Acknowledgements

Thanks go to the many organizations, agencies, and individuals who have contributed materials for this *Sourcebook* and to medical consultant Dr. David Cooke and document engineer Bruce Bellenir. Special thanks go to managing editor Karen Bellenir and permissions coordinator Liz Collins for their help and support.

About the Health Reference Series

The *Health Reference Series* is designed to provide basic medical information for patients, families, caregivers, and the general public. Each volume takes a particular topic and provides comprehensive coverage. This is especially important for people who may be dealing with a newly diagnosed disease or a chronic disorder in themselves or in a family member. People looking for preventive guidance, information about disease warning signs, medical statistics, and risk factors for health problems will also find answers to their questions in the *Health Reference Series*. The *Series*, however, is not intended to serve as a tool for diagnosing illness, in prescribing treatments, or as a substitute for the physician/patient relationship. All people concerned about medical symptoms or the possibility of disease are encouraged to seek professional care from an appropriate health care provider.

Locating Information within the Health Reference Series

The *Health Reference Series* contains a wealth of information about a wide variety of medical topics. Ensuring easy access to all the fact sheets, research reports, in-depth discussions, and other material contained within the individual books of the series remains one of our highest priorities. As the *Series* continues to grow in size and scope, however, locating the precise information needed by a reader may become more challenging.

A Contents Guide to the Health Reference Series was developed to direct readers to the specific volumes that address their concerns. It presents an extensive list of diseases, treatments, and other topics of general interest compiled from the Tables of Contents and major index headings. To access *A Contents Guide to the Health Reference Series*, visit www.healthreferenceseries.com.

Medical Consultant

Medical consultation services are provided to the *Health Reference Series* editors by David A. Cooke, M.D. Dr. Cooke is a graduate of Brandeis University, and he received his M.D. degree from the University of Michigan. He completed residency training at the University of Wisconsin Hospital and Clinics. He is board-certified in Internal Medicine. Dr. Cooke currently works as part of the University of Michigan Health System and practices in Ann Arbor, MI. In his free time, he enjoys writing, science fiction, and spending time with his family.

Our Advisory Board

We would like to thank the following board members for providing guidance to the development of this series:

Dr. Lynda Baker, Associate Professor of Library and Information Science, Wayne State University, Detroit, MI

Nancy Bulgarelli, William Beaumont Hospital Library, Royal Oak, MI

Karen Imarisio, Bloomfield Township Public Library, Bloomfield Township, MI

Karen Morgan, Mardigian Library, University of Michigan-Dearborn, Dearborn, MI

Rosemary Orlando, St. Clair Shores Public Library, St. Clair Shores, MI

Health Reference Series *Update Policy*

The inaugural book in the *Health Reference Series* was the first edition of *Cancer Sourcebook* published in 1989. Since then, the *Series* has been enthusiastically received by librarians and in the medical community. In order to maintain the standard of providing high-quality health information for the layperson the editorial staff at Omnigraphics felt it was necessary to implement a policy of updating volumes when warranted.

Medical researchers have been making tremendous strides, and it is the purpose of the *Health Reference Series* to stay current with the most recent advances. Each decision to update a volume is made on an individual basis. Some of the considerations include how much new information is available and the feedback we receive from people who use the books. If there is a topic you would like to see added to the update list, or an area of medical concern you feel has not been adequately addressed, please write to:

Editor
Health Reference Series
Omnigraphics, Inc.
615 Griswold Street
Detroit, MI 48226
E-mail: editorial@omnigraphics.com

Part One

Prenatal Concerns and Preventing Birth Defects

Chapter 1

Birth Defects: An Overview

About 120,000 babies (1 in 33) in the United States are born each year with birth defects.[1] A birth defect is an abnormality of structure, function, or metabolism (body chemistry) present at birth that results in physical or mental disabilities or death. Several thousand different birth defects have been identified. Birth defects are the leading cause of death in the first year of life.[2]

What causes birth defects?

Both genetic and environmental factors, or a combination of these factors, can cause birth defects. However, the causes of about 70 percent of birth defects are unknown.[1]

Single Gene Defects: In many cases, a single gene change can cause birth defects. Every human being has about 20,000 to 25,000 genes that determine traits like eye and hair color.[3] Genes also direct the growth and development of every part of our physical and biochemical systems. Genes are packaged into each of the forty-six chromosomes inside our cells.

Chromosomal Birth Defects: Abnormalities in the number or structure of chromosomes can cause many birth defects. Chromosomal abnormalities usually result from an error that occurred when an egg or sperm cell was developing. As a result of this error, a baby can be born with too many or too few chromosomes, or with one or more chromosomes that are broken or rearranged.

Environmental Factors: Environmental substances that can cause birth defects are called teratogens. These include alcohol, certain drugs/medications, infections, and certain chemicals.

Each year between one thousand and six thousand babies are born with fetal alcohol syndrome (FAS) in this country.[4] FAS is a pattern of mental and physical birth defects that is common in babies of mothers who drink heavily during pregnancy. Women who are pregnant or planning pregnancy should not drink any alcohol. Even moderate or light drinking during pregnancy may harm the baby.

Some drugs and medications can contribute to birth defects. For example, the acne drug isotretinoin (sold under the brand names Accutane, Amnesteem, Claravis, and Sotret) poses a high risk of serious birth defects. A woman who is pregnant or who could become pregnant should never use this drug. Illicit drugs such as cocaine also may pose a risk.

Certain infections can result in birth defects when a woman contracts them during pregnancy. About forty thousand babies a year (about 1 percent of all newborns in this country) are born with a viral infection called cytomegalovirus (CMV).[5] About one in ten infected babies develop serious disabilities, including mental retardation and loss of vision and hearing.[5] Pregnant women often get CMV from young children who have few or no symptoms.

Sexually transmitted infections in the mother also can endanger the fetus and newborn. For example, untreated syphilis can result in stillbirth, newborn death, or bone defects. About 412 babies were affected by congenital syphilis in 2002.[6]

Multi-Factorial Birth Defects: Some birth defects appear to be caused by a combination of one or more genes and environmental exposures. This is called "multi-factorial inheritance." In some cases, an individual may inherit one or more genes that make him more likely to have a birth defect if he is exposed to certain environmental substances (such as cigarette smoke). These individuals have a genetic predisposition to a birth defect. But if the individual is not exposed to the environmental substance before birth, he probably won't have the birth defect. Examples of multi-factorial birth defects are as follows:

- Cleft lip/palate (opening in the lip and/or roof of the mouth)
- Neural tube defects (serious birth defects of the brain and spinal cord, including spina bifida and anencephaly)
- Heart defects

What are the most common birth defects?

Cleft lip/palate and Down syndrome are among the most common birth defects in the United States.[7] About 6,800 babies are born with cleft lip/palate each year.[7] Cleft lip/palate can cause problems with eating, speech, and language. Some affected babies have a small cleft that can be corrected with one surgical procedure, while others have severe clefts and need multiple surgeries. About 5,500 babies are born each year with Down syndrome.[7]

About 1,900 babies are born with a serious heart defect called transposition of the great arteries each year.[7] Many more babies are born with other serious heart defects. While advances in surgery have dramatically improved the outlook for affected babies, heart defects remain the leading cause of birth defect-related infant deaths.[8] Health care providers usually do not know what causes a baby's heart to form abnormally, although both genetic and environmental factors play a role.

Spina bifida (open spine) occurs in about 1,300 babies each year.[9] Affected babies have varying degrees of paralysis and bladder and bowel problems. Both genetic and environmental factors (including insufficient amounts of a vitamin called folic acid) appear to play a role.

Other common birth defects include musculoskeletal defects (including arm and leg defects), gastrointestinal defects (including defects of the esophagus, stomach, and intestines), and eye defects.[7] These birth defects usually are multi-factorial.

What are birth defects of body chemistry?

In 2002, about 3,000 babies were born with disorders affecting body chemistry (metabolic disorders).[10] These disorders are not visible, but they can be harmful or even fatal.

Most disorders of body chemistry are recessive genetic diseases. These diseases result from the inability of cells to produce enzymes (proteins) needed to change certain chemicals into others, or to carry substances from one place to another.

Can birth defects be prevented?

There are a number of steps a woman can take to reduce her risk of having a baby with a birth defect. One important step is a preconception visit with her health care provider. During this visit, the provider can identify, and often treat, health conditions that can pose a risk in pregnancy, such as high blood pressure or diabetes. The provider can provide advice on lifestyle factors, such as quitting smoking and avoiding alcohol, and occupational exposures that can pose pregnancy risks. The provider also can make sure that any medications a woman takes are safe during pregnancy. All of these steps help prevent birth defects.

A preconception visit is especially crucial for women with chronic health conditions, like diabetes, high blood pressure, and epilepsy, which can affect pregnancy. For example, women with diabetes who have poor blood sugar control are several times more likely than women without diabetes to have a baby with a serious birth defect. However, if their blood sugar levels are well controlled starting before pregnancy, they are almost as likely to have a healthy baby as women without diabetes.[11]

At a preconception visit, the provider can check to see if a woman's vaccinations are up to date. If she is not immune to rubella and chickenpox, she should be vaccinated before pregnancy. With widespread childhood vaccination, rubella is now uncommon. However, if a pregnant woman comes down with the disease, it poses a high risk of birth defects. Chickenpox also can cause birth defects, though the risk is low. A woman should wait for one month after being vaccinated before trying to become pregnant.

The provider also will ask a woman about her health history, as well as that of her partner and her family. This may help the provider identify risk factors for birth defects or inherited genetic conditions. The provider may refer couples with risk factors to a genetic counselor. A genetic counselor can discuss the risks of birth defects in their children and arrange for blood tests (such as carrier tests), when needed.

All women who could become pregnant should take a daily multivitamin containing 400 micrograms of the B-vitamin folic acid. Studies show that taking this vitamin before and during early pregnancy reduces the risk of having a baby with neural tube defects (spina bifida and anencephaly). If a woman already has had a pregnancy affected by one of these birth defects, she should consult her provider before pregnancy about how much folic acid to take. Generally a higher dose,

4 milligrams, is recommended.[12] Women with diabetes or epilepsy or who are obese are at increased risk of these birth defects. They should ask their providers before pregnancy about whether they should take the larger dose of folic acid.

A woman who is pregnant or planning pregnancy should avoid drinking alcohol, smoking, and using drugs. All of these can cause birth defects and other pregnancy complications. She should not take any medication (prescription, over-the-counter, or herbal) without first checking with her health care provider. She should also avoid changing the cat's litter box or eating raw or undercooked meat. These are possible sources of an infection called toxoplasmosis that can cause birth defects.

Can some birth defects be diagnosed before birth?

Some birth defects can be diagnosed before birth using one or more prenatal tests, including ultrasound, amniocentesis, and chorionic villus sampling (CVS). Ultrasound can help diagnose structural birth defects, such as spina bifida, heart defects, and some urinary tract defects. Amniocentesis and CVS are used to diagnose or rule out chromosomal abnormalities, such as Down syndrome, and numerous genetic birth defects. Most women have screening tests (blood tests) to see if they are at increased risk of certain birth defects, including Down syndrome and spina bifida. These screening tests cannot diagnose a condition, but they can suggest that further diagnostic testing is needed.

Can birth defects be treated before birth?

A small percentage of couples learn through prenatal diagnosis that their baby has a birth defect. While this news can be devastating, prenatal diagnosis sometimes can improve the outlook for the baby. It is now possible to treat some birth defects before birth. For example, biotin dependence and methylmalonic academia (two life-threatening inherited disorders of body chemistry) have been diagnosed by amniocentesis and treated in the womb, resulting in the births of healthy babies.

Prenatal surgery has saved babies with urinary tract blockages and rare tumors of the lung. More than three hundred babies have undergone experimental prenatal surgery to repair spina bifida before birth.[13] Prenatal surgery poses a number of serious risks for mother and baby, including preterm birth. (The National Institutes of Health

7

is currently conducting a study through 2007 to compare the safety and effectiveness of surgery before and after birth for babies with spina bifida. For information contact www.spinabifidamoms.com.) Doctors also have saved babies with serious heart rhythm disturbances by treating the pregnant woman with medications.

However, even when a fetus has a condition for which prenatal treatment is not yet possible, prenatal diagnosis permits parents to prepare themselves emotionally, and to plan with their provider the safest timing, hospital facility, and method of delivery.

Couples who have had a baby with a birth defect, or who have a family history of birth defects, should consider consulting a genetic counselor. These health professionals help families understand what is known about the causes of a birth defect, and the chances of the birth defect recurring in another pregnancy. Genetic counselors can provide referrals to medical experts as well as to appropriate support groups in the community. The National Society of Genetic Counselors provides the names and contact information of genetic counselors.

References

1. Centers for Disease Control and Prevention (CDC). *Birth Defects: Frequently Asked Questions*. March 21, 2006.

2. Martin, J.A., et al. Annual Summary of Vital Statistics—2003. *Pediatrics*, 115, no. 3 (March 2005): 619–34.

3. National Institutes of Health (NIH). International Human Genome Sequencing Consortium Describes Finished Genome Sequence. *NIH News*, October 20, 2004.

4. Centers for Disease Control and Prevention (CDC). *Fetal Alcohol Information*. Updated 8/5/04.

5. American Academy of Pediatrics. Cytomegalovirus, in Pickering, L.K. (ed.), *Red Book: 2003 Report of the Committee on Infectious Diseases*, 26th edition. Elk Grove Village, IL: American Academy of Pediatrics, 2003, 259–62.

6. Centers for Disease Control and Prevention (CDC). *Syphilis: CDC Fact Sheet*. Accessed 6/7/05.

7. Centers for Disease Control and Prevention (CDC). Improved National Prevalence Estimates for 18 Selected Major Birth Defects—United States, 1999–2001. *Morbidity and Mortality Weekly Report*, 54 (51&52), January 6, 2006, 1301–5.

8. Kochanek, K.D., et al. Deaths: Final Data for 2002. *National Vital Statistics Reports*, 53, no. 5, October 12, 2004.

9. Centers for Disease Control and Prevention (CDC). Spina Bifida and Anencephaly Before and After Folic Acid Mandate—United States, 1995–1996 and 1999–2000. *Morbidity and Mortality Weekly Report*, 53, no. 17 (May 7, 2004): 362–65.

10. National Newborn Screening and Genetics Resource Center, published in General Accounting Office, *Newborn Screening: Characteristics of State Programs*. Washington, DC: U.S. General Accounting Office, 2003, publication GAO-03-449.

11. American College of Obstetricians and Gynecologists (ACOG). Pregestational Diabetes Mellitus. *ACOG Practice Bulletin* 60 (March 2005).

12. Centers for Disease Control and Prevention (CDC). *Folic Acid: Frequently Asked Questions*. Updated 9/25/03.

13. Bennett, K.A., et al. Fetal Surgery for Myelomeningocele, in Wyszynski, D. (ed.): *Neural Tube Defects: From Origin to Treatment*. New York: Oxford University Press, 2006, 217–30.

Chapter 2

Prenatal Care and the Prevention of Birth Defects

Chapter Contents

Section 2.1—Prenatal Care: What to Expect 12
Section 2.2—Understanding Prenatal Tests 17
Section 2.3—Pregnancy and a Healthy Diet 33
Section 2.4—Folic Acid 39

Section 2.1

Prenatal Care: What to Expect

Reprinted from "Prenatal Care," National Women's Health Information Center, U.S. Department of Health and Human Services, April 2006.

What is prenatal care?

Prenatal care is the health care you get while you are pregnant. Take care of yourself and your baby by doing the following:

- Get early prenatal care. If you know you're pregnant, or think you might be, call your doctor to schedule a visit.

- Get regular prenatal care. Your doctor will schedule you for many appointments over the course of your pregnancy. Don't miss any—they are all important.

- Follow your doctor's advice.

Why do I need prenatal care?

Prenatal care can help keep you and your baby healthy. Babies of mothers who do not get prenatal care are three times more likely to have a low birth weight and five times more likely to die than those born to mothers who do get care.

Doctors can spot health problems early when they see mothers regularly. This allows doctors to treat them early. Early treatment can cure many problems and prevent others. Regular health care is best for you and your baby.

I am thinking about getting pregnant. How can I take care of myself?

You should start taking care of yourself before you start trying to get pregnant. By staying active, eating right, and taking a multivitamin, you can help keep yourself and your baby healthy even before it is conceived. This will help you have a healthy pregnancy and lower your chances of having a baby born with a birth defect.

Here are some ways to take care of yourself before you get pregnant:

- Eat healthy foods, exercise regularly (thirty minutes per day most days of the week is best), and get enough rest and sleep. Talk to your doctor about what kinds of food and exercise are best for you.

- Get 400 micrograms (mcg) of folic acid (one of the B vitamins) every day. The best way to do this is to take a daily multivitamin with this amount of folic acid. Getting enough folic acid every day before you get pregnant and during early pregnancy can help prevent certain birth defects. Many breakfast cereals and other grain products are enriched with folic acid. But only some products contain 400 mcg of folic acid per serving. Always check the labels to be sure you're getting your daily dose.

- See your doctor for a complete checkup. Make sure that you've had all your shots, especially for rubella (German measles). Rubella can cause serious birth defects. Chickenpox can also be dangerous during pregnancy. If you've had chickenpox and rubella in the past, you should be immune to them. If not, talk to your doctor about the vaccines.

- Tell your doctor about any prescription or over-the-counter medicines (including herbal remedies) you are taking. Some medicines are not safe to take during pregnancy.

- Stop smoking cigarettes, drinking alcohol, or taking drugs. Ask your doctor for help. Members of your faith community, counselors, or friends can also give support.

I'm pregnant. What should I do or avoid for a healthy baby?

Some things you can do to take care of yourself and the precious life growing inside you include the following:

- Take a multivitamin or prenatal vitamin with 400 micrograms (mcg) of folic acid every day.

- Get early and regular prenatal care. Whether this is your first pregnancy or third, health care is extremely important. Your doctor will check to make sure you and the baby are healthy at each visit. If there are any problems, early action will help you and the baby.

- Eat a healthy diet that includes fruits, vegetables, grains, and calcium-rich foods. Choose foods low in saturated fat.

- Unless your doctor tells you not to, try to be active for thirty minutes, most days of the week. If you don't have much time, get your exercise in ten-minute segments, three times a day.

- If you smoke, drink alcohol, or use drugs, **stop!** These can cause long-term harm to your baby. Ask your doctor for help.

- Ask your doctor before taking any medicine. Some are not safe during pregnancy. Remember that even over-the-counter medicines and herbal products may cause side effects or other problems. So ask your doctor before taking these products too.

- Avoid hot tubs, saunas, and x-rays.

- If you have a cat, ask your doctor about toxoplasmosis. This infection is caused by a parasite sometimes found in cat feces. When left untreated toxoplasmosis can cause birth defects. Your doctor may suggest avoiding cat litter and working in garden areas used by cats.

- Don't eat uncooked or undercooked meats or fish.

- Stay away from chemicals like insecticides, solvents (like some cleaners or paint thinners), lead, and mercury. Not all products have pregnancy warnings on their labels. If you're unsure if a product is safe, ask your doctor before using it.

- Avoid or control caffeine in your diet. Pregnant women should have no more than two servings of caffeine per day. Remember that teas, sodas, and chocolate may contain caffeine.

- Stay active. Most women continue working through pregnancy. Few jobs are unsafe for pregnant women. But if you're worried about the safety of your job, talk with your doctor.

- Get informed. Read books, watch videos, go to a childbirth class, and talk with experienced moms.

- Ask your doctor about childbirth education classes for you and your partner. Classes can help you prepare for the birth of your baby.

I don't want to get pregnant right now. But should I still take folic acid every day?

Experts recommend that all women of childbearing age get 400 micrograms (mcg) of folic acid every day. Even women with very little chance of getting pregnant should get their daily dose of folic acid. This is because many pregnancies are not planned. Often women don't know they are pregnant for a number of weeks, and some birth defects happen during this very early part of pregnancy.

Taking 400 mcg of folic acid every day will help prevent some birth defects that happen in early pregnancy. If a woman doesn't start taking vitamins until the second or third month of pregnancy, it may be too late to prevent birth defects. Folic acid may also have other health benefits for women.

How often should I see my doctor during pregnancy?

Your doctor will give you a schedule of all the doctor's visits you should have while pregnant. As your pregnancy progresses, you'll see the doctor more often. Most experts suggest the following schedule:

- See your doctor about once each month for the first six months of pregnancy.
- See your doctor every two weeks during the seventh and eighth months of pregnancy.
- See your doctor every week after this until the baby is born.

If you are over thirty-five or your pregnancy is high risk because of health problems (like diabetes or high blood pressure), you'll probably see your doctor more often.

What happens during prenatal visits?

During the first prenatal visit, you can expect your doctor or nurse to do the following:

- ask about your health history, including diseases, operations, or prior pregnancies
- ask about your family's health history
- do a complete physical exam
- do a pelvic exam with a Pap test
- order tests of your blood and urine
- check your blood pressure, urine, height, and weight
- figure out your expected due date
- answer your questions

15

At the first visit, you should ask questions and discuss any issues related to your pregnancy. Find out all you can about how to stay healthy.

Later prenatal visits will probably be shorter. Your doctor will check on your health and make sure the baby is growing as expected. Most prenatal visits will include the following:

- checking the baby's heart rate
- checking your blood pressure
- checking your urine for signs of diabetes
- measuring your weight gain

While you're pregnant your doctor or midwife may suggest a number of laboratory tests, ultrasound exams, and other screening tests.

I am in my late thirties and I want to get pregnant. Should I do anything special?

As you age, you have an increasing chance of having a baby born with a birth defect. Yet most women in their late thirties and early forties have healthy babies. See your doctor regularly before you even start trying to get pregnant. He or she will be able to help you prepare your body for pregnancy. He or she will also be able to tell you about how age can affect pregnancy.

During your pregnancy, seeing your doctor regularly is very important. Because of your age, your doctor will probably suggest some additional tests to check on your baby's health.

More and more women are waiting until they are in their thirties and forties to have children. While many women of this age have no problems getting pregnant, fertility does decline with age. Women over forty who don't get pregnant after six months of trying should see their doctors for a fertility evaluation.

Experts define infertility as the inability to become pregnant after trying for one year. If you think you or your partner may be infertile, talk to your doctor. She or he will be able to suggest treatments such as drugs, surgery, or assisted reproductive technology.

Where can I go to get free or reduced-cost prenatal care?

Women in every state can get help to pay for medical care during their pregnancies. This prenatal care can help you have a healthy baby. Every state in the United States has a program to help. Programs give medical care, information, advice, and other services important for a healthy pregnancy.

To find out about the program in your state:

- Call 800-311-BABY (800-311-2229). This toll-free telephone number will connect you to the health department in your area code.

- For information in Spanish, call 800-504-7081.

- Call or contact your local health department.

Section 2.2

Understanding Prenatal Tests

Reprinted from "Prenatal Tests," This information was provided by KidsHealth, one of the largest resources online for medically reviewed health information written for parents, kids, and teens. For more articles like this one, visit www.KidsHealth.org, or www.TeensHealth.org. © 2005 The Nemours Center for Children's Health Media, a division of The Nemours Foundation.

Every parent-to-be hopes for a healthy baby. But these dreams often are accompanied by moments of worry. What if the baby has a serious or untreatable health problem? What would I do? Would it be my fault?

Concerns like these are completely natural. Fortunately, though, a wide array of prenatal tests for pregnant women can help to reassure them and keep them informed throughout their pregnancies.

Prenatal tests can serve a useful function in terms of identifying— and sometimes treating—health problems that could endanger both you and your unborn child. However, they do have limitations. As an expectant parent, it's important to take the time to educate yourself about these tests and to think about what you would do if a health problem is detected in either you or your baby.

Why Are Prenatal Tests Performed?

Prenatal tests can identify several different things:

- treatable health problems in the mother that can affect the baby's health
- characteristics of the baby, including size, sex, age, and placement in the uterus
- the chance that a baby has certain congenital, genetic, or chromosomal problems
- certain types of fetal abnormalities, including heart problems

The last two items on this list may seem the same, but there's a key difference. Some prenatal tests are screening tests and reveal only the possibility of a problem existing. Other prenatal tests are diagnostic, which means they can determine—with a fair degree of certainty—whether a fetus has a specific problem. In the interest of making the more specific determination, the screening test may be followed by a diagnostic test.

Prenatal testing is further complicated by the fact that approximately 250 birth defects can be diagnosed in a fetus—many more than can be treated or cured.

What Do Prenatal Tests Find?

Among other things, routine prenatal tests can determine key things about the mother's health:

- her blood type
- whether she has gestational diabetes
- her immunity to certain diseases
- whether she has a sexually transmitted disease (STD) or cervical cancer

All of these conditions can affect the health of the fetus.

Prenatal tests also can determine things about the fetus's health, including whether it's one of the 2 to 3 percent of babies in the United States that the American College of Obstetricians and Gynecologists (ACOG) says have major congenital birth defects. The different categories of defects screened by prenatal tests are as follows.

Dominant Gene Disorders

In dominant gene disorders, there's a 50-50 chance a child will inherit the gene from the affected parent and have the disorder. Dominant gene disorders include:

- **Achondroplasia:** a rare abnormality of the skeleton that causes a form of dwarfism.

- **Huntington disease**: a disease of the nervous system that causes a combination of mental deterioration and a movement disorder affecting people in their thirties and forties.

Recessive Gene Disorders

Because there are so many genes in each cell, everyone carries some abnormal genes, but most people don't have a defect because the normal gene overrules the abnormal recessive one. But if a fetus has a pair of abnormal recessive genes (one from each parent), the child will have the disorder. It's more likely for this to happen in children born to certain ethnic groups. Recessive gene disorders include:

- **Cystic fibrosis:** a disease most common among people of northern European descent that is life threatening and causes severe lung damage and nutritional deficiencies.

- **Sickle cell disease:** a disease most common among people of African descent in which red blood cells form a "sickle" shape (rather than the typical donut shape), which can get caught in blood vessels and cause damage to organs and tissues.

- **Tay-Sachs disease:** a disorder most common among people of European (Ashkenazi) Jewish descent that causes mental retardation, blindness, seizures, and death.

- **Beta thalassemia**: a disorder most common among people of Mediterranean descent that causes anemia.

X-Linked Disorders

These disorders are determined by genes on the X chromosome. The X and Y chromosomes are the chromosomes that determine sex. These disorders are much more common in boys because the pair of sex chromosomes in males contains only one X chromosome (the other is a Y chromosome). If the disease gene is present on the one X chromosome, the X-linked disease shows up because there's no other paired

19

gene to "overrule" the disease gene. One such X-linked disorder is hemophilia, which prevents the blood from clotting properly.

Chromosomal Disorders

Some chromosomal disorders are inherited but most are caused by a random error in the genetics of the egg or sperm. The chance of a child having these disorders increases with the age of the mother. For example, according to ACOG, 1 in 1,667 live babies born to twenty-year-olds have Down syndrome, which causes mental retardation and physical defects. That number changes to 1 in 378 for thirty-five-year-olds and 1 in 106 for forty-year-olds.

Multifactorial Disorders

This final category includes disorders that are caused by a mix of genetic and environmental factors. Their frequency varies from country to country, and some can be detected during pregnancy.

Multifactorial disorders include neural tube defects, which occur when the tube enclosing the spinal cord doesn't form properly. Neural tube defects, which often can be prevented by taking folic acid during the early part of pregnancy, include:

- **Spina bifida**: Also called "open spine," this defect happens when the lower part of the neural tube doesn't close during embryo development, leaving the spinal cord and nerve bundles exposed.

- **Anencephaly:** This defect occurs when the brain and head don't develop properly, and the top half of the brain is completely absent.

Other multifactorial disorders include:

- congenital heart defects;
- obesity;
- diabetes;
- cancer.

Who Has Prenatal Tests?

Certain prenatal tests are considered routine—that is, almost all pregnant women receiving prenatal care get them. Other nonroutine tests are recommended only for certain women, especially those with high-risk pregnancies. These include women who:

- are age thirty-five or older;
- have had a premature baby;
- have had a baby with a birth defect—especially heart or genetic problems;
- have high blood pressure, diabetes, lupus, asthma, or a seizure disorder;
- have an ethnic background in which genetic disorders are common (or a partner who does);
- have a family history of mental retardation (or a partner who does).

Although your health care provider (which may be your OB-GYN, family doctor, or a certified nurse-midwife) may recommend these tests, it's ultimately up to you to decide whether to have them.

Also, if you or your partner have a family history of genetic problems, you may want to consult with a genetic counselor to help you construct a family tree going back as far as three generations.

To decide which tests are right for you, it's important to carefully discuss with your health care provider:

- what these tests are supposed to measure;
- how reliable they are;
- the potential risks;
- your options and plans if the results indicate a disorder or defect.

Prenatal Tests during the First Visit

During your first visit to your health care provider for prenatal care, you can expect to have a full physical, including a pelvic and rectal examination, and you'll undergo certain tests regardless of your age or genetic background.

Blood tests check for:

- Your blood type and Rh factor. If your blood is Rh negative and your partner's is Rh positive, you may develop antibodies that prove dangerous to your fetus. This can be treated through a course of injections.

21

- Anemia (a low red blood cell count) to make sure you're not iron deficient).

- Hepatitis B, syphilis, and human immunodeficiency virus (HIV).

- Immunity to German measles (rubella) and chickenpox (varicella).

- Cystic fibrosis. Health care providers now routinely check for this even when there's no family history of the disorder.

Cervical tests (also called Pap smears) check for:

- Sexually transmitted diseases (STDs) such as chlamydia and gonorrhea;

- Cervical cancer.

To do a Pap smear, your health care provider uses what looks like a very long mascara wand or cotton swab to gently scrape the inside of your cervix (the opening to the uterus that's located at the very top of the vagina). This doesn't hurt at all; some women say they feel a little twinge, but it only lasts a second.

Prenatal Tests Performed Throughout or Later in Pregnancy

After the initial visit, your health care provider will order other tests based on, among other things, your personal medical history and needs. Some of these tests may include:

- **Urine tests for sugar, protein, and signs of infection:** The sugar in urine indicates gestational diabetes—diabetes that occurs during pregnancy; the protein can indicate preeclampsia—a condition that develops in late pregnancy and is characterized by a sudden rise in blood pressure and excessive weight gain, with fluid retention and protein in the urine.

- **Test for group B streptococcus (GBS) infection:** GBS bacteria are found naturally in the vaginas of many women and can cause serious infections in newborns. This test involves swabbing the vagina, usually between the thirty-fifth and thirty-seventh weeks of pregnancy.

- **Sickle cell trait tests:** For women of African or Mediterranean descent, who are at higher risk for having sickle cell anemia—a chronic blood disease—or carrying the trait, which can be passed on to their children.

Other Tests

Following is a list of other tests that are now performed almost routinely in the United States as well as those that are performed only in high-risk pregnancies or if the health care provider suspects an abnormality in the fetus.

Ultrasound

Why is this test performed? In this test, sound waves are bounced off the baby's bones and tissues to construct an image showing the baby's shape and position in the uterus. Ultrasounds were once used only in high-risk pregnancies but have become so common that they're often part of routine prenatal care.

Also called a sonogram, sonograph, echogram, or ultrasonogram, an ultrasound is used:

- to determine whether the fetus is growing at a normal rate;
- to verify the expected date of delivery;
- to record fetal heartbeat or breathing movements;
- to see whether there might be more than one fetus;
- to identify a variety of abnormalities that might affect the remainder of the pregnancy or delivery;
- to make sure the amount of amniotic fluid in the uterus is adequate;
- to indicate the position of the placenta in late pregnancy (which may be blocking the baby's way out of the uterus);
- to detect pregnancies outside the uterus;
- as a guide during other tests such as amniocentesis.

Ultrasounds also are used to detect:

- structural defects such as spina bifida and anencephaly;
- congenital heart defects;
- gastrointestinal and kidney malformations;
- cleft lip or palate.

23

Should I have this test? Most women have at least one ultrasound. The test is considered to be safe; however, it is wise to find out from your health care provider if it's the most appropriate test for you.

When should I have this test? An ultrasound is usually performed at eighteen to twenty weeks to look at your baby's anatomy. If you want to know your baby's gender, you may be able to find out during this time—that is, if his or her genitals are in a visible position.

Ultrasounds also can be done sooner or later and sometimes more than once, depending on the health care provider. For example, some will order an ultrasound to date the pregnancy, usually during the first two months. And others may want to order one during late pregnancy to make sure the baby's turned the right way before delivery.

Women with high-risk pregnancies may need to have multiple ultrasounds using more sophisticated equipment. Results can be confirmed when needed using special three-dimensional (3-D) equipment that allows the technician to get a more detailed look at the baby.

How is this test performed? Women need to have a full bladder for a transabdominal ultrasound (an ultrasound of the belly) to be performed in the early months—you may be asked to drink a lot of water and not urinate. You'll lie on an examining table and your abdomen will be coated with a special ultrasound gel. A technician will pass a wand-like instrument called a transducer back and forth over your abdomen. High-frequency sound waves "echo" off your body and create a picture of the fetus inside on a computer screen.

You may want to ask to have the picture interpreted for you, even in late pregnancy—it often doesn't look like a baby to the untrained eye.

Sometimes, if the technician isn't getting a good enough image from the ultrasound, he or she will determine that a transvaginal ultrasound is necessary. This is especially common in early pregnancy. For this procedure, your bladder should be empty. Instead of a transducer being moved over your abdomen, a slender probe called an endovaginal transducer is placed inside your vagina. This technique often provides improved images of the uterus and ovaries.

Some health care providers may have the equipment and trained personnel necessary to provide in-office ultrasounds, whereas others may have you go to a local hospital or radiology center. Depending on where you have the ultrasound done, you may be able to get a printed picture (or multiple pictures) of your baby and/or a disc of images you can view on your computer and even send to friends and family.

When are the results available? Immediately, but a full evaluation may take up to one week. A radiologist (a physician experienced in obstetric ultrasound) will analyze the images and send a signed report with his or her interpretation to your doctor.

Depending on where you have the ultrasound done, the technician may be able to tell you that day whether everything looks ok. However, most radiology centers or health care providers prefer that technicians not comment until a specialist has taken a look—especially if an abnormality is detected, but even when everything is ok.

Glucose Screening

Why is this test performed? Glucose screening checks for gestational diabetes, a short-term form of diabetes that develops in some women during pregnancy. Gestational diabetes occurs in 1 to 3 percent of pregnancies and can cause health problems for the baby.

Should I have this test? Most women have this test.

When should I have this test? Screening for gestational diabetes usually takes place at twelve weeks for women at higher risk of having the condition, including those who:

- have previously had a baby that weighs more than nine pounds (4.1 kilograms);
- have a family history of diabetes;
- are obese;
- are older than age thirty.

All other pregnant women are tested for diabetes at around twenty-four to twenty-eight weeks. But if you've had high sugar in two routine urine tests, your health care provider may order it earlier.

How is the test performed? This test involves drinking a sugary liquid and then having your blood drawn after an hour. If the sugar level in the blood is high, you'll have a glucose-tolerance test, which means you'll drink a glucose solution on an empty stomach and have your blood drawn once every hour for three hours. The

25

American Diabetes Association suggests that in order to confirm diabetes, these tests be performed at different times.

When are the results available? The results are usually available within a day, although your health care provider probably won't call you unless the reading is high and you need to come in for another test.

Chorionic Villus Sampling (CVS)

Why is this test performed? Chorionic villi are tiny finger-like units that make up the placenta (a disk-like structure that sticks to the inner lining of the uterus and provides nutrients from the mother to the fetus through the umbilical cord). They have the same chromosomes and genetic makeup as the fetus.

This newer alternative to an amniocentesis removes some of the chorionic villi and tests them for chromosomal abnormalities, such as Down syndrome. Its advantage over an amniocentesis is that it can be performed earlier, allowing more time for expectant parents to receive counseling and make decisions.

Should I have this test? Your health care provider may recommend this test if you:

- are older than age thirty-five;
- have a family history of genetic disorders (or a partner who does);
- have a previous child with a birth defect;
- have had an earlier screening test that indicates that there may be a concern.

Possible risks of this test include:

- between 0.5% and 1% risk of miscarriage;
- prematurity;
- early labor;
- infection;
- spotting or bleeding (this is more common with the transcervical method—see below).

When should I have this test? At ten to twelve weeks.

How is this test performed? This test is done in one of two ways:

- Transcervical: Using ultrasound as a guide, a thin tube is passed from the vagina into the cervix. Gentle suction removes a sample of tissue from the chorionic villi. No anesthetic is used, although some women do experience a pinch and cramping.

- Transabdominal: A needle is inserted through the abdominal wall—this minimizes the chances of intrauterine infection, and in a woman whose uterus is in a bent position, reduces the chance of miscarriage. After the sample is taken, the doctor will check the fetus's heart rate. You should rest for several hours afterward.

When are the results available? Less than one week for Down syndrome and about two weeks for a thorough analysis.

Maternal Blood Screening/Triple Screen/Quadruple Screen

Why is this test performed? Doctors use this to test the mother's blood only for alpha-fetoprotein (AFP). AFP is the protein produced by the fetus, and it appears in varying amounts in the mother's blood and the amniotic fluid at different times during pregnancy. A certain level in the mother's blood is considered normal, but higher or lower levels may indicate a problem. The test typically is used to determine risk for Down syndrome.

This test has been expanded, however, to also detect two pregnancy hormones—estriol and human chorionic gonadotropin (HCG)—which is why it's now sometimes called a "triple screen" or "triple marker." The test is called a "quadruple screen" ("quad screen") or "quadruple marker" ("quad marker") when the level of an additional substance—inhibin-A—is also measured. The greater number of markers increases the accuracy of the screening and better identifies the possibility of a birth defect.

This test, which also is called a multiple-marker screening or maternal serum screening, calculates a woman's individual risk of birth defects based on the levels of the three (or more) substances plus:

- her age;
- her weight;
- her race;
- whether she has diabetes requiring insulin treatment.

It's important to note, though, that this screening test determines risk only—it doesn't diagnose a condition.

Should I have this test? All women are offered this test. Remember that this is a screening, not a definitive test—it indicates whether a woman is likely to be carrying an affected fetus. It's also not foolproof—spina bifida may go undetected, and some women with high levels have been found to be carrying a healthy baby. Further testing is recommended to confirm a positive result.

When should I have this test? At sixteen to eighteen weeks.

How is the test performed? Blood is drawn from the mother.

When are the results available? In three to five days, although it may take up two weeks.

Amniocentesis

Why is this test performed? This test is most often used to detect:

- Down syndrome and other chromosome abnormalities;
- structural defects such as spina bifida and anencephaly;
- inherited metabolic disorders.

Late in the pregnancy, this test can reveal if a baby's lungs are strong enough to allow the baby to breathe normally after birth. This can help the health care provider make decisions about inducing labor or trying to prevent labor, depending on the situation. For instance, if a mother's water breaks early, the health care provider may want to try to hold off on delivering the baby as long as possible to allow for the baby's lungs to mature.

Other common birth defects, such as heart disorders and cleft lip and palate, can't be determined using this test.

Should I have this test? Your health care provider may recommend this test if you:

- are older than age thirty-five;
- have a family history of genetic disorders (or a partner who does);
- have a previous child with a birth defect.

This test can be very accurate—close to 100 percent—but only certain disorders can be detected. According to the Centers for Disease Control and Prevention (CDC), the rate of miscarriage with this procedure is between 1 in 400 and 1 in 200. The procedure also carries a low risk of uterine infection (less than 1 in 1,000), which can cause miscarriage.

When should I have this test? At sixteen to eighteen weeks.

How is the test performed? A needle is inserted through the abdominal wall into the uterus to remove some (about one ounce) of the amniotic fluid. A local anesthetic may be used. Some women report that they experience cramping when the needle enters the uterus or pressure while the doctor retrieves the sample.

The doctor will check the fetus's heartbeat after the procedure to make sure it's normal. Most doctors recommend rest for several hours after the procedure.

The cells in the withdrawn fluid are grown in a special culture and then analyzed (the specific tests conducted on the fluid depend on personal and family medical history).

When are the results available? Timing varies; it can take up to one month, with the possibility that the lab will ask for a repeat. Tests of lung maturity are available immediately.

Nonstress Test

Why is this test performed? A nonstress test (NST) can determine if the baby is responding normally to a stimulus. Used mostly in high-risk pregnancies or when a health care provider is uncertain of fetal movement, an NST can be performed at any point in the pregnancy after the twenty-sixth to twenty-eighth week when fetal heart rate can appropriately respond by accelerating and decelerating.

If you've gone beyond your due date, this test also uses external fetal monitoring to determine fetal movement. The NST can help a doctor make sure that the baby is receiving enough oxygen and that the nervous system is responding. However, a nonresponsive baby doesn't necessarily mean that the baby is in danger.

Should I have this test? Your health care provider may recommend this if you have a high-risk pregnancy or if you have a low-risk pregnancy but are past your due date.

When should I have this test? At one week after the due date.

How is the test performed? The health care provider will measure the response of the fetus's heart rate to each movement the fetus makes as reported by the mother or observed by the doctor on an ultrasound screen. If the fetus doesn't move during the test, he or she may be asleep and the health care provider may use a buzzer to wake the baby.

When are the results available? Immediately.

Contraction Stress Test

Why is this test performed? This test stimulates the uterus with Pitocin, a synthetic form of oxytocin (a hormone secreted during childbirth), to determine the effect of contractions on fetal heart rate. It's usually recommended when a nonstress test indicates a problem and can determine whether the baby's heart rate remains stable during contractions.

Should I have this test? This test is usually ordered if the nonstress test indicates a problem. It does have a high false-positive rate, though, and can induce labor.

When should I have this test? Your doctor will schedule it if he or she is concerned about how the baby will respond to contractions or feels that it is the appropriate test to determine the fetal heart rate response to a stimulus.

How is the test performed? Mild contractions are brought on either by injections of Pitocin or by squeezing the mother's nipples (which causes oxytocin to be secreted). The fetus's heart rate is then monitored.

When are the results available? Immediately.

Percutaneous Umbilical Blood Sampling (PUBS)

Why is this test performed? This test obtains fetal blood by guiding a needle into the umbilical vein. It's primarily used in addition to an ultrasound and amniocentesis if your health care provider needs to quickly check your baby's chromosomes for defects or disorders or if he or she is concerned that your baby may be anemic.

The advantage to this test is its speed. There are situations (such as when a fetus shows signs of distress) in which it's helpful to know whether the fetus has a fatal chromosomal defect. If the fetus is suspected to be anemic or to have a platelet disorder, this test is the only way to confirm this because it provides a blood sample rather than amniotic fluid. It also allows transfusion of blood or needed fluids into the baby while the needle is in place.

Should I have this test? This test is used:

- after an abnormality has been noted on an ultrasound;
- when amniocentesis results aren't conclusive;
- if the fetus may have Rh disease;
- if you've been exposed to an infectious disease that could potentially affect fetal development.

When should I have this test? Between eighteen and thirty-six weeks.

How is the test performed? A fine needle is passed through your abdomen and uterus into the fetal vein in the umbilical cord and blood is withdrawn for testing.

When are the results available? In three days.

Talking to Your Health Care Provider

Some prenatal tests can be stressful, and because many aren't definitive, even a negative result may not ease any anxiety you may be experiencing. Because many women who have abnormal tests end up having healthy babies and because many of the problems that are detected can't be treated, some women decide not to have some of the tests.

One important thing to consider is what you'll do in the event that a birth defect is discovered. Your health care provider or a genetic counselor can help you establish priorities, give you the facts, and discuss your options.

It's also important to remember that tests are offered to women— they are not mandatory. You should feel free to ask your health care provider why he or she is ordering a certain test, what the risks and benefits are, and, most important, what the results will—and won't— tell you.

If you think that your health care provider isn't answering your questions adequately, you should say so. You don't have to accept the answer, "I do this test on all of my patients." Things you might want to ask include:

- How accurate is this test?
- What are you looking to get from these test results?/What do you hope to learn?
- How long before I get the results?
- Is the procedure painful?
- Is the procedure dangerous to me or the fetus?
- Do the potential benefits outweigh the risks?
- What could happen if I don't undergo this test?
- How much will the test cost?
- Will the test be covered by insurance?
- What do I need to do to prepare?

You also can ask your health care provider for literature about each type of test.

Preventing Birth Defects

The best thing that mothers-to-be can do to avoid birth defects is to take care of their bodies during pregnancy by:

- not smoking (and avoiding secondhand smoke);
- avoiding alcohol;
- eating a healthy diet;
- taking prenatal vitamins;
- getting exercise;
- getting plenty of rest;
- getting prenatal care.

Section 2.3

Pregnancy and a Healthy Diet

Reprinted from "Eating During Pregnancy." This information was provided by KidsHealth, one of the largest resources online for medically reviewed health information written for parents, kids, and teens. For more articles like this one, visit www.KidsHealth.org, or www.TeensHealth.org. © 2004 The Nemours Center for Children's Health Media, a division of The Nemours Foundation.

To eat well during pregnancy you must do more than simply increase how much you eat. You must also consider what you eat. Although you need about three extra calories a day—especially later in your pregnancy, when your baby grows quickly—those calories should come from nutritious foods so they can contribute to your baby's growth and development.

Why It's Important to Eat Well When You're Pregnant

Do you wonder how it's reasonable to gain twenty-five to thirty-five pounds (on average) during your pregnancy when a newborn baby weighs only a fraction of that? Although it varies from woman to woman, this is how those pounds may add up:

- 7.5 pounds: average baby's weight
- 7 pounds: your body's extra stored protein, fat, and other nutrients
- 4 pounds: your extra blood
- 4 pounds: your other extra body fluids
- 2 pounds: breast enlargement
- 2 pounds: enlargement of your uterus
- 2 pounds: amniotic fluid surrounding your baby
- 1.5 pounds: the placenta

Of course, patterns of weight gain during pregnancy vary. It's normal to gain less if you start out heavier and more if you're having twins or triplets—or if you were underweight before becoming pregnant. More important than how much weight you gain is what makes up those extra pounds.

When you're pregnant, what you eat and drink is the main source of nourishment for your baby. In fact, the link between what you consume and the health of your baby is much stronger than once thought. That's why doctors now say, for example, that no amount of alcohol consumption should be considered safe during pregnancy.

The extra food you eat shouldn't just be empty calories—it should provide the nutrients your growing baby needs. For example, calcium helps make and keep bones and teeth strong. While you're pregnant, you still need calcium for your body, plus extra calcium for your developing baby. Similarly, you require more of all the essential nutrients than you did before you became pregnant.

A Nutrition Primer for Expectant Mothers

Whether or not you're pregnant, a healthy diet includes proteins, carbohydrates, fats, vitamins, minerals, and plenty of water. The U.S. government publishes dietary guidelines that can help you determine how many servings of each kind of food to eat every day. Eating a variety of foods in the proportions indicated is a good step toward staying healthy.

Food labels can tell you what kinds of nutrients are in the foods you eat. The letters RDA, which you find on food labeling, stand for recommended daily allowance, or the amount of a nutrient recommended for your daily diet. When you're pregnant, the RDAs for most nutrients are higher.

Table 2.1 shows some of the most common nutrients you need and the foods that contain them.

Scientists know that your diet can affect your baby's health—even before you become pregnant. For example, recent research shows that folic acid helps prevent neural tube defects (including spina bifida) from occurring during the earliest stages of fetal development—so it's important for you to consume plenty of it before you become pregnant and during the early weeks of your pregnancy.

Even though lots of foods, particularly breakfast cereals, are fortified with folic acid, doctors now encourage women to take folic acid supplements before and throughout pregnancy (especially for the first twenty-eight days). Be sure to ask your doctor about folic acid if you're considering becoming pregnant.

Calcium is another important nutrient for pregnant women. Because your growing baby's calcium demands are high, you should increase your calcium consumption to prevent a loss of calcium from your own bones. Your doctor will also likely prescribe prenatal vitamins for you, which contain some extra calcium.

Your best food sources of calcium are milk and other dairy products. However, if you have lactose intolerance or dislike milk and milk

Table 2.1. Common Nutrients and the Foods that Contain Them

Nutrient	Needed for	Best sources
Protein	Cell growth and blood production	Lean meat, fish, poultry, egg whites, beans, peanut butter, tofu
Carbohydrates	Daily energy production	Breads, cereals, rice, potatoes, pasta, fruits, vegetables
Calcium	Strong bones and teeth, muscle contraction, nerve function	Milk, cheese, yogurt, sardines or salmon with bones, spinach
Iron	Red blood cell production (needed to prevent anemia)	Lean red meat, spinach, iron-fortified whole-grain breads and cereals
Vitamin A	Healthy skin, good eyesight, growing bones	Carrots, dark leafy greens, sweet potatoes
Vitamin C	Healthy gums, teeth, and bones; assistance with iron absorption	Citrus fruit, broccoli, tomatoes, fortified fruit juices
Vitamin B_6	Red blood cell formation; effective use of protein, fat, and carbohydrates	Pork, ham, whole-grain cereals, bananas
Vitamin B_{12}	Formation of red blood cells, maintaining nervous system health	Meat, fish, poultry, milk (Note: vegetarians who don't eat dairy products need supplemental B_{12})
Vitamin D	Healthy bones and teeth; aids absorption of calcium	Fortified milk, dairy products, cereals, and breads
Folic acid	Blood and protein production, effective enzyme function	Green leafy vegetables, dark yellow fruits and vegetables, beans, peas, nuts
Fat	Body energy stores	Meat, whole-milk dairy products, nuts, peanut butter, margarine, vegetable oils (Note: limit fat intake to 30 percent or less of your total daily calorie intake)

products, ask your doctor about a calcium supplement. (Signs of lactose intolerance include diarrhea, bloating, or gas after eating milk or milk products. Taking a lactase capsule or pill, or using lactose-free milk products may help.) Other calcium-rich foods include sardines or salmon with bones, tofu, broccoli, spinach, and calcium-fortified juices and foods.

Doctors don't usually recommend starting a strict vegan diet when you become pregnant. However, if you already follow a vegetarian diet, you can continue to do so during your pregnancy—but do it carefully. Be sure your doctor knows about your diet. It's challenging to get the nutrition you need if you don't eat fish and chicken, or milk, cheese, or eggs. You'll likely need supplemental protein and may also need to take vitamin B_{12} and D supplements. To ensure that you and your baby receive adequate nutrition, consult a registered dietitian for help with planning meals.

What Do Food Cravings during Pregnancy Mean?

You've probably known women who craved specific foods during pregnancy, or perhaps you've had such cravings yourself. Researchers have tried to determine whether a hunger for a particular type of food indicates that a woman's body lacks the nutrients that food contains. Although this isn't the case, it's still unclear why these urges occur.

Some pregnant women crave chocolate, spicy foods, fruits, and comfort foods, such as mashed potatoes, cereals, and toasted white bread. Other women crave nonfood items, such as clay and cornstarch. The craving and eating of nonfood items is known as pica. Consuming things that aren't food can be dangerous to both you and your baby. If you have urges to eat nonfood items, notify your doctor.

But following your cravings is fine, as long as you crave foods and these foods contribute to a healthy diet. Frequently, these cravings diminish about three months into the pregnancy.

What Should You Avoid Eating and Drinking during Pregnancy?

As mentioned earlier, avoid alcohol. No level of alcohol consumption is considered safe during pregnancy. Also, check with your doctor before you take any vitamins or herbal products. Some of these can be harmful to the developing fetus.

Although many doctors feel that one or two six- to eight-ounce cups per day of coffee, tea, or soda with caffeine won't harm your baby, it's probably wise to avoid caffeine altogether if you can. High caffeine consumption has been linked to an increased risk of miscarriage, so limit your intake or switch to decaffeinated products.

When you're pregnant, it's also important to avoid food-borne illnesses, such as listeriosis and toxoplasmosis, which can be life-threatening to an unborn baby and may cause birth defects or miscarriage. Foods you'll want to steer clear of include:

- soft, unpasteurized cheeses (often advertised as "fresh") such as feta, goat, Brie, Camembert, and blue cheese;

- unpasteurized milk, juices, and apple cider;

- raw eggs or foods containing raw eggs, including mousse and tiramisu;

- raw or undercooked meats, fish, or shellfish;

- processed meats such as hot dogs and deli meats (these should be well cooked).

If you've eaten these foods at some point during your pregnancy, try not to worry too much about it now; just avoid them for the remainder of the pregnancy. If you're really concerned, talk to your doctor.

You'll also want to avoid eating shark, swordfish, king mackerel, or tilefish, as well as limit the amount of other kinds of fish that you eat. Although fish and shellfish can be an extremely healthy part of your pregnancy diet (they contain beneficial omega-3 fatty acids, and are high in protein and low in saturated fat), these types of fish may contain high levels of mercury. Because mercury can cause damage to the developing brain of a fetus or growing child, the U.S. Food and Drug Administration (FDA) and the U.S. Environmental Protection Agency (EPA) say that these fish should not be eaten at all by pregnant women, women who may become pregnant, nursing mothers, and young children.

Mercury, which occurs naturally in the environment, can also be released into the air through industrial pollution and can accumulate in streams and oceans, where it turns into methylmercury in the water. The methylmercury builds up in fish, especially larger fish that eat other smaller fish.

If you're pregnant and eat shark, swordfish, king mackerel, or tilefish, even occasionally, it's a good idea to stop. Although almost all fish and shellfish contain small amounts of mercury, you can enjoy some with lower mercury levels (shrimp, canned light tuna, salmon, pollock, and catfish) in moderation (no more than twelve ounces a week, say the FDA and EPA). Because albacore (or white) tuna or tuna steaks are higher in mercury than canned light tuna, it's recommended that you eat no more than six ounces a week.

Avoiding Some Common Problems

Because the iron in prenatal vitamins and other factors may cause constipation during pregnancy, it's a good idea to consume more fiber than you did before you became pregnant. Try to eat about 20 to 30 grams of fiber a day. Your best sources are fresh fruits and vegetables and whole-grain breads, cereals, or muffins.

Some people also use fiber tablets or drinks or other high-fiber products available at your pharmacy, but check with your doctor before trying them. (Don't use laxatives while you're pregnant unless your doctor advises you to do so. And avoid the old wives' remedy—castor oil—because it can actually interfere with your body's ability to absorb nutrients.)

If constipation is a problem for you, your doctor may prescribe a stool softener. Be sure to drink plenty of fluids, especially water, when increasing fiber intake, or you can make your constipation worse. One of the best ways to avoid constipation is to get more exercise. You should also drink plenty of water between meals each day to help soften your stools and move food through your digestive system. Sometimes hot tea, soups, or broth can help. Also, keep dried fruits handy for snacking.

Some pregnant women find that broccoli, spinach, cauliflower, and fried foods give them heartburn or gas. You can plan a balanced diet to avoid these foods. Carbonated drinks also cause gas or heartburn for some women, although others find they calm the digestive system.

If you're frequently nauseated, eat small amounts of bland foods, like toast or crackers, throughout the day. If nothing else sounds good, try cereal with milk or a sweet piece of fruit. To help combat nausea, you can also do the following:

- Take your prenatal vitamin before going to bed after you've eaten a snack—not on an empty stomach.

- Eat a small snack when you get up to go to the bathroom early in the morning.

- Suck on hard candy.

How Can You Know If You're Eating Well during Pregnancy?

The key is to eat foods from the different food groups in approximately the recommended proportions. If nausea or lack of appetite cause you to eat less at times, don't worry—it's unlikely to cause fetal harm because your baby gets first crack at the nutrients you consume. And although it's generally recommended that a woman of normal weight gain approximately twenty-five to thirty-five pounds during pregnancy (most gain four to six pounds during the first trimester and one pound a week during the second and third trimesters), don't fixate on the scale. Instead, focus on eating a good variety and balance of nutritious foods to keep both you and your baby healthy.

Section 2.4

Folic Acid

Reprinted from "Folic Acid Basics" and "Folic Acid: Frequently Asked Questions," National Center on Birth Defects and Developmental Disabilities, Centers for Disease Control and Prevention, November 16, 2005.

The Basics about Folic Acid

The B vitamin folic acid helps prevent birth defects. If a woman has enough folic acid in her body before and while she is pregnant, her baby is less likely to have a major birth defect of the brain or spine.

Most women do not know how important folic acid is for their bodies and for the health of a baby they might have in the future. They also do not know that a woman needs to take folic acid every day, starting before she is pregnant, for it to work to prevent birth defects.

Birth defects of a baby's brain or spine happen in the first few weeks of pregnancy, often before a woman knows that she is pregnant. That is why it is important for a woman to get enough folic acid each day, starting before she is pregnant.

A woman's body uses folic acid to make healthy new cells for her baby. Scientists are not sure how folic acid works to prevent birth defects, but they do know that it is needed for making the cells that will form a baby's brain, spine, organs, skin, and bones.

Every woman needs folic acid for the healthy new cells her body makes every day . . . even if she is not planning to get pregnant.

Frequently Asked Questions about Folic Acid

What are neural tube defects (NTDs)?

Neural tube defects (NTDs) are major birth defects of a baby's brain or spine. They happen when the neural tube (that later turns into the brain and spine) doesn't form right, and the baby's brain or spine is damaged. This happens within the first few weeks a woman is pregnant, often before a woman knows that she is pregnant.

The two most common NTDs are spina bifida (spi-na bif-a-da) and anencephaly (an-en-sef-a-lee). These birth defects can cause lifelong disability or death.

Many NTDs (up to 70 percent) can be prevented by getting enough of the B vitamin folic acid every day, starting before a woman gets pregnant.

What are spina bifida and anencephaly?

Spina bifida and anencephaly are two common types of NTDs. About three thousand pregnancies in the United States are affected by spina bifida or anencephaly each year. Many of these defects could be prevented if all women got enough of the B vitamin folic acid every day starting before they get pregnant.

Spina bifida occurs when the spine and backbones do not close all the way. When this happens, the spinal cord and backbones do not form as they should. A sac of fluid comes through an opening in the baby's back. Much of the time, part of the spinal cord is in this sac and it is damaged. Most children born with spina bifida live full lives, but they often have lifelong disabilities and need many surgeries. They may have many problems:

- Not being able to move lower parts of their body. Some might need to use crutches, braces, or wheelchairs to get around.

- Loss of bowel and bladder control. Some have to wear protective clothing. Others learn new ways to empty their bladders and bowels.

- Fluid building up and putting pressure on the brain (hydro-cephalus), a condition that needs to be fixed with an operation.

- Learning disabilities

- Allergy to latex (a created material found in some rubber-type products such as balloons or hospital gloves).

Children born with spina bifida don't all have the same needs. Some children's problems are much more severe than others. Even so, with the right care, most of these children will grow up to lead full and productive lives.

Anencephaly occurs when the brain and skull bones do not form properly. When this happens, part or all of the brain and skull bones might be missing. Babies with this defect die before birth (miscarriage) or shortly after birth.

Who can have a baby with a neural tube defect in the United States?

Any woman in the United States can have a baby with an NTD. If a woman can get pregnant, she is at risk for having an NTD-affected pregnancy. No one can predict which women will have a pregnancy affected by an NTD. All women are at risk.

Some things can increase a woman's chance of having a baby with an NTD:

- Previous NTD-affected pregnancy

- Diabetes when the blood sugar is out of control

- Some medicines (like some of those that treat epilepsy)

- Obesity

- High temperatures in early pregnancy (such as fever that lasts a while, or using hot tubs and saunas)

- Hispanic ethnicity (Hispanic women tend to have more babies affected by NTDs)

What are the costs linked with NTDs?

The average cost of caring for a child born with spina bifida for life is about $636,000.00 per child. This is only an average cost, and for many families the total cost might be well above $1,000,000. And it's not just the money. The physical and emotional tolls upon the families

41

affected are high as well. That's why it's so important that women take folic acid every day to help prevent these birth defects.

What is folic acid and where can I get it?

Folic acid is a B vitamin that the body needs to make healthy new cells. If a woman has enough folic acid in her body before and during pregnancy, her baby is less likely to have an NTD. Women need to take folic acid every day, starting before they get pregnant.

Every woman who could possibly get pregnant should take 400 micrograms (400 mcg or 0.4 mg) of folic acid daily in a vitamin or in foods that have been enriched with folic acid.

There are two simple ways to be sure to get enough each day:

- Take one vitamin with folic acid each day. Most multivitamins sold in the United States have the amount of folic acid women need each day. Women can also choose to take a small pill that has only folic acid in it each day. Both types of vitamins can be found at most local pharmacy, grocery, or discount stores.

OR

- Eat a bowl of a breakfast cereal that has 100 percent of the daily value (DV) of folic acid per serving every day. Total, Product 19, Cheerios Plus, Special K Plus, Life, and Smart Start are some examples. The label on the side of the box should say "100%" next to folic acid.

Along with taking a vitamin or eating a cereal that has 100 percent DV of folic acid, women should always eat a healthy diet that has lots of fresh fruits and vegetables and other healthy foods.

Scientists don't know how folic acid works to prevent birth defects. But they do know that folic acid is needed to make healthy new cells, like the ones that make up a baby's brain and spine. Taking folic acid every day, starting before and during pregnancy, can reduce the risk for these serious birth defects by 50 to 70 percent.

Are women getting enough folic acid?

Most women in the United States do not get enough folic acid to help prevent birth defects. The average woman gets less than the amount needed from her diet alone. That's why all women who can get pregnant are urged to take a vitamin with folic acid or eat a serving of fully fortified breakfast cereal each day.

Can women get too much folic acid?

It's unlikely that women will be hurt from getting too much folic acid. We don't know of an amount that is dangerous. Yet, for most women, consuming more than 1,000 mcg of folic acid daily is of no benefit. Unless their doctor advises them to take more, most women should limit the amount they take to 1,000 mcg a day.

Why can't I wait until I'm pregnant or planning to get pregnant to start taking folic acid?

Birth defects of the brain and spine happen in the first few weeks of pregnancy, often before a woman finds out she is pregnant. By the time she realizes she is pregnant, it might be too late to prevent those birth defects. Also, half of all pregnancies in the United States are unplanned. These are two reasons why it is important for all women who can get pregnant to be sure to get 400 mcg of folic acid every day, even if they aren't planning a pregnancy any time soon.

I can't swallow large pills. How can I take a vitamin with folic acid?

A woman can get her vitamin with folic acid in one of several ways. She can take a multivitamin or a small single supplement of folic acid. These days, multivitamins with folic acid come in chewable chocolate or fruit flavors, liquids, and large oval or smaller round pills. A single serving of many breakfast cereals also has the amount of folic acid that a woman needs each day. Check the label! Look for cereals that have 100 percent daily value (DV) of folic acid in a serving.

Vitamins cost too much. How can I get the vitamin with folic acid that I need?

Many stores offer a single folic acid supplement for just pennies a day. Another good choice is a store brand multivitamin, which includes more of the vitamins a woman needs each day. Unless her doctor suggests a special type, she does not have to choose among vitamins for women or active people, or even one to go with a low carbohydrate diet. A basic multivitamin meets the needs of most women.

How can I remember to take a vitamin with folic acid every day?

A woman may combine taking her vitamin with another habit. Taking a vitamin when she brushes her teeth, has her morning coffee, finishes her shower, or brushes her hair may make it easier to remember. Seeing the vitamin bottle on the bathroom or kitchen counter could help her remember it. She might even take a vitamin when her children take theirs. That sets a good example!

Are there other health benefits of taking folic acid?

Folic acid might help to prevent some other birth defects, such as cleft lip and palate and some heart defects. There might also be other health benefits of taking folic acid for both women and men. More research is needed to confirm these other health benefits.

Chapter 3

Smoking and Pregnancy

Frequently Asked Questions about Smoking and Pregnancy

Smoking rates are going down among Americans. However, the smoking rates among women are going down more slowly than smoking rates among men. In fact, smoking among high school senior girls was the same in 2000 as in 1998.

When young women who smoke start to think about having children, they also need to think about quitting smoking. The best time to quit is when a woman is planning to get pregnant in the near future, or after she finds out that she is already pregnant. This will be better for her own health and for that of her baby.

Pregnancy is a great time to quit smoking and stay quit after the baby is born.

Don't some mothers smoke during pregnancy and have healthy babies?

They are the lucky ones! If a woman smokes during pregnancy she takes a big chance with her baby's health. There is a greater chance

---

This chapter begins with "Frequently Asked Questions about Smoking and Pregnancy" from "There's Never Been a Better Time to Quit." Reprinted with permission © 2006 American Lung Association. For more information about the American Lung Association or to support the work it does, call 800-LUNG-USA (800-586-4872) or log on to http://www.lungusa.org. "Smoking during Pregnancy May Affect Baby's Fingers and Toes" is © 2006 The Children's Hospital of Philadelphia. All rights reserved. Reprinted with permission.

that she will lose the baby during pregnancy. The baby could also be born too early, before the lungs are ready, so he or she will have trouble breathing. Why take a chance when there is so much to lose?

Babies often weigh less when the mother smokes. Isn't it easier to deliver a small baby?

It is not always easier to deliver a low-birth-weight baby. And a baby that weighs too little is often sick with lots of health problems. Smaller babies are more likely to need special care and stay longer in the hospital. Some may die either at birth or within the first year.

Does cigarette smoke get through to the unborn baby?

Yes, when the mother smokes, so does the baby. Smokers take in poisons such as nicotine and carbon monoxide (the same gas that comes out of a car's exhaust pipe). These poisons get into the placenta, which is the tissue that connects the mother and the baby before it is born. These poisons keep the unborn baby from getting the food and oxygen needed to grow.

Will a woman gain extra weight if she quits smoking during pregnancy?

A woman needs to gain weight during pregnancy. An unborn baby depends on the mother to eat the right foods. So, if she stays away from junk foods and sweets, the mother's weight gain will be fine. And she needs to exercise. Her doctor can help her plan how to keep active; brisk walking is good for most women.

Even if a pregnant woman gains a few extra pounds, she can lose it after the baby's born. And speaking of how she looks, the woman can think about how smoking stains her teeth and fingers. It makes her clothes and her breath smell bad. And smoking may even add more skin wrinkles.

How about cutting down on cigarettes rather than quitting for good?

The only way to really protect your unborn baby is to quit. Cutting down is better than doing nothing but it may not make things much better for the baby.

If a pregnant woman cuts down or switches to low-tar cigarettes, she must be careful not to inhale more deeply or take more puffs to get the same amount of nicotine as before.

Does it matter when the pregnant woman quits smoking?

The best time to quit is when the woman thinks she will get pregnant in the near future. If she does quit, her baby will probably weigh the same as the baby of a woman who has never smoked. If she quits within the first three or four months of her pregnancy she can lower her baby's chance of being born too small and with lots of health problems.

Many women are able to quit during pregnancy. It is easier than other times when they tried to quit. They can quit now for their babies as well as for themselves.

If the woman feels sick in the first couple of months, cigarettes may taste bad, and so it is easier to quit.

Even if a woman quits at the end of her pregnancy, she can help her baby get more oxygen and have a better chance of making it. It's never too late to quit, but the earlier the better for both the mother and her baby!

What about other people smoking around the pregnant woman?

New studies show that if a woman's partner smokes near her during her pregnancy, there are added risks. She has a greater chance of having a baby that weighs too little and may have health problems. So, a pregnant woman should ask her partner, and other people as well, not to smoke near her.

Does quitting smoking provide benefits for the woman as well as for her baby?

Pregnancy is a great time for a woman to quit. No matter how long she has been smoking, her body benefits from quitting. She will feel better and have more energy to go through the pregnancy and to care for her new baby.

Of course, she will also avoid many of the future health risks of smoking, such as heart disease, cancer, and other lung problems. Furthermore, she will save money that she can spend on herself and her new baby.

If a woman quits smoking during pregnancy, will she have a hard time handling the stress?

She can learn to relax in other ways that are much better for her and the unborn baby. When she feels tense, she can take some deep breaths or chew sugarless gum. She can also do something with her hands like sew something for the baby or call a friend.

These are safer ways to handle stress. She can also remind herself that smoking will not make things any better.

If a mother who smokes breast feeds her baby, does the nicotine get into her milk?

Breast feeding is a good way to feed a new baby but smoking may cause problems. Nicotine is a poison in cigarettes. So if the mother smokes, the baby drinks the poison in her breast milk.

Are there any long-term harmful effects on the baby if the mother smokes during pregnancy?

Yes, there can be. Smoking during pregnancy may mean that after the child is born it will have more colds and other lung problems.

These children may also be slower learners in school. And they may be shorter and smaller than children of nonsmokers. And, of course, they are more likely to smoke when they get older because they see their parents smoking.

We know that a woman should not smoke during pregnancy, but is it all right to go back to smoking after the baby is born?

It makes no sense at all for her to go back to smoking! Even after the baby is born, her smoking can hurt the baby.

Babies have very small lungs and airways which get even smaller when they breathe smoke-filled air. Smoking can make it hard for the baby to breathe. It can cause lung problems like bronchitis and pneumonia that could put the baby back in the hospital.

Babies of smokers also get more colds and coughs and middle-ear infections. Mothers should also ask people like family, friends, baby sitters, and day care workers not to smoke in any areas near the baby.

How can the pregnant smoker get help in quitting?

Here are some ways to get started:

- She can ask for help from her doctor or nurse and from family and friends.

- She can make a list of her reasons for wanting to quit, for herself as well as for her baby.

- Set a quit-date; the sooner the better. If a woman is not ready to set a date, she can begin to cut down on smoking. Then, she can make a plan to stop all smoking in the near future.

- Ask for stop-smoking materials and read them. A smoker needs to learn about her own smoking habit and plan ways to cope with urges to smoke after she quits. She can try the four D's: delay, deep breathe, drink water, and do something else.

If a woman slips and goes back to smoking, she should first find out what caused the slip and then she can keep trying to quit again until she makes it for good. The only failure is if she stops trying.

When she stops smoking, she shows that she wants to raise her baby in a smoke-free world.

Smoking during Pregnancy May Affect Baby's Fingers and Toes

There's one more reason not to smoke during pregnancy. A mother's cigarette smoking increases the risk that her newborn may have extra, webbed, or missing fingers or toes, according to a study in the January 2006 issue of *Plastic and Reconstructive Surgery*.

Although the overall risk of these abnormalities in fingers and toes is relatively low, just half a pack of cigarettes per day increases the risk to the baby by 29 percent, compared to nonsmokers. Because limbs develop very early in pregnancy, the effect may occur even before a woman knows she is pregnant.

"We found that the more a woman smoked, the higher the risk became that the baby would have these defects," said study leader Benjamin Chang, M.D., pediatric plastic and reconstructive surgeon at the Children's Hospital of Philadelphia. Dr. Chang and coauthor Li-Xing Man, M.Sc., both of Children's Hospital and the University of Pennsylvania, reviewed the records of more than 6.8 million live births listed in the U.S. Natality database from 2001 and 2002. It was the largest study of its kind, covering 84 percent of U.S. births.

The researchers divided the study population into four groups: nonsmokers, those who smoked one to ten cigarettes daily, those who smoked eleven to twenty cigarettes daily, and those who smoked twenty-one or more cigarettes per day. There was a statistically significant dose-response effect, with increased odds of having a newborn with a congenital digital anomaly with increased maternal cigarette smoking during pregnancy. Women who smoked up to half a pack a day were 29 percent more likely to have babies with digital anomalies, and women who smoked more than a pack of cigarettes a day during pregnancy were 78 percent more likely to have babies with digital anomalies.

Of the total 6.8 million births, the researchers found 5,171 children born with digital anomalies whose mother smoked during pregnancy. "Overall, the likelihood of having a digital anomaly is relatively low, about one in 2,000 to 2,500 live births, and compared to other public health issues, is a very small problem," said Dr. Chang. "Usually surgery can restore full or nearly full function to children with these anomalies."

Digital anomalies include polydactyly (presence of more than five fingers or toes on a hand or foot), adactyly (the absence of fingers or toes), and syndactyly (fused or webbed fingers or toes).

Limbs begin to develop between four and eight weeks of gestation and advance from a tiny nub to nearly fully formed fingers and toes. Many women only discover they are pregnant during this period.

Missing digits are twice as likely to occur in boys and are more common in Caucasians than African-Americans; more than five digits on hands and feet is ten times more common in African-Americans and only slightly more common in boys.

Nevertheless, the majority of isolated congenital digital anomalies occur spontaneously without any family history. The increased number of cases involving these diagnoses in their own practices led researchers to investigate environmental factors that might be associated with these conditions.

Although the current study does not prove that prenatal exposure to cigarettes causes digital anomalies, says Dr. Chang, there is a strong association, the population studied is very large, and the dose-response effect is significant (higher exposure is linked to higher risk). "Although the overall risk of having these defects is rather small, the increase in risk posed by tobacco exposure has the potential to affect thousands of children," he added. "Health professionals should increase their efforts to remind women of the dangers of smoking."

Chapter 4

Alcohol Use during Pregnancy

Chapter Contents

Section 4.1—What You Should Know about Fetal Alcohol
                Syndrome 52
Section 4.2—Alcohol in Pregnancy May Cause Permanent
                Fetal Nerve Damage 54
Section 4.3—Fetal Alcohol Spectrum Disorders through the
                Lifespan 56

Section 4.1

What You Should Know about Fetal Alcohol Syndrome

Reprinted from "Fetal Alcohol Syndrome,"
National Women's Health Information Center, August 2002.

Is it okay to drink a little alcohol during pregnancy?

There is no known safe level of alcohol a pregnant woman can drink and not affect her baby. It is best to drink no alcohol at all:

• if you are trying to get pregnant,

• if there is a chance you could possibly be pregnant, or

• if you are pregnant.

Not all women who drink alcohol during pregnancy will have a child born with fetal alcohol syndrome (FAS). But not drinking alcohol is the only sure way to protect your baby from FAS, alcohol-related birth defects (ARBD), and alcohol-related neurodevelopmental disorder (ARND). If you are pregnant and have been drinking, stop drinking now to protect your baby. If you need help to stop drinking, talk with your health care provider.

What is fetal alcohol syndrome?

Fetal alcohol syndrome (FAS) is a group of birth defects caused by drinking alcohol during pregnancy. Children with FAS have many physical, mental, and behavioral problems and may be mentally retarded. They are small, underweight babies. As they get older, they often have trouble with learning, attention, memory, and problem solving. They may have poor coordination, be impulsive, and have speech and hearing problems.

The effects of FAS last a lifetime. Most children with FAS have trouble with work and with personal relationships when they become adults. Many have legal problems.

FAS cannot be reversed, but it can be prevented by not drinking alcohol when pregnant.

What are the most common birth defects or problems of FAS?

Children with FAS have many different problems:

- **Facial features that are not normal:** A thin upper lip, short nose, short eye openings, and flat cheeks and philtrum (the groove in the middle of the upper lip).

- **Growth retardation:** They are small and underweight from birth.

- **Brain damage:** They may be mentally retarded or have problems with development, learning, and behavior.

All of these birth defects are caused by drinking alcohol in pregnancy.

If a child has some but not all of the alcohol-related problems of FAS, he or she is sometimes said to have fetal alcohol effects (FAE). There are two types of FAE:

- **Alcohol-related birth defects (ARBD):** This term is used when a child does not have FAS, but does have one or more physical birth defects caused by alcohol. These may be physical defects of the face, eyes, ears, heart, brain, or limbs.

- **Alcohol-related neurodevelopmental disorder (ARND):** This term is used when a child does not have FAS, but does have some brain damage caused by alcohol. Children with ARND are harder to identify than children with ARBD or FAS. They often have trouble in school and have behavior problems.

How does alcohol cause these problems?

When a pregnant woman drinks beer, wine, hard liquor, or other alcoholic beverages, alcohol gets into her blood. The alcohol in the mother's blood goes to her baby through the umbilical cord. When the alcohol enters the baby's body, it can cause birth defects. Drinking alcohol in the early stages of pregnancy can cause the facial and other physical defects of FAS. Drinking alcohol at any time during pregnancy can slow down the baby's growth and affect the baby's brain.

There is no time during pregnancy when there is no chance at all of hurting your baby if you drink alcohol.

Can FAS be cured?

No. But children with FAS can be helped. They may need hearing aids or eyeglasses. They should get regular medical care. When they go to school, they need special help. As children with FAS get older, they may need special services and support to help them live on their own.

Section 4.2

Alcohol in Pregnancy May Cause Permanent Fetal Nerve Damage

Reprinted from "New Study Finds Babies Born to Mothers Who Drink Alcohol Heavily May Suffer Permanent Nerve Damage," *NIH News,* National Institutes of Health, March 8, 2004.

Newborns whose mothers drank alcohol heavily during pregnancy had damage to the nerves in the arms and legs, according to a study by researchers at the National Institute of Child Health and Human Development (NICHD), one of the National Institutes of Health. The study was conducted in collaboration with researchers at the University of Chile.

The nerve damage was still present when the children were reexamined at one year of age.

The study is the first to examine whether exposure to alcohol before birth affects the developing peripheral nervous system—the nerves in the arms and legs, rather than in the brain or spinal cord. The study appears in the March 2004 issue of the *Journal of Pediatrics.*

"Infants born to mothers who drink heavily during pregnancy are known to be at risk for mental retardation and birth defects," said Duane Alexander, M.D., director of the NICHD. "This is the first study to show that these infants may suffer peripheral nerve damage as well."

The Problem

Adults who drink excessive amounts of alcohol can experience peripheral neuropathy, a condition that occurs when nerves involved in communication between the central nervous system (the brain and spinal cord) and the rest of the body are damaged. This can lead to tingling sensations, numbness, pain, or weakness.

The Study

The NICHD-University of Chile Alcohol and Pregnancy Study compared seventeen full-term, newborn infants whose mothers drank heavily during pregnancy to thirteen newborns not exposed to alcohol in the womb. "Heavy drinking" is defined as having four standard drinks per day (one standard drink is equivalent to one can of beer, one glass of wine or one mixed drink). All women identified as heavy drinkers were advised that their drinking habits were potentially dangerous to their fetus and were offered help from an alcohol counseling clinic to stop drinking alcohol or to cut down on their drinking.

All of the children underwent a complete neurological exam followed by testing of the nerves in their upper and lower limbs. The researchers stimulated the nerves using a machine that passed a very mild electric current through the skin and then recorded the electrical activity of the nerves to determine if they were normal or damaged. (The procedure uses a current mild enough not to cause pain.) The nerve studies were performed when the children were about one month old and again when they were twelve to fourteen months old.

The Results

The children exposed to alcohol before they were born experienced significant problems in conducting a message through the nerves—both at one month and at one year of age. The alcohol-exposed children did not experience any catch-up or improvement in nerve function by the time they reached their first birthday.

"The finding that the nerve damage persisted when the children were a year old suggests that alcohol may cause permanent damage to developing nerves," said James L. Mills, M.D., M.S., director of the study and chief of the Pediatric Epidemiology Section in the Division of Epidemiology, Statistics and Prevention Research at the NICHD. "Because the children were evaluated before they could talk, they were unable to tell us if they had symptoms such as pain or numbness. We are continuing to follow these children to determine what effect this nerve damage will have on normal nerve function and whether it will lead to weakness or problems with touch sensation or fine motor skills later in life."

Section 4.3

Fetal Alcohol Spectrum Disorders through the Lifespan

Fetal alcohol syndrome (FAS) and fetal alcohol spectrum disorders (FASD) have lifelong implications. There are a broad range of characteristics to watch for at different ages:

- **Infants:** low birth weight; irritability; sensitivity to light, noises, and touch; poor sucking; slow development; poor sleep-wake cycles; and increased ear infections

- **Toddlers:** poor memory capability; hyperactivity; lack of fear; no sense of boundaries; and a need for excessive physical contact

- **Grade-school years:** short attention span; poor coordination; and difficulty with both fine and gross motor skills

- **Older children:** trouble keeping up with school; low self-esteem from recognizing they are different from their peers

- **Teenagers:** poor impulse control; difficulty distinguishing between public and private behaviors; a need for reminders about concepts on a daily basis

- **Adults:** difficulties with many daily obstacles, such as affordable and appropriate housing, transportation, employment, and money handling

Strategies for Living

Establish a relationship with a pediatrician and consult him or her with any problems or questions. Here are some other helpful tips.

Infants

- **Poor sleep-wake cycles/irritability:** Play soft music and sing to your baby. Rocking, frequent holding, low lights, automatic swings, and wrapping them snugly in a soft blanket also can be helpful.

- **Poor weight gain:** Consult a nutritionist to develop a food plan or discuss supplement use.

- **Chronic ear infections:** Speak to a specialist about evaluating your child's hearing and effectively treating infections.

- **Delays in rolling over, crawling, walking:** See an occupational therapist for assistance. Also help your baby in crawling, grabbing, and pulling.

- **Speech delays:** Consult a speech therapist and purchase tapes or toys that are specifically designed for children with delays. Speak and read aloud expressively to your baby.

Toddlers

- **Continued motor skill delays:** Work with an occupational or physical therapist. Use toys that focus on manipulating joints and muscles.

- **Distraction:** Establish a routine and use structure. Simplify rooms in the home and reduce noises or other stimulation.

- **Dental problems:** Consult a pediatric dentist. Your child may not be able to sit still, so be sure to prepare your child for the exam and allow more time for the appointment.

- **Small appetites or sensitivity to food texture:** Serve small portions that are lukewarm or cool and have some texture. Allow plenty of time during meals and decrease distractions such as television, radio, or multiple conversations.

School Age

- **Bedtime:** If your child cannot sleep at night, shorten naps or cut them out completely.

- **Making and keeping friends:** Pair your child with another who is one or two years younger. Provide activities that are short and fun.

- **Boundary issues:** Create a stable, structured home with clear routines and plenty of repetition.

- **Attention problems:** Medication may be helpful. Keep the child's environment as simple as possible and structure time with brief activities.

- **Frustration and tantrums:** Remove your child from the situation and use calming techniques such as sitting in a rocker, giving a warm bath, or playing quiet music.

- **Difficulty understanding cause and effect:** Repetition, consistency, and clear consequences for behavior are important.

Adolescence

- **Anxiety and depression:** Medication may be helpful, as well as counseling or encouraging your child to participate in sports, clubs, or other structured activities.

- **Victimization:** Monitor the activities of your child and discuss dealing with strangers.

- **Lying, stealing, or antisocial behavior:** Family counseling is helpful, as well as setting simple and consistent rules with immediate consequences.

Adulthood

- **Housing:** Finding appropriate housing for adults affected by FAS/FASD is extremely challenging. Contact your state's department of disabilities to pursue residential funding and get on every waiting list you can find that offers housing options.

- **Poor peer or social relations:** Enroll your child in classes or social clubs for adults with disabilities.

- **Mental health issues:** Provide structure, routine, and plenty of activities. Investigate medication options and counseling.

- **Handling money:** Many FAS adults need the family to handle all financial matters.

- **Difficulty obtaining or keeping jobs:** Investigate trade schools, job training programs, or job coaches. Be sure to select jobs that offer structured, routine activities that won't cause overload or stress.

More Tips

Routine

- Keep the family's routine as much the same each day as you can.
- If the family's routine or schedule changes, remind your child about changes.

Behavior

- Learn how to tell when your child is getting frustrated, and help out early.
- Make sure your child understands the rules at home.
- Tell your child about what will happen if he or she has good behavior or bad behavior at home.
- Let your child know when he or she has good behavior.
- Teach self-talk to help your child develop self-control. Use specific, short phrases such as "stop and think."
- Repeat everything you say and give your child many chances to do what you ask.
- Be patient.
- Give directions one step at a time. Wait for your child to do the first step in the directions before telling your child the second step.
- Tell your child before you touch him or her.
- Be sure your child understands your rules, and be firm and consistent with them.

Chapter 5

Illicit Drug Use during Pregnancy

When you are pregnant it is important that you watch what you put into your body. Consumption of illegal drugs is not safe for the unborn baby or for the mother. Studies have shown that consumption of illegal drugs during pregnancy can result in miscarriage, low birthweight, premature labor, placental abruption, fetal death, and even maternal death.

Marijuana

Common slang names: Pot, weed, grass, and reefer.

What happens when a pregnant woman smokes marijuana: Marijuana crosses the placenta to your baby. Marijuana, like cigarette smoke, contains toxins that keep your baby from getting the proper supply of oxygen that he or she needs to grow.

How can marijuana affect the unborn baby: Studies of marijuana in pregnancy are inconclusive since many women who smoke marijuana also use tobacco and alcohol. Smoking marijuana increases the levels of carbon monoxide and carbon dioxide in the blood, which reduces the oxygen supply to the baby. Smoking marijuana during pregnancy can increase the chance of miscarriage, low birth weight, premature births, developmental delays, and behavioral and learning problems.

What if I smoked marijuana before I knew I was pregnant: According to Dr. Richard S. Abram, author of *Will it Hurt the Baby*, "occasional use of marijuana during the first trimester is unlikely to cause birth defects." Once you are aware you are pregnant, you should stop smoking. Doing this will decrease the chances of harming your baby.

Cocaine

Common slang names: Bump, toot, C, coke, crack, flake, snow, and candy.

What happens when a pregnant woman consumes cocaine: Cocaine crosses the placenta and enters your baby's circulation. The elimination of cocaine is slower in the fetus than in an adult. This means that cocaine remains in the baby's body much longer than in you.

How can cocaine affect my unborn baby: According to the Organization of Teratology Information Services (OTIS), during the early months of pregnancy cocaine exposure may increase the risk of miscarriage. Later in pregnancy, cocaine use can cause placental abruption. Placental abruption can lead to severe bleeding, preterm birth, and fetal death. OTIS also states that the risk of a birth defect appears to be greater when the mother has used cocaine frequently during pregnancy. According to the American College of Obstetricians and Gynecology (ACOG), women who use cocaine during their pregnancy have a 25 percent increased chance of premature labor. Babies born to mothers who use cocaine throughout their pregnancy may also have a smaller head and their growth may be hindered. Babies who are exposed to cocaine later in pregnancy may be born dependent and suffer from withdrawal symptoms such as tremors, sleeplessness, muscle spasms, and difficulty feeding. Some experts believe that learning difficulties may result as the child gets older. Defects of the genitals, kidneys, and brain are also possibilities.

What if I consumed cocaine before I knew I was pregnant: There have not been any conclusive studies done on single doses of cocaine during pregnancy. Birth defects and other side effects are usually a result of prolonged use but since studies are inconclusive it is best to just stay away from cocaine altogether. Cocaine is a very addictive drug and it is easier not to abuse if you don't experiment.

Heroin

Common slang names: Horse, smack, junk, and H-stuff.

What happens when a pregnant woman uses heroin: Heroin is a very addictive drug that crosses the placenta to the baby. Because this drug is so addictive, the unborn baby can become dependent on the drug.

How can heroin affect my unborn baby: Using heroin during pregnancy increases the chance of premature birth, low birth weight, breathing difficulties, low blood sugar (hypoglycemia), bleeding within the brain (intracranial hemorrhage), and infant death. Babies can also be born addicted to heroin and can suffer from withdrawal symptoms. Withdrawal symptoms include irritability, convulsions, diarrhea, fever, sleep abnormalities, and joint stiffness. Mothers who inject narcotics are more susceptible to HIV, and HIV-infected women run a high risk of passing HIV to their unborn child.

What if I am addicted to heroin and I am pregnant: Treating an addiction to heroin can be complicated, especially when you are pregnant. Your doctor may prescribe methadone as a form of treatment. It is best that you communicate with your doctor so he or she can provide the best treatment for you and your baby.

PCP and LSD

What happens when a pregnant woman takes PCP and LSD: PCP and LSD are hallucinogens. Both PCP and LSD users can have violent behavior, which may cause harm to the baby if the mother hurts herself.

How can PCP and LSD affect my unborn baby: PCP use during pregnancy can lead to low birth weight, poor muscle control, brain damage, and withdrawal syndrome if used frequently. Withdrawal symptoms include lethargy, alternating with tremors. LSD can lead to birth defects if used frequently.

What if I experimented with LSD or PCP before I knew I was pregnant: No conclusive studies have been done on one-time use effects of these drugs on the fetus. It is best not to experiment if you are trying to get pregnant or think you may have a chance of being pregnant.

Speed

What happens when a pregnant woman takes speed: Speed is an amphetamine, which causes the heart rate of the mother and baby to increase.

How can speed affect my unborn baby: Taking speed during pregnancy can result in problems similar to those seen with the use of cocaine in pregnancy. The use of speed can cause the baby to get less oxygen, which can lead to a small baby at birth. Speed can also increase the likelihood of premature labor, miscarriage, and placental abruption. Babies can be born addicted to speed and suffer withdrawal symptoms that include tremors, sleeplessness, muscle spasms, and difficulty feeding. Some experts believe that learning difficulties may result as the child gets older.

What if I experimented with speed before I knew I was pregnant: There have not been any significant studies done on the effect of one-time use of speed during pregnancy. It is best not to experiment if you are trying to get pregnant or think you may have a chance of being pregnant.

What Does the Law Say?

Currently there is only one state, South Carolina, that holds prenatal substance abuse as a criminal act of child abuse and neglect. Other states have their own way of dealing with prenatal substance abuse:

- Iowa, Minnesota, and North Dakota's health care professionals are required to report prenatal drug exposure.

- Arizona, Illinois, Massachusetts, Michigan, Utah, Virginia, and Rhode Island's health care professionals are required to report and test for prenatal exposure. Reporting and testing can be evidence used in child welfare proceedings.

- Some states consider prenatal substance abuse as part of their child welfare laws. Therefore prenatal drug exposure can provide grounds for terminating parental rights because of child abuse or neglect. These states include: Florida, Illinois, Indiana, Maryland, Minnesota, Nevada, Ohio, Rhode Island, South Carolina, South Dakota, Texas, Virginia, and Wisconsin

- Some states have policies that enforce admission to an inpatient treatment program for pregnant women who use drugs. These states include: Minnesota, South Carolina, and Wisconsin

- A 2004 Texas law made it a felony to smoke marijuana while pregnant, resulting in a prison sentence of two to twenty years.

How Can I Get Help?

You can get help from counseling, support groups, and treatment programs. Popular groups include the twelve-step program. Numbers that can help you locate a treatment center include:

- National Drug Help Hotline 1-800-662-4357

- National Alcohol and Drug Abuse 1-800-234-1253

Chapter 6

Pregnancy and Medication

Chapter Contents

Section 6.1—Medication Use during Pregnancy: An
    Overview 68
Section 6.2—Risk of Birth Defects with Accutane 72
Section 6.3—Risk of Birth Defects with Angiotensin
    Converting Enzyme (ACE) Inhibitors 77
Section 6.4—Risk of Birth Defects with Paxil 78
Section 6.5—Risk of Birth Defects with Thalidomide 80
Section 6.6—Vaccines and Pregnancy 82

Section 6.1

Medication Use during Pregnancy: An Overview

Reprinted from "Pregnancy and Medications," National Women's Health Information Center, U.S. Department of Health and Human Services, November 2002.

Is it safe to take medicine while you are pregnant?

It can be hard to plan exactly when you will get pregnant, in order to avoid taking any medicine. Most of the time, medicine a pregnant woman is taking does not enter the fetus. But sometimes it can, causing damage or birth defects. The risk of damage being done to a fetus is the greatest in the first few weeks of pregnancy, when major organs are developing. But researchers also do not know if taking medicines during pregnancy also will have negative effects on the baby later.

Many drugs that you can buy over the counter (OTC) in drug and discount stores, and drugs your health care provider prescribes, are thought to be safe to take during pregnancy, although there are no medicines that are proven to be absolutely safe when you are pregnant. Many of these products tell you on the label if they are thought to be safe during pregnancy. If you are not sure you can take an OTC product, ask your health care provider.

Some drugs are not safe to take during pregnancy. Even drugs prescribed to you by your health care provider before you became pregnant might be harmful to both you and the growing fetus during pregnancy. Make sure all of your health care providers know you are pregnant, and never take any drugs during pregnancy unless they tell you to.

Also, keep in mind that other things like caffeine, vitamins, and herbal teas and remedies can affect the growing fetus. Talk with your health care provider about cutting down on caffeine and the type of vitamins you need to take. Never use any herbal product without talking to your health care provider first.

What over-the-counter and prescription drugs are not safe to take during pregnancy?

The Food and Drug Administration (FDA) has a system to rate drugs in terms of their safety during pregnancy. This system rates both over-the-counter (OTC) drugs you can buy in a drug or discount store and drugs your health care provider prescribes. But most medicines have not been studied in pregnant women to see if they cause damage to the growing fetus. Always talk with your health care provider if you have questions or concerns.

The FDA system ranks drugs in the following categories:

- **Category A:** Drugs that have been tested for safety during pregnancy and have been found to be safe. This includes drugs such as folic acid, vitamin B6, and thyroid medicine in moderation, or in prescribed doses.

- **Category B:** Drugs that have been used a lot during pregnancy and do not appear to cause major birth defects or other problems. This includes drugs such as some antibiotics, acetaminophen (Tylenol), aspartame (artificial sweetener), famotidine (Pepcid), prednisone (cortisone), insulin (for diabetes), and ibuprofen (Advil, Motrin) before the third trimester. Pregnant women should not take ibuprofen during the last three months of pregnancy.

- **Category C:** Drugs that are more likely to cause problems for the mother or fetus. Also includes drugs for which safety studies have not been finished. The majority of these drugs do not have safety studies in progress. These drugs often come with a warning that they should be used only if the benefits of taking them outweigh the risks. This is something a woman would need to carefully discuss with her doctor. These drugs include prochlorperazine (Compazine), Sudafed, fluconazole (Diflucan), and ciprofloxacin (Cipro). Some antidepressants are also included in this group.

- **Category D:** Drugs that have clear health risks for the fetus. These include alcohol, lithium (used to treat manic depression), phenytoin (Dilantin), and most chemotherapy drugs to treat cancer. In some cases, chemotherapy drugs are given during pregnancy.

- **Category X:** Drugs that have been shown to cause birth defects and should never be taken during pregnancy. These include drugs to treat skin conditions like cystic acne (Accutane) and psoriasis (Tegison or Soriatane); a sedative (thalidomide); and a drug to prevent miscarriage used up until 1971 in the United States and 1983 in Europe (diethylstilbestrol or DES).

Aspirin and other drugs containing salicylate are not recommended during pregnancy, especially during the last three months. In rare cases, a woman's health care provider may want her to use these type of drugs under close watch. Acetylsalicylate, a common ingredient in many OTC painkillers, may make a pregnancy last longer and may cause severe bleeding before and after delivery.

Will there be studies in the future that will look at whether certain medicines or products are safe in pregnant women?

To help women make informed and educated decisions about using medicines during pregnancy, it is necessary to find out the effect of these medicines on the unborn baby. Pregnancy registries are one way to do this. A pregnancy registry is a study that enrolls pregnant women after they have been taking medicine and before the birth of the baby. Babies born to women taking a particular medicine are compared with babies of women not taking the medicine. Researchers must look at a large number of women and babies in order to find out the effect of the medicine on the babies.

If you are pregnant and currently taking medicine—or have been exposed to a medicine during your pregnancy—you may be able to join and help with this needed information. The Food and Drug Administration's (FDA) web site (http://www.fda.gov/womens/registries/) has a list of pregnancy registries that are enrolling pregnant women.

Should I avoid taking any medicine while I am pregnant?

Whether or not you should continue taking medicine during pregnancy is a serious question. But, if you stop taking medicine that you need, this could harm both you and your baby. An example of this is if you have an infection called toxoplasmosis, which you can get from handling cat feces or eating infected meat. It can cause problems with the brain, eyes, heart, and other organs of a growing fetus. This infection requires treatment with antibiotics.

For pregnant women living with HIV, the Centers for Disease Control and Prevention (CDC) recommends the drug zidovudine (AZT). Studies have found that HIV-positive women who take AZT during pregnancy decrease by two-thirds the risk of passing HIV to their babies. If a diabetic woman does not take her medicine during pregnancy, she increases her risk for miscarriage and stillbirth. If asthma or high blood pressure is not controlled during pregnancy, problems with the fetus may result. Talk with your health care provider about whether the benefits of taking a medication outweigh the risk for you and your baby.

What about taking natural medications, or herbal remedies, when you are pregnant?

While some herbal remedies say they will help with pregnancy, there have been no studies to figure out if these claims are true. Likewise, there have been very few studies to look at how safe and effective herbal remedies are. Echinacea, gingko biloba, and St. John's wort have been popular herbs, to name a few. Do not take any herbal products without talking to your health care provider first. These products may contain agents that could harm you and the growing fetus, and cause problems with your pregnancy.

I have heard that some women who were pregnant between 1938 and 1971 were given a drug called DES to prevent miscarriages that is now known to cause cancers. Would I be affected if my mother took this drug?

The synthetic (or manmade) estrogen, diethylstilbestrol or DES, was made in London in 1938. DES was used in the United States between 1938 and 1971 to prevent miscarriage (losing a pregnancy). Many women who had problems with earlier pregnancies were given DES because it was thought to be both safe and effective. Over time, it was found that not only did DES not prevent miscarriage, it also caused cancers of the vagina (birth canal) and cervix (opening to the uterus or womb).

While many women were given DES over this time, many mothers do not remember what they were given by their health care providers when they were pregnant. Some prescription prenatal vitamins also contained DES. If your mother is not sure whether she took DES, you can talk with the health care provider she went to when she was pregnant with you or contact the hospital for a copy of her medical records.

DES can affect both the pregnant woman and the child (both daughters and sons). Daughters born to women who took DES are more at risk for cancer of the vagina and cervix. Sons born to women who took DES are more at risk for noncancerous growths on the testicles and underdeveloped testicles. Women who took DES may have a higher risk for breast cancer.

If you think or know that your mother took DES when she was pregnant with you, talk with your health care provider right away. Ask her or him about what types of tests you may need, how often they need to be done, and anything else you may need to do to make sure you don't develop any problems.

Section 6.2

Risk of Birth Defects with Accutane

Reprinted from "Accutane (Isotretinoin) and Pregnancy," © 2006 Organization of Teratology Information Services (OTIS). Reprinted with permission. Member programs of OTIS are located throughout the U.S. and Canada. To find the Teratogen Information Service in your area, call OTIS toll-free at 866-626-OTIS (866-626-6847), or visit their website at www .otispregnancy.org.

Any woman who gets pregnant has a 3 to 5 percent chance of having a baby with a birth defect. The information below will help you to determine if your exposure to isotretinoin during pregnancy increases your risk above this background risk. This information should not be used as a substitute for the medical care and advice of your health care provider.

What is Accutane?

Accutane is a prescription medication taken by mouth to treat severe disfiguring cystic acne that has not responded to other treatments. Accutane is a man-made form of Vitamin A. Its generic name is isotretinoin. Other drug companies are now allowed to make and sell isotretinoin under different names, such as Amnesteem, Claravis, and Sotret.

How long does isotretinoin stay in the body? How long after a woman stops taking isotretinoin should she wait to become pregnant?

The time it takes isotretinoin to be cleared from the blood varies. This is because some women use higher doses and some women may not be using the medicine as prescribed. Isotretinoin is not found in a woman's blood four to five days after the last dose. Most of its by-products should be gone within ten days after the last dose. It is recommend that a woman wait one month after stopping isotretinoin before trying to become pregnant.

Can isotretinoin make it more difficult to get pregnant?

There have been reports of irregular menstrual periods in some women taking isotretinoin. There are no reports of problems getting pregnant while taking isotretinoin. Women who are trying to become pregnant should not be taking isotretinoin!

Does exposure to isotretinoin cause an increased risk for miscarriage or infant death?

Yes. The risk for having a miscarriage may be as high as 40 percent when a woman takes isotretinoin in early pregnancy.

Can taking isotretinoin during pregnancy cause birth defects?

Yes. Isotretinoin causes a pattern of birth defects in more than 35 percent of infants whose mothers take the drug during pregnancy. Most of the infants with birth defects will have small or absent ears and hearing and eyesight problems. Some will have a small jaw, small head, and cleft palate and some will be born with a small or missing thymus gland. Life-threatening heart defects and fluid around the brain are seen in almost half of the exposed infants.

Will taking isotretinoin have an effect on a baby's behavior and development?

Yes. Many of the exposed children will have moderate to severe mental retardation. These difficulties are not noticed at birth, but are discovered in childhood. The long-term effects on any exposed child are still unknown.

If a woman gets pregnant while taking isotretinoin, what should she do?

Stop taking the medicine right away! As soon as possible, call the doctor who prescribed the isotretinoin and the doctor who will be taking care of you during your pregnancy. Your doctors can tell you what the risks are and testing that may be done. A special ultrasound done in the second trimester of pregnancy may be able to see if a birth defect has been caused by exposure to isotretinoin. Ultrasound can detect many birth defects but it cannot tell if a child may have learning or developmental problems.

Can a woman ever safely use isotretinoin?

Yes. Isotretinoin can be prescribed under a special program called iPLEDGE™. Women must adhere to all requirements of the iPLEDGE program. Following are a few of the requirements:

- Women must be able to understand that severe birth defects can occur with use of isotretinoin.

- Women must receive and be able to understand safety information about isotretinoin and the iPLEDGE requirements.

- Women must sign an informed consent form that contains warnings about the risks of using isotretinoin.

- Women must not be pregnant or be breastfeeding.

- Women must have two negative pregnancy tests before starting isotretinoin.

- Women must have a pregnancy test every month during treatment, and a negative test a month after treatment.

- Women must use two different forms of birth control at all times (unless woman agrees not to have sex) starting one month before treatment, continuing during treatment, and for one month after treatment.

- Women must fill their prescription within seven days after the doctor visit.

- Women must agree to see their doctor every month during treatment for a health check and to get a new prescription.

For more information about the iPLEDGE program call 866-495-0654 or visit the iPLEDGE website: https://www.ipledgeprogram.com.

The Organization of Teratology Information Specialists recommends that women who are not sexually active still talk to their health care provider about using a safe and effective birth control method because almost 50 percent of all pregnancies are unplanned or unintended.

Can isotretinoin be taken while breastfeeding?

There have been no studies looking at taking isotretinoin during breastfeeding. It is not known if isotretinoin can get into breast milk but other similar medications can. We do not know what effect exposure to isotretinoin through the breast milk can have on a nursing infant. Until more is known, women who are breastfeeding should not take isotretinoin.

Isotretinoin is a man-made vitamin A. Are there other vitamin A–related medicines that women should avoid prior to or during pregnancy?

Yes. Tegison (etretinate), Soriatane (acitretin), and high-dose Vitamin A (more than 20,000 IU per day) are medications used to treat skin problems. They should never be used by women of childbearing age and can cause birth defects similar to isotretinoin.

References

Adams J and Lammer EJ. (1991) Relationship between dysmorphology and neuropsychological function in children exposed to isotretinoin "in utero." In: T. Fujii and G. J. Boer (eds), *Functional Neuroteratology of Short Term Exposure to Drugs.* Tokyo: Teikyo University Press. pp.159–70.

Adams J and Lammer EJ. Neurobehavioral teratology of isotretinoin. *Reprod Toxicol*. 7(2):175–77, 1993.

Adams J. Similarities in genetic mental retardation and neuroteratogenic syndromes. *Pharmacol Biochem Behav*. Dec; 55(4):683–90, 1996.

Committee on Drugs, American Academy of Pediatrics: Retinoid therapy for severe dermatological disorders. *Pediatrics* 90:119–20, 1992.

Dai WS, Hsu M-A, Itri LM: Safety of pregnancy after discontinuation of isotretinoin. *Arch Dermatol* 125:362–65, 1989.

Dai WS, LaBraico JM, Stern RS: Epidemiology of isotretinoin exposure during pregnancy. *J Am Acad Dermatol* 26:599–606, 1992.

DiGiovanna JJ, Zech LA, Ruddel ME, et al.: Etretinate: Persistent serum levels of a potent teratogen. *Clin Res* 32:579A, 1984.

Goldsmith LA, Bolognia JL, Callen JP, Chen SC, Feldman SR, Lim HW, Lucky AW, Reed BR, Siegfried EC, Thiboutot DM, Wheeland RG; American Academy of Dermatology. American Academy of Dermatology Consensus Conference on the safe and optimal use of isotretinoin: summary and recommendations. 1: *J Am Acad Dermatol.* 2004 Jun; 50(6):900–906. [Erratum in: *J Am Acad Dermatol.* 2004 Sep; 51(3):348. dosage error in text.]

Lammer EJ, Hayes EM, Schunior A, Holmes LB (1987). Risk for major malformation among human fetuses exposed to isotretinoin (13-cisretinoic acid). *Teratology*, 35, 68A.

Lammer EJ, Chen DT, Hoar RM, Agnish SO, Benke PJ, Brown JT, Curry CJ, Fernhoff PM, Grix AW, Loft IT, Richard JM, Sun SC. (1985). Retinoic acid embryopathy. *New Engl. J. Medicine*, 313, 837–41.

Mitchell AA: Oral retinoids. What should the prescriber know about their teratogenic hazards among women of child-bearing potential? *Drug Saf* 7(2):79–85, 1992.

Recommendations for isotretinoin use in women of childbearing potential. *Teratology* 44:1–6, 1991.

Rosa FW: Teratogenicity of isotretinoin. *Lancet* 2:513, 1983. https://www.ipledgeprogram.com/AboutiPLEDGE.aspx ©iPLEDGE 2005 [accessed December 20, 2005].

Section 6.3

Risk of Birth Defects with Angiotensin Converting Enzyme (ACE) Inhibitors

Background

Use of angiotensin converting enzyme (ACE) inhibitors during the second and third trimesters of pregnancy is contraindicated because of their association with an increased risk of fetopathy [disease in the fetus]. In contrast, first-trimester use of ACE inhibitors has not been linked to adverse fetal outcomes. We conducted a study to assess the association between exposure to ACE inhibitors during the first trimester of pregnancy only and the risk of congenital malformations.

Methods

We studied a cohort of 29,507 infants enrolled in Tennessee Medicaid and born between 1985 and 2000 for whom there was no evidence of maternal diabetes. We identified 209 infants with exposure to ACE inhibitors in the first trimester alone, 202 infants with exposure to other antihypertensive medications in the first trimester alone, and 29,096 infants with no exposure to antihypertensive drugs at any time during gestation. Major congenital malformations were identified from linked vital records and hospitalization claims during the first year of life and confirmed by review of medical records.

Results

Infants with only first-trimester exposure to ACE inhibitors had an increased risk of major congenital malformations (risk ratio, 2.71; 95 percent confidence interval, 1.72 to 4.27) as compared with infants who had no exposure to antihypertensive medications. In contrast, fetal exposure to other antihypertensive medications during only the first trimester did not confer an increased risk (risk ratio, 0.66; 95 percent confidence interval, 0.25 to 1.75). Infants exposed to ACE inhibitors were at increased risk for malformations of the cardiovascular system (risk ratio, 3.72; 95 percent confidence interval, 1.89 to 7.30) and the central nervous system (risk ratio, 4.39; 95 percent confidence interval, 1.37 to 14.02).

Conclusions

Exposure to ACE inhibitors during the first trimester cannot be considered safe and should be avoided.

Section 6.4

Risk of Birth Defects with Paxil

Reprinted from "FDA Advising of Risk of Birth Defects with Paxil," *FDA News,* U.S. Food and Drug Administration, December 8, 2005.

The Food and Drug Administration is alerting health care professionals and patients about early results of new studies for Paxil (paroxetine) suggesting that the drug increases the risk for birth defects, particularly heart defects, when women take it during the first three months of pregnancy. Paxil is approved for the treatment of depression and several other psychiatric disorders. FDA is currently gathering additional data and waiting for the final results of the recent studies in order to better understand the higher risk for birth defects that has been seen with Paxil.

FDA is advising health care professionals to discuss the potential risk of birth defects with patients taking Paxil who plan to become pregnant or are in their first three months of pregnancy. Health care professionals should consider discontinuing Paxil (and switching to another antidepressant if indicated) in these patients. In some patients, the benefits of continuing Paxil may be greater than the potential risk to the fetus. FDA is advising health care professionals not to prescribe Paxil in women who are in the first three months of pregnancy or are planning pregnancy, unless other treatment options are not appropriate.

FDA is advising patients that this drug should usually not be taken during pregnancy, but for some women who have already been taking Paxil, the benefits of continuing may be greater than the potential risk to the fetus. Women taking Paxil who are pregnant or plan to become pregnant should talk to their physicians about the potential risks of taking the drug during pregnancy. Women taking Paxil should not stop taking it without first talking with their physician.

The early results of two studies showed that women who took Paxil during the first three months of pregnancy were about one and a half to two times as likely to have a baby with a heart defect as women who received other antidepressants or women in the general population. Most of the heart defects reported in these studies were atrial and ventricular septal defects (holes in the walls of the chambers of the heart). In general, these types of defects range in severity from those that are minor and may resolve without treatment to those that cause serious symptoms and may need to be repaired surgically.

In one of the studies, the risk of heart defects in babies whose mothers had taken Paxil early in pregnancy was about 2 percent, compared to a 1 percent risk in the whole population. In the other study, the risk of heart defects in babies whose mothers had taken Paxil in the first three months of pregnancy was 1.5 percent, compared to 1 percent in babies whose mothers had taken other antidepressants in the first three months of pregnancy.

FDA has asked the manufacturer, Glaxo Smith Kline (GSK), to change the pregnancy category from C to D, a stronger warning. Category D means that studies in pregnant women (controlled or observational) have demonstrated a risk to the fetus. However, the benefits of therapy may outweigh the potential risks to the fetus.

Based on results of the preliminary data, GSK updated the drug's labeling in September 2005 to add data from one study. As additional data have become available, the label has now been changed to reflect the latest data from the two studies and to change the pregnancy category.

Section 6.5

Risk of Birth Defects with Thalidomide

Excerpted from "Frequently Asked Questions Concerning Thalidomide,"
U.S. Food and Drug Administration, 2003.

What is thalidomide?

Thalidomide is a drug that was marketed outside of the United States in the late 1950s and early 1960s. It was used as a sleeping pill, and to treat morning sickness during pregnancy. However, its use by pregnant women resulted in the birth of thousands of deformed babies.

Is thalidomide approved in any other countries? If so, which countries?

Yes, thalidomide is approved in Brazil and Mexico.

What is thalidomide approved for in the United States?

Thalomid (thalidomide) is approved to treat the painful, disfiguring skin sores associated with leprosy, and to prevent and control the return of these skin sores.

Is Thalomid (thalidomide) use safe during pregnancy, or if I plan to get pregnant?

No. A pregnant woman or any woman thinking about becoming pregnant must not take Thalomid (thalidomide), because it is known to cause severe birth defects or death to an unborn baby, even after taking just one dose. When a woman of childbearing age has no other appropriate treatment choice and must take Thalomid (thalidomide), there are many precautions that must be taken to avoid pregnancy. Some of these precautions are as follows:

- A pregnancy test twenty-four hours before taking Thalomid (thalidomide) and then weekly during the first month of use; then monthly in women with regular menstrual cycles, or every two weeks if menstrual cycles are irregular, as long as you are taking Thalomid (thalidomide).

- Committing to either not having heterosexual sexual intercourse, or to using two methods of birth control starting four weeks before your first dose of Thalomid (thalidomide) and continuing for four weeks after your last dose of Thalomid (thalidomide).

Can I breast-feed while taking Thalomid (thalidomide)?

No. You must not breast-feed a baby while taking Thalomid (thalidomide) because of possible side effects to the infant.

Can I donate blood or sperm while being treated with Thalomid (thalidomide)?

No. You must not donate blood or sperm while you are taking Thalomid (thalidomide).

Are there any side effects with Thalomid (thalidomide)?

The most serious side effect known with Thalomid (thalidomide) is its risk of severe birth defects or death to an unborn baby, even after taking one dose. Therefore, if you are pregnant or trying to get pregnant, you must not take Thalomid (thalidomide).

Thalomid (thalidomide) is also associated with the following adverse events:

- **Nerve damage that can be severe and permanent:** If you notice any numbness, tingling, or pain or a burning sensation in your hands and feet, stop taking Thalomid (thalidomide) and call your health care provider.
- **Allergic reactions:** Signs may include rash, fever, a fast heartbeat, or very low blood pressure. Call your health care provider if you have any of these symptoms.
- **Increase in viral load for HIV-positive patients**
- **Drowsiness:** Use caution when driving or operating heavy machinery.
- **Dizziness or a drop in blood pressure:** Sit upright for a few minutes before standing up from a lying down or seated position to avoid falling.
- **Rash**
- **Low white blood count**

Section 6.6

Vaccines and Pregnancy

Reprinted from "Vaccines and Pregnancy," © 2005 Organization of Teratology Information Services (OTIS). Reprinted with permission. Member
programs of OTIS are located throughout the U.S. and Canada. To find
the Teratogen Information Service in your area, call OTIS toll-free at 866-
626-OTIS (866-626-6847), or visit their website at www.otispregnancy.org.

Any woman who gets pregnant has a 3 to 5 percent chance of having a baby with a birth defect. The information below will help you to
determine if your exposure to vaccines during pregnancy increases your
risk above this background risk. This information should not be used
as a substitute for the medical care and advice of your health care provider.

What are vaccines?

Vaccines are medicines that can be given to help protect you from
various diseases. They are made from killed or weakened bacteria or
virus. In this form they act like the disease without actually causing
the illness. Vaccines cause your body's immune system to make antibodies. Once these antibodies are made they protect you if you are
exposed to that disease in the future.

*What is the difference between a live and an inactivated
vaccine?*

A "live vaccine" is made from a live virus or bacteria that has been
weakened. This causes the body to make protective antibodies but does
not usually cause the infection. Live vaccines generally provide long-
lasting protection with a single dose. Given the slight possibility that
that a live vaccine could cause the disease itself, live vaccines are not
routinely given to pregnant women.

An "inactivated vaccine" is made from a virus or bacteria that has
been killed. An inactivated vaccine cannot cause the disease that it
is given to prevent. Inactivated vaccines may require multiple doses
and periodic boosters to provide protection.

Which vaccines can be given safely in pregnancy? Which vaccines should not be given in pregnancy?

Vaccination of a pregnant woman with inactivated vaccines has not been shown to cause an increase risk to the fetus. Live vaccines are usually not given in pregnancy due to the potential risk of causing the disease in the fetus. However, when the likelihood of disease exposure is high or when infection would pose a risk to the mother or fetus, then vaccination with a live vaccine is generally recommended.

What if a live vaccine is accidentally given during pregnancy? Does this mean that the pregnancy should be terminated?

No. This alone would not be considered a medical reason to end a pregnancy because the chance of the fetus being infected is generally very low. Counseling by a knowledgeable healthcare provider would be recommended.

Are there any vaccines that are recommended in pregnancy?

Yes. It is recommended that you get the inactivated flu vaccine (flu shot) if you will be pregnant during flu season. If you get the flu during pregnancy you are at a greater risk of flu-related complications. You can get the flu vaccine anytime during your pregnancy but it is best to get the flu shot before the flu season begins for the best protection.

FluMist® is made from live virus and has not been studied for use in pregnancy. As discussed, live vaccines are not recommended during pregnancy.

Diseases such as rabies and tetanus are fatal. Clearly the benefit of vaccination in an exposed pregnancy would outweigh any risks that may be associated with the vaccine.

The need for vaccination with other vaccines during pregnancy will vary and the issue should be discussed with your doctor.

Is it safe for my child to be vaccinated while I am pregnant?

Yes. Inactivated vaccines cannot cause disease. Even if your child or other close contact has a vaccine reaction, there is no chance that you will get the disease that the vaccine was given to prevent. Though unlikely, live vaccines could cause the disease they are trying to prevent. Being in the same household with a healthy child who has been vaccinated with a live vaccine is still not likely to increase the risk to a pregnant woman or her fetus.

Is it safe to breast-feed if I have been vaccinated?

Yes. The use of most vaccines in breast-feeding women is generally considered safe.

Should men delay fathering a child after they have been vaccinated?

No. There is no evidence to suggest that inactivated or live vaccines affect the sperm or are transmitted to the developing embryo through the semen following vaccination in men.

References

National Immunization Program. 2005. *Guidelines for vaccinating pregnant women.* Available at: http://www.cdc.gov/nip/publications/preg_guide.htm

Centers for Disease Control & Prevention. 2005. *Epidemiology and Prevention of Vaccine-preventable Diseases.* Eighth edition. Washington, D.C.: Public Health Foundation. 295 p.

Atkinson WL, Pickering LK, Schwartz B, et al. 2002. Recommendations of the Advisory Committee on Immunization Practices (ACIP) and the American Academy of Family Physicians (AAFP). *MMWR* 51(RR-2): 18–19.

Chapter 7

X-Rays, Pregnancy, and You

Pregnancy is a time to take good care of yourself and your unborn child. Many things are especially important during pregnancy, such as eating right, cutting out cigarettes and alcohol, and being careful about the prescription and over-the-counter drugs you take. Diagnostic x-rays and other medical radiation procedures of the abdominal area also deserve extra attention during pregnancy. This chapter will help you understand the issues concerning x-ray exposure during pregnancy.

Diagnostic x-rays can give the doctor important and even life-saving information about a person's medical condition. But like many things, diagnostic x-rays have risks as well as benefits. They should be used only when they will give the doctor information needed to treat you.

You'll probably never need an abdominal x-ray during pregnancy. Yet sometimes, because of a particular medical condition, your physician may feel that a diagnostic x-ray of your abdomen or lower torso is needed. If this should happen, don't be upset. The risk to you and your unborn child is very small, and the benefit of finding out about your medical condition is far greater. In fact, the risk of not having a needed x-ray could be much greater than the risk from the radiation. Yet even small risks should not be taken if they're unnecessary.

Reprinted from "X-Rays, Pregnancy and You," U.S. Food and Drug Administration, HHS Publication No. (FDA) 94-8087, May 11, 2001.

You can reduce those risks by telling your doctor if you are, or think you might be, pregnant whenever an abdominal x-ray is prescribed. If you are pregnant, the doctor may decide that it would be best to cancel the x-ray examination, to postpone it, or to modify it to reduce the amount of radiation. Or, depending on your medical needs, and realizing that the risk is very small, the doctor may feel that it is best to proceed with the x-ray as planned. In any case, you should feel free to discuss the decision with your doctor.

What kind of x-rays can affect the unborn child?

During most x-ray examinations—like those of the arms, legs, head, teeth, or chest—your reproductive organs are not exposed to the direct x-ray beam. So these kinds of procedures, when properly done, do not involve any risk to the unborn child. However, x-rays of the mother's lower torso—abdomen, stomach, pelvis, lower back, or kidneys—may expose the unborn child to the direct x-ray beam. They are of more concern.

What are the possible effects of x-rays?

There is scientific disagreement about whether the small amounts of radiation used in diagnostic radiology can actually harm the unborn child, but it is known that the unborn child is very sensitive to the effects of things like radiation, certain drugs, excess alcohol, and infection. This is true, in part, because the cells are rapidly dividing and growing into specialized cells and tissues. If radiation or other agents were to cause changes in these cells, there could be a slightly increased chance of birth defects or certain illnesses, such as leukemia, later in life.

It should be pointed out, however, that the majority of birth defects and childhood diseases occur even if the mother is not exposed to any known harmful agent during pregnancy. Scientists believe that heredity and random errors in the developmental process are responsible for most of these problems.

What if I'm x-rayed before I know I'm pregnant?

Don't be alarmed. Remember that the possibility of any harm to you and your unborn child from an x-ray is very small. There are, however, rare situations in which a woman who is unaware of her pregnancy may receive a very large number of abdominal x-rays over a short period. Or she may receive radiation treatment of the lower torso. Under these circumstances, the woman should discuss the possible risks with her doctor.

How can I help minimize the risks?

- Most important, tell your physician if you are pregnant or think you might be. This is important for many medical decisions, such as drug prescriptions and nuclear medicine procedures, as well as x-rays. And remember, this is true even in the very early weeks of pregnancy.

- Occasionally, a woman may mistake the symptoms of pregnancy for the symptoms of a disease. If you have any of the symptoms of pregnancy—nausea, vomiting, breast tenderness, fatigue—consider whether you might be pregnant and tell your doctor or x-ray technologist (the person doing the examination) before having an x-ray of the lower torso. A pregnancy test may be called for.

- If you are pregnant, or think you might be, do not hold a child who is being x-rayed. If you are not pregnant and you are asked to hold a child during an x-ray, be sure to ask for a lead apron to protect your reproductive organs. This is to prevent damage to your genes that could be passed on and cause harmful effects in your future descendants.

- Whenever an x-ray is requested, tell your doctor about any similar x-rays you have had recently. It may not be necessary to do another. It is a good idea to keep a record of the x-ray examinations you and your family have had taken so you can provide this kind of information accurately.

- Feel free to talk with your doctor about the need for an x-ray examination. You should understand the reason x-rays are requested in your particular case.

Chapter 8

Chemical and Other Environmental Risks and Pregnancy

There are more than four million chemical mixtures in homes and businesses in this country, with little information on the effects of most of them during pregnancy. However, a few are known to be harmful to an unborn baby. Most of these are found in the workplace, but certain environmental pollutants found in air and water, as well as chemicals used at home, may pose a risk during pregnancy.

A pregnant woman can inhale these chemicals, ingest them in food or drink, or, in some cases, absorb them through the skin. For most hazardous substances, a pregnant woman would have to be exposed to a large amount for a long time in order for them to harm her baby. Most workplaces have preventive measures to help make sure this doesn't happen. Pregnant women can take steps to help protect themselves and their babies from pollutants and potentially risky chemicals used at home.

What are the risks of lead exposure during pregnancy?

Lead is a naturally occurring metal that was found for many years in gasoline, paint, and other products used in homes and businesses. While lead is still present in the environment, the amounts continue to decrease since the Environmental Protection Agency (EPA) banned its use in these products in the 1970s.

Lead poses health risks for everyone, but young children and unborn babies are at greatest risk. Exposure to high levels of lead during pregnancy contributes to miscarriage, preterm delivery, low birth weight, and developmental delays in the infant. Lead toxicity in children is characterized by behavioral and learning problems and anemia. Few pregnant women in the United States are exposed to high levels of lead. However, even low levels of exposure may cause subtle learning and behavioral problems in the child.

Women who live in older homes may be exposed to higher levels of lead due to deteriorating lead-based paint. About 80 percent of homes built before 1978 were painted with lead-based paint. As long as paint is not crumbling or peeling, it poses little risk. However, if lead-based paint needs to be removed from a home, pregnant women and children should stay out of the home until the project is complete. Sanding or scraping leaded paint produces lead dust. Only experts should remove leaded paint, using proper precautions.

Occasionally, a pregnant woman is exposed to significant amounts of lead in her drinking water if her home has lead pipes, lead solder on copper pipes, or brass faucets. Pregnant women can contact their state health department to find out how to get their pipes tested for lead. The EPA recommends running water for thirty seconds before using it for drinking or cooking to help reduce lead levels. A pregnant woman should use water from only the cold water pipe, which contains less lead than hot water, for cooking, drinking, and preparing baby formula. Many home filters do not remove lead, so a pregnant woman should read the label on her filter carefully and change the filter as recommended.

Lead crystal glassware and some ceramic dishes may contain lead, and pregnant women and children should avoid frequent use of these items. Commercial ceramics are safer than those made by craftspeople. Other unexpected sources of lead in the home may include the wicks of scented candles (which release lead particles into the air when burned) and the plastic (polyvinyl chloride) grips on some hand tools.

Some arts and crafts materials (e.g., oil paints, ceramic glazes, and stained glass materials) contain lead. A woman should try to stick with lead-free alternatives (such as acrylic or watercolor paints) during pregnancy and breastfeeding.

If anyone in the home is exposed to lead on the job (such as painters and those working in smelters, auto repair shops, battery manufacturing plants, or certain types of construction), they should change their clothing and shower at work to avoid bringing lead into the home. They should wash contaminated clothing at work, if possible, or wash it at home separately from the rest of the family's clothing.

Does mercury exposure pose a risk in pregnancy?

Mercury is another metal that is present naturally in the environment. Pregnant women are most often exposed to mercury by eating contaminated fish. Mercury enters the environment from natural and man-made sources (such as coal-burning or other industrial pollution). It is converted by bacteria to a more dangerous form (methylmercury) that accumulates in the fatty tissues of fish. While trace amounts of mercury are present in many types of fish, mercury is most concentrated in large fish that eat other fish, such as swordfish and sharks.

In 2004, the U.S. Food and Drug Administration (FDA) and the Environmental Protection Agency (EPA) made three recommendations for women who might become pregnant, women who are pregnant, and nursing mothers. By following these recommendations, women can get the benefits of eating fish and shellfish and be confident that they have reduced their exposure to the harmful effects of mercury.

1. Do not eat shark, swordfish, king mackerel, or tilefish because they contain high levels of mercury.

2. Eat up to twelve ounces (two average meals) a week of a variety of fish and shellfish that are lower in mercury. Five of the most commonly eaten fish that are low in mercury are shrimp, canned light tuna, salmon, pollock, and catfish. Another commonly eaten fish, albacore ("white") tuna, has more mercury than canned light tuna. When choosing two meals of fish and shellfish, women may eat up to six ounces (one average meal) of albacore tuna per week.

3. Check local advisories about the safety of fish caught by family and friends in local lakes, rivers, and coastal areas. If no advice is available, women may eat up to six ounces (one average meal) per week of fish caught from local waters, but they should not consume any other fish during that week.

Game fish also may be contaminated with other industrial pollutants such as polychlorinated biphenyls (PCBs); a pregnant woman's exposure to PCBs may contribute to a child's learning problems, reduced IQ, and low birth weight. Pregnant women or women who could become pregnant should not consume any game fish without checking with their state or local health department or the EPA to find out which fish are safe to eat.

It's less certain whether exposure to elemental mercury, which is used in thermometers, dental fillings, and batteries, poses a risk in pregnancy. Some studies have found an increased risk of miscarriage in women working in dental offices. Women who work with mercury should take all recommended precautions to reduce their exposure.

What other metals pose a risk in pregnancy?

Arsenic and cadmium are two other metals that are suspected of posing pregnancy risks. These metals enter the environment through natural (weathering of rock and forest fires) and man-made (mining and burning of fossil fuels and waste) forces.

While arsenic is a well-known poison, the small amounts normally found in the environment are unlikely to harm a fetus. However, certain women may be exposed to higher levels of arsenic that could pose a risk. Several studies suggest that women working at or living near metal smelters may be at increased risk of miscarriage and stillbirth. Women who live in agricultural areas where arsenic fertilizers (now banned) were used on crops or who live near hazardous waste sites or incinerators also may be exposed to higher-than-normal levels of arsenic. They can help protect themselves by having their water tested for arsenic or by drinking bottled water and limiting contact with soil. Because arsenic also is used as part of a preservative in pressure-treated lumber, pregnant women should avoid wood dust from home construction projects. Anyone who works with arsenic (semiconductor manufacturing, metal smelting, herbicide application) should avoid bringing the metal home on clothing.

Scientists suspect that cadmium may pose a risk in pregnancy. One study suggests that cadmium may damage the placenta and reduce birth weight. This metal is used in many occupations, including semiconductor manufacturing, welding, soldering, ceramics, and painting. Women who work with cadmium should take all recommended precautions and avoid bringing it home on clothing. Pregnant women also may want to consider eliminating sources of cadmium from the house, such as fungicides containing cadmium chloride, certain fabric dyes and ceramic and glass glazes, and some fertilizers.

Can pesticides harm an unborn baby?

Pregnant women should avoid pesticides, whenever possible. There is no proof that exposure to pest-control products at levels commonly used at home pose a risk to the fetus. However, all insecticides are to some extent poisonous and some studies have suggested that high levels of exposure to pesticides may contribute to miscarriage, preterm delivery, and birth defects. Certain pesticides and other chemicals, including PCBs, have weak, estrogen-like qualities called endocrine disrupters that some scientists suspect may affect development of the fetus's reproductive system.

A pregnant woman can reduce her exposure to pesticides by controlling pest problems with less toxic products such as boric acid (use the blue form available at hardware stores). If she must have her home or property treated with pesticides, a pregnant woman should:

- Have someone else apply the chemicals and leave the area for the amount of time indicated on the package instructions

- Remove food, dishes, and utensils from the area before the pesticide is applied. Afterward, have someone open the windows and wash off all surfaces on which food is prepared.

- Close all windows and turn off air conditioning, when pesticides are used outdoors, so fumes aren't drawn into the house

- Wear rubber gloves when gardening to prevent skin contact with pesticides

Health care providers also have some concerns about the use of insect repellants during pregnancy. The insect repellant DEET (diethyltoluamide) is among the most effective at keeping bugs from biting; however, its safety during pregnancy has not been fully assessed. If a pregnant woman uses DEET, she should not apply it to her skin. Instead, she should place small amounts on her socks and shoes and outer clothes, using gloves or an applicator to avoid contact with her fingers.

What are organic solvents?

Organic solvents are chemicals that dissolve other substances. Common organic solvents include alcohols, degreasers, paint thinners, and varnish removers. Lacquers, silk-screening inks, and paints also contain these chemicals. A 1999 Canadian study found that women who were exposed to solvents on the job during their first trimester of pregnancy were about thirteen times more likely than unexposed women to have a baby with a major birth defect, like spina bifida (open spine), clubfoot, heart defects, and deafness. The women in the study included factory workers, laboratory technicians, artists, graphic designers, and printing industry workers.

Other studies have found that women workers in semiconductor plants exposed to high levels of solvents called glycol ethers were almost three times more likely to miscarry than unexposed women. Glycol ethers also are used in jobs that involve photography, dyes, and silk-screen printing.

Pregnant women who work with solvents, including women who do arts and crafts at home, should minimize their exposure by making sure their workplace is well ventilated and by wearing appropriate protective equipment, including gloves and a face mask. They should never eat or drink in their work area. To learn more about the chemicals she works with, a woman can ask her employer for the Material Safety Data Sheets for the products she uses or contact the National Institute for Occupational Safety and Health or visit http://www.msdssearch.com.

Is drinking chlorinated tap water safe during pregnancy?

In recent years, media reports have raised concerns about possible pregnancy risks from by-products of chlorinated drinking water. Chlorine is added to drinking water to kill disease-causing microbes. However, when chlorine combines with other materials in water, it forms chloroform and related chemicals called trihalomethanes. The level of these chemicals in water supplies varies. A few studies suggest that the risk of miscarriage and poor fetal growth may be increased when levels of these chemicals are high, while other studies have not found an increased risk. Scientists continue to study the safety of these chemicals during pregnancy. Until we know more, pregnant women who are concerned about chlorine may choose to drink bottled water.

Drinking water also can become contaminated with pesticides, lead, or other metals. Women who suspect their water supply may be affected can have their water tested or drink bottled water.

Do household cleaning products pose a risk in pregnancy?

While some household cleansers contain solvents, there are many safe alternatives. Pregnant women should read labels carefully and avoid products (such as some oven cleaners) whose labels indicate they're toxic.

Products that contain ammonia or chlorine are unlikely to harm an unborn baby, though their odors may trigger nausea in a pregnant woman. A pregnant woman should open windows and doors and wear rubber gloves when using these products. She should never mix ammonia and chlorine products because the combination produces fumes that are dangerous for anyone.

A pregnant woman who is worried about commercial cleansers or bothered by their odors can substitute safe, natural products. For example, baking soda can be used as a powdered cleanser to scrub greasy areas, pots and pans, sinks, tubs, and ovens. A solution of vinegar and water can effectively clean many surfaces such as countertops.

Does the March of Dimes support research on environmental risks in pregnancy?

The March of Dimes has long supported studies seeking to identify environmental exposures that may pose a risk in pregnancy. One grantee found that a combination of genetic susceptibility with workplace exposure to the solvent benzene appeared to shorten pregnancy. This finding may eventually make it possible to identify high-risk women so that they can take steps to reduce their risk. Another grantee is hoping to provide better dietary counseling to pregnant women by studying the levels of mercury and PCBs in fish that may contribute to learning problems in children. Others are looking at how early environmental exposures may disrupt embryonic development, possibly leading to birth defects of the heart, brain, and other organs.

References

Agency for Toxic Substances and Disease Registry. *Public Health Statement for Arsenic*. Centers for Disease Control and Prevention, updated 9/00, accessed 1/14/03.

Correa, Adolfo, et al. Ethylene Glycol Ethers and Risks of Spontaneous Abortion and Subfertility. *American Journal of Epidemiology*, volume 143, number 7, 1996, pages 707–17.

Department of Health and Human Services and Environmental Protection Agency. *FDA and EPA announce the revised consumer advisory on methylmercury in fish*, March 19, 2004.

Farley, D. Dangers of Lead Still Linger. *FDA Consumer Magazine*, January/February 1998.

Khattak, S., et al. Pregnancy Outcome Following Gestational Exposure to Organic Solvents: A Prospective Controlled Study. *Journal of the American Medical Association*, volume 281, number 12, March 24/ 31, 1999, pages 1106–9.

Lappe, M. and Chalfin, N. *Identifying Toxic Risks Before and During Pregnancy: A Decision Tree Action Plan*. Report to the March of Dimes, Center for Ethics and Toxics (CETOS), Gualala, CA, April 15, 2002.

Reproductive Toxicology Center. *Diethyltoluamide* (revised 4/1/00), *Arsenic* (revised 9/1/01), *Cadmium* (revised 5/1/01), *Trihalomethanes* (revised 2/1/01), *Chlorine* (revised 10/1/01), *Chloroform* (revised 6/1/ 01), *Tapwater* (revised 7/1/01); all accessed 1/23/03.

U.S. Environmental Protection Agency. *Lead in Paint, Dust, and Soil*. Updated 12/23/02, accessed 1/23/03.

U.S. Environmental Protection Agency Air Toxics Program. *The Integrated Urban Strategy: Report to Congress*. July 2000, accessed 1/24/ 03.

Chapter 9

Fetal Risks Associated with Maternal Conditions

Chapter Contents

Section 9.1—Maternal Asthma 98
Section 9.2—Maternal Cancer 101
Section 9.3—Maternal Diabetes 104
Section 9.4—Maternal High Blood Pressure 113
Section 9.5—Maternal Obesity 119
Section 9.6—Maternal Phenylketonuria (PKU) 121

Section 9.1

Maternal Asthma

Excerpted from "New Treatment Guidelines for Pregnant Women with Asthma: Monitoring and Managing Asthma Important for Healthy Mother and Baby," *NIH News*, National Heart, Lung, and Blood Institute (NHLBI), National Institutes of Health, January 11, 2005.

In January 2005, the National Asthma Education and Prevention Program (NAEPP) issued the first new guidelines in more than a decade for managing asthma during pregnancy. The report reflects new medications that have emerged and updates treatment recommendations for pregnant women with asthma based on a systematic review of data on the safety of asthma medications during pregnancy. An executive summary of the guidelines is published in the January 2005 issue of the *Journal of Allergy and Clinical Immunology.*

Poorly controlled asthma can lead to serious medical problems for pregnant women and their fetuses. The guidelines emphasize that controlling asthma during pregnancy is important for the health and well-being of the mother as well as for the healthy development of the fetus. A stepwise approach to asthma care similar to that used in the NAEPP general asthma treatment guidelines for children and nonpregnant adults is recommended. Under this approach, medication is stepped up in intensity if needed, and stepped down when possible, depending on asthma severity. Because asthma severity changes during pregnancy for most women, the guidelines also recommend that clinicians who provide obstetric care monitor asthma severity during prenatal visits of their patients who have asthma.

"The guidelines review the evidence on asthma medications used by pregnant patients," said Barbara Alving, M.D., acting director of the National Heart, Lung, and Blood Institute (NHLBI), which administers the NAEPP. "The evidence is reassuring, and suggests that it is safer to take medications than to have asthma exacerbations. The guidelines should be a useful tool for physicians to develop optimal asthma management plans for pregnant women."

"Simply put, when a pregnant patient has trouble breathing, her fetus also has trouble getting the oxygen it needs," added William W.

Busse, M.D., professor of medicine at the University of Wisconsin Medical School, and chair of the NAEPP multidisciplinary expert panel that developed the guidelines. "There are many ways we can help pregnant women control their asthma, and it is imperative that providers and their patients work together to do so."

Asthma affects over twenty million Americans and is one of the most common potentially serious medical conditions to complicate pregnancy. Maternal asthma is associated with increased risk of infant death, preeclampsia (a serious condition marked by high blood pressure, which can cause seizures in the mother or fetus), premature birth, and low birth weight. These risks are linked to asthma severity—more severe asthma increases risk, while better-controlled asthma is tied to decreased risks.

Asthma worsens in approximately 30 percent of women who have mild asthma at the beginning of their pregnancy, according to a recent study by the National Institute of Child Health and Human Development Maternal-Fetal Medicine Units Network and co-funded by NHLBI. The study also found that, conversely, asthma improved in 23 percent of the women who initially had moderate or severe asthma.

"We cannot predict who will worsen during pregnancy, so the new guidelines recommend that pregnant patients with persistent asthma have their asthma checked at least monthly by a healthcare provider," explained Mitchell Dombrowski, M.D., chief of obstetrics and gynecology for St. John Hospital in Detroit, and a member of the NAEPP expert panel. "Clinicians who provide obstetric care should be part of the patient's asthma management team, working with the patient and her asthma care provider to adjust her medications if needed to keep her asthma under control and to lower the risk of complications from asthma for her and her baby."

Key recommendations from the guidelines regarding medications include the following:

- Albuterol, a short-acting inhaled beta$_2$-agonist, should be used as a quick-relief medication to treat asthma symptoms. Pregnant women with asthma should have this medication available at all times.

- Women who have symptoms at least two days a week or two nights a month have persistent asthma and need daily medication for long-term care of their asthma and to prevent exacerbations. Inhaled corticosteroids are the preferred medication to control the underlying inflammation in pregnant women with persistent asthma. The guidelines note that there are more data on the safety of budesonide use during pregnancy than on other inhaled corticosteroids; however, there are no data indicating that other inhaled corticosteroids are unsafe during pregnancy, and other inhaled corticosteroids may be continued if they effectively control a patient's asthma. Alternative daily medications are leukotriene receptor antagonists, cromolyn, or theophylline.

- For patients whose persistent asthma is not well controlled on low doses of inhaled corticosteroids alone, the guidelines recommend either increasing the dose of inhaled corticosteroid or adding another medication—a long-acting beta agonist. The expert panel concluded that data are insufficient to indicate a preference of one option over the other.

- Oral corticosteroids may be required for the treatment of severe asthma. The guidelines note that there are conflicting data regarding the safety of oral corticosteroids during pregnancy; however, severe, uncontrolled asthma poses a definite risk to the mother and fetus; and use of oral corticosteroids may be warranted.

"Several studies have shown that taking inhaled corticosteroids improves lung function during pregnancy and reduces asthma exacerbations—and other large, prospective studies found no relation between taking inhaled corticosteroids and congenital abnormalities or other adverse pregnancy outcomes," said Michael Schatz, M.D., M.S., chief of the Department of Allergy for Kaiser Permanente San Diego Medical Center. Schatz is also a member of the NAEPP expert panel on asthma during pregnancy and author of an editorial accompanying the guidelines report.

The guidelines highlight other important aspects of asthma management during pregnancy, such as identifying and limiting exposure to asthma triggers. Similarly, women with other conditions that can worsen asthma, such as allergic rhinitis, sinusitis, and gastroesophageal reflux, should have those conditions treated as well. Such conditions often become more troublesome during pregnancy.

"As important as medications are for controlling asthma, a pregnant woman can reduce how much medication is needed by identifying and avoiding the factors that make her asthma worse, such as tobacco smoke or allergens like dust mites," added Dr. Schatz.

Section 9.2

Maternal Cancer

Cancer during pregnancy is fortunately rare. Little research is available to guide patients and doctors. It is known that in some cases a pregnant woman with cancer is capable of giving birth to a healthy baby and that certain cancer treatments are safe during pregnancy.

Prevalence

Cancer occurs in approximately one out of every one thousand pregnancies. However, pregnancy itself does not cause cancer, and pregnant women are not more susceptible to cancer than other women. The cancers that tend to occur during pregnancy are those that are more common in younger people, such as cervical cancer, breast cancer, Hodgkin lymphoma, malignant melanoma, and thyroid cancer. Because age is the most significant risk factor for cancer, doctors expect the rate of cancer during pregnancy to increase as more women are waiting until they are older to have children.

Diagnosis

Being pregnant can delay a cancer diagnosis. Symptoms such as abdominal bloating, frequent headaches, or rectal bleeding might suggest ovarian, brain, or colon cancer. These symptoms are also common during pregnancy and are not considered suspicious. In rare cases in which these symptoms are related to cancer, diagnosis of the cancer is likely to be delayed.

Breast cancer is the most common cancer in pregnant women, affecting approximately one in three thousand pregnancies. Pregnancy-related breast enlargement makes it difficult to detect small breast tumors, and mammograms are not routinely done during pregnancy.

If cancer is suspected during pregnancy, women and their doctors may be concerned about diagnostic tests such as x-rays. However, research has shown that the level of radiation in diagnostic x-rays is too low to harm the fetus. When possible, a lead shield covering the abdomen offers extra protection. Other diagnostic tests, such as magnetic resonance imaging tests (MRIs), ultrasounds, and biopsies, are also considered safe during pregnancy because they don't use radiation.

Sometimes, pregnancy can uncover cancer that had previously gone undetected. A Pap test performed as part of routine, early prenatal care can detect cervical cancer. Similarly, routine ultrasounds performed during pregnancy can often detect ovarian cancer that might otherwise go undiagnosed.

Treatment

Treatment for cancer during pregnancy means balancing optimal treatment for the mother against possible risk to the fetus. The type of treatment given will depend on many factors, including how far the pregnancy has progressed; the type, location, size, and stage of the cancer; and the wishes of the expectant mother and family. Because some cancer treatments can harm the fetus, especially during the first trimester (the first three months of pregnancy), treatment may be delayed until the second or third trimesters. When cancer is diagnosed later in pregnancy, doctors may wait to start treatment until after the baby is born, or they may consider inducing labor early. In some cases, such as early stage (stage 0 or 1A) cervical cancer, doctors may wait to treat the cancer until after delivery.

Cancer treatments used during pregnancy may include surgery, chemotherapy, and in some cases, radiation therapy, but only after careful consideration and treatment planning to ensure maternal and fetal safety.

Surgery poses little risk to the fetus and is considered the safest cancer treatment option during pregnancy. In some instances, more extensive surgery can be done to avoid having to use chemotherapy or radiation therapy.

Chemotherapy is the use of drugs to kill cancer cells. Chemotherapy is toxic and capable of harming the fetus, particularly if given during the first trimester of pregnancy when the fetus's organs are still developing. Chemotherapy during the first trimester can cause birth defects or miscarriage (early pregnancy loss). During the second and third trimesters, chemotherapy can be taken without harming the fetus. The placenta (the organ that develops during pregnancy) acts as a barrier between the mother and the fetus that most chemotherapy cannot pass through. When the standard chemotherapy regimen includes a drug that is not safe during any stage of pregnancy, another drug can usually be substituted.

Although chemotherapy later in pregnancy may not directly harm the fetus, chemotherapy can cause health problems for the mother that can indirectly harm the fetus, such as malnutrition and anemia (low red blood cell count). Chemotherapy given during the second and third trimesters can cause early labor and low birth weight, both of which may lead to further complications, such as problems with breastfeeding, gaining weight, and fighting infections.

Radiation therapy involves high-energy x-rays to destroy cancer cells and shrink cancerous tumors. Because radiation therapy can harm the fetus, particularly during the first trimester, this treatment is generally not recommended. The use of radiation therapy in the second or third trimesters depends on the dose of radiation and the area of the body being treated.

Prognosis and Fetal Outcome

In most cases, the prognosis (chance of recovery) for a pregnant woman with cancer is the same as for another woman of the same age with the same type and stage of cancer. However, if diagnosis is delayed during pregnancy, women tend to have a worse overall prognosis than nonpregnant women diagnosed with cancer. In addition, pregnancy can affect the behavior of some cancers. For example, there is some evidence to suggest that the hormonal changes of pregnancy may stimulate the growth of malignant melanoma.

Cancer rarely affects the fetus directly. Although some cancers can metastasize to the placenta, most cancers cannot metastasize to the fetus itself. In rare cases, malignant melanoma is capable of spreading to the placenta and the fetus.

Breastfeeding

Although cancer cells cannot pass to the infant through breast milk, women who are being treated for cancer are generally advised not to breastfeed. Chemotherapy can be especially dangerous, as it can build up in breast milk and harm the infant. Similarly, radioactive components that are taken internally, such as radioactive iodine used in treating thyroid cancer, also cross into breast milk and can harm the infant.

Pregnancy after Cancer

As more young people are surviving cancer, more women are considering whether they should have a baby after having cancer. In general, pregnancy after cancer is considered safe for both the mother and the baby, and pregnancy does not appear to increase the chances of cancer recurring. However, since some cancers do recur, women are usually advised to wait a number of years after completing cancer treatment until the risk of recurrence has decreased. The amount of time you will be advised to wait before becoming pregnant depends on the type and stage of cancer and course of treatment.

In some cases, cancer treatments can cause damage to areas of the body such as the heart or lungs. Before becoming pregnant, these organs may need to be evaluated to be sure that the pregnancy will be safe.

Unfortunately, some cancer treatments can also cause infertility, making it difficult or impossible for some women to have children.

Section 9.3

Maternal Diabetes

"Diabetes and Pregnancy: Frequently Asked Questions" is reprinted from the Centers for Disease Control and Prevention, October 5, 2005. "Multivitamin Supplements and Diabetes-Associated Birth Defects" is reprinted from "Do Multivitamin Supplements Reduce the Risk for Diabetes-Associated Birth Defects?" Centers for Disease Control and Prevention, May 5, 2003.

Diabetes and Pregnancy: Frequently Asked Questions

Diabetes is often detected in women during their childbearing years and can affect the health of both the mother and her unborn child. Poor control of diabetes in a woman who is pregnant increases the chances for birth defects and other problems for the baby. It might cause serious complications for the woman, also. Proper health care before and during pregnancy will help prevent birth defects and other poor outcomes, such as miscarriage or stillbirth.

What is diabetes?

Diabetes is a condition in which the body cannot use the sugars and starches (carbohydrates) it takes in as food to make energy. The body either makes too little insulin in the pancreas or cannot use the insulin it makes to change those sugars and starches into energy. As a result, the body collects extra sugar in the blood and gets rid of some sugar in the urine. The extra sugar in the blood can damage organs of the body, such as the heart, eyes, and kidneys, if it is allowed to collect in the body too long. The three most common types of diabetes are type I, type II, and gestational:

- Type I diabetes is a condition in which the pancreas makes so little insulin that the body can't use blood sugar for energy. Type I diabetes must be controlled with daily insulin shots.

- Type II diabetes is a condition in which the body either makes too little insulin or can't use the insulin it makes to use blood sugar for energy. Often type II diabetes can be controlled through eating a proper diet and exercising regularly. Some people with type II diabetes have to take diabetes pills or insulin or both.

- Gestational diabetes is a type of diabetes that occurs in a pregnant woman who did not have diabetes before she was pregnant. Often gestational diabetes can be controlled through eating a proper diet and exercising regularly, but sometimes a woman with gestational diabetes must also take insulin shots. Usually gestational diabetes goes away after pregnancy, but sometimes it doesn't. Also, many women who have had gestational diabetes develop type II diabetes later in life.

What are some common problems caused by diabetes?

People with diabetes can suffer from high blood pressure, kidney disease, nerve damage, heart disease, and blindness. Young women with diabetes might not have these problems yet. The damage caused by these problems often happens in people whose blood sugar has been out of control for years. Keeping blood sugar under control can help prevent the damage from happening.

People with diabetes can go into "diabetic coma" if their blood sugar is too high. They can also develop blood sugar that is too low (hypoglycemia) if they don't get enough food or they exercise too much without adjusting insulin or food. Both diabetic coma and hypoglycemia can be very serious, and even fatal, if not treated quickly. Closely watching blood sugar, being aware of the early signs and symptoms of blood sugar that is too high or too low, and treating those conditions early can prevent these problems from becoming too serious.

How does a person get diabetes?

We don't know exactly how people get diabetes. However, it appears that both genetics and personal lifestyle play a role in who gets diabetes. Some people have diabetes that "runs" in the family. Lack of exercise, poor eating habits, and obesity seem to increase the risk of developing type II diabetes in other people. In some but not all cases, type II diabetes can be controlled if people lose weight, eat right, and exercise regularly.

Can a person prevent problems from diabetes?

A person with diabetes who keeps her blood sugar as close to normal as possible has fewer problems than a person who does not keep his blood sugar in "tight control." A woman with diabetes who can get pregnant should watch her blood sugar closely to prevent problems if she should get pregnant. To keep blood sugar in tight control, a person can manage her diabetes with a strict plan:

- Eat healthy foods from personal diabetes meal plan.
- Exercise regularly.
- Monitor blood sugar often.
- Take medications on time, including insulin if ordered by the doctor.
- Know how to adjust food intake, exercise, and insulin depending on the results of blood sugar tests.
- Control or treat low blood sugar and high blood sugar.
- Follow up with health care provider regularly

How does gestational diabetes differ from type I or type II diabetes?

Gestational diabetes happens in a woman who develops diabetes during pregnancy. Some women have more than one pregnancy affected by diabetes that disappears after the pregnancy ends. About half of the women with gestational diabetes will develop type II diabetes later.

If not controlled, gestational diabetes can cause the baby to grow extra large and lead to problems with delivery for the mother and the baby. Gestational diabetes might be controlled with diet and exercise, or it might take insulin as well as diet and exercise to get control.

Type I and type II diabetes often are present before a woman gets pregnant. If not controlled before and during pregnancy, type I and type II diabetes can cause the baby to have birth defects and cause the mother to have problems (or her problems to worsen if they are already present), such as high blood pressure, kidney disease, nerve damage, heart disease, or blindness. Type I diabetes must be controlled with a balance of diet, exercise, and insulin. Type II diabetes might be controlled with diet and exercise, or it might take diabetes pills or insulin or both as well as diet and exercise to get control.

Will my baby have diabetes?

Babies born to mothers with diabetes do not come into the world with diabetes. However, if the mother's diabetes was not controlled during pregnancy, the baby can very quickly develop low blood sugar after birth and must be watched very closely until his or her body adjusts the amount of insulin it makes.

Extra-large babies are more likely to become obese and to develop type II diabetes later in life. They especially need to develop healthy eating and regular exercise habits as they grow up to lessen the chance of obesity and type II diabetes.

If the father of the developing baby has diabetes, does his diabetes affect the pregnancy?

Diabetes in the father does not affect the developing baby during pregnancy. However, depending on the type of diabetes the father has, the baby might have a greater chance of developing diabetes later in life.

What can happen to a woman with type I or type II diabetes who becomes pregnant?

Pregnancy is a time when a woman's body goes through lots of changes as it nurtures a developing baby. All women need more nutrients, rest, and energy to grow the baby when they are pregnant. They also need to be physically active. When a woman with diabetes is pregnant, changes happen in her blood sugar, often quickly. If a woman with diabetes does not keep good control of her blood sugar, she might get some of the common problems of diabetes, or those problems might get worse if she already has them. Out-of-control blood sugar could lead to a woman having a miscarriage. Out-of-control blood sugar might also cause high blood pressure in a woman during pregnancy, and she will need extra visits to the doctor. High blood pressure during pregnancy might lead to a baby being born early and also could cause seizures or a stroke (a blood clot in the brain that can lead to brain damage) in the woman during labor and delivery. Sometimes, out-of-control blood sugar causes a woman to make extra-large amounts of amniotic fluid around the baby, which might lead to preterm (early) labor. Another problem common to a pregnant woman with uncontrolled diabetes is that her baby grows too large. Besides causing discomfort to the woman during the last few months of pregnancy, an extra-large baby can lead to problems during delivery for both the mother and the baby.

What can happen to the baby of a woman with type I or type II diabetes during pregnancy?

Diabetes in a pregnant woman can cause the baby to have birth defects, miscarry, be born early and have a low birth weight, be stillborn, or grow extra large and have a hard delivery.

A woman who has type I or type II diabetes that is not tightly controlled has a higher chance of having a baby with a birth defect than does a woman without diabetes. The organs of the baby form during the first two months of pregnancy, often before a woman knows that she is pregnant. Out-of-control blood sugar can affect those organs while they are being formed and cause serious birth defects, such as those of the brain, spine, and heart, or can lead to miscarriage of the developing baby.

If the woman's blood sugar remains out of control throughout the pregnancy, the baby likely will grow extra large. Out-of-control diabetes causes the baby's blood sugar to be high. The baby makes more insulin and uses the extra calories or stores them as fat. The baby is "overfed" and grows extra large. Extra-large babies can occur in women with any out-of-control diabetes, including type I, type II, and gestational. The extra-large baby can cause problems during and after delivery. Nerve damage to the baby can happen from pressure on the baby's shoulder during delivery. A newborn might have quickly changing blood sugars after delivery. A large baby born to a woman with diabetes might have a greater chance of being obese and/or developing type II diabetes later in life.

If the woman with diabetes has problems that lead to a preterm birth, the baby might have breathing problems, heart problems, bleeding into the brain, intestinal problems, and vision problems. A woman with diabetes might have a baby born on time with low birth weight. A baby with low birth weight might have problems with eating, gaining weight, fighting off infections, and staying warm.

What can happen to a pregnant woman with gestational diabetes?

A pregnant woman who does not have diabetes can develop "gestational diabetes" later in pregnancy. A woman with gestational diabetes will need to watch her blood sugar closely and balance food intake, exercise, and, if needed, insulin shots to keep her blood sugar in control. If a woman with gestational diabetes does not keep her blood sugar in good control, she could have several problems. She might have an extra-large baby, have high blood pressure, deliver too early, or need to have a cesarean section (an operation to get the baby out of the mother through her abdomen). The extra-large baby might cause the woman to feel uncomfortable during the last months of pregnancy. Also, it could lead to problems for both the woman and the baby during delivery. When the baby is delivered surgically by a cesarean section (C-section), it takes longer for the woman to recover from childbirth. High blood pressure when a woman is pregnant might lead to an early delivery and could cause seizures or a stroke in the woman.

Sometimes gestational diabetes in women does not go away after delivery. These women have converted to type II diabetes. A woman whose diabetes does not go away after delivery will need to manage her diabetes for the rest of her life.

What can happen to the baby of a woman with gestational diabetes?

A woman who has gestational diabetes has less chance of having a baby with a birth defect than does a woman with type I or type II diabetes. Since gestational diabetes develops later in pregnancy, the baby's organs are already formed. If her blood sugar is not controlled, a woman with gestational diabetes still has a greater chance of having a stillborn baby than a woman who doesn't have diabetes.

If the woman's blood sugar remains out of control throughout the pregnancy, the baby likely will grow extra large. Out-of-control diabetes causes the baby's blood sugar to be high. The baby makes more insulin and uses the extra calories or stores them as fat. The baby is "overfed" and grows extra large. Extra-large babies can occur in women with any out-of-control diabetes, including type I, type II, and gestational.

The extra-large baby can cause problems during and after delivery. Nerve damage to the baby can happen from pressure on the baby's shoulder during delivery. A newborn might have quickly changing blood sugars after delivery. A large baby born to a woman with diabetes might have a greater chance of being obese and/or developing type II diabetes later in life.

If the woman with diabetes has problems that lead to a preterm birth, the baby might have breathing problems, heart problems, bleeding into the brain, intestinal problems, and vision problems. A woman with diabetes might have a baby born on time with low birth weight. A baby with low birth weight might have problems with eating, gaining weight, fighting off infections, and staying warm.

Can a woman with diabetes prevent the problems to herself and to her baby during pregnancy?

If a woman with diabetes keeps her blood sugar in tight control before and during pregnancy, she can lessen her risk of having a baby with a birth defect to that of a woman who doesn't have diabetes. Controlling her blood sugar also reduces the risk that a woman will develop common problems of diabetes, or that the problems will get worse during pregnancy. The baby is less likely to grow extra large during her pregnancy if a woman keeps her blood sugar in tight control.

How can a woman with diabetes who wants to get pregnant prevent problems to herself and her baby?

There are several steps she can take:

- **Plan the pregnancy.** Unplanned pregnancies are more common among women with diabetes than among women who do not have diabetes. About 70 percent of women with diabetes don't plan their pregnancies, as compared to about 50 percent of women who don't have diabetes. It is very important for a woman with diabetes to get her body ready before she becomes pregnant.

- **See her doctor.** Her doctor needs to look at the effects that diabetes has had on her body already, talk with her about getting and keeping control of her blood sugar, change medications if needed, and plan for frequent follow-up. Her doctor will remind her about the usual steps to get ready for pregnancy, such as to take prenatal vitamins (with folic acid), stop smoking, avoid alcohol, eat right, exercise, and avoid stress.

- **Eat healthy foods from a meal plan made for her as a person with diabetes.** If a woman is overweight, she might try to lose weight before getting pregnant as part of her plan to get her blood sugar in control. A dietitian can help her plan a good diet for a person with diabetes, especially if she plans to lose weight before she gets pregnant. A dietitian can also help her learn how to control her blood sugar while she is pregnant.

- **Exercise regularly.** Exercise is another way to keep blood sugar under control. Exercise helps to balance food intake. A woman should begin a regular exercise plan before she gets pregnant and stick with the exercise plan both while she is pregnant and after the baby comes.

- **Monitor blood sugar often.** Because pregnancy causes the body's need for energy to change, blood sugar levels can change very quickly. A pregnant woman with diabetes needs to check her blood sugar more often, sometimes six to eight times a day, which might be higher than when she is not pregnant. Checking blood sugar levels often can help a woman keep her blood sugar in control.

- **Take medications on time.** If insulin is ordered by a doctor, a pregnant woman with diabetes should take it when it's needed. She should know how to adjust food intake, exercise, and insulin, depending on the results of her blood sugar tests, to keep the blood sugar in the range of tight control.

- **Control and treat low blood sugar quickly.** Keeping tight blood sugar control can lead to a chance of low blood sugar at times. A pregnant woman with diabetes should have a ready source of carbohydrates, such as glucose tablets or gel, on hand at all times. It's helpful to teach family members and close co-workers or friends how to help in case of a severe low blood sugar reaction.

- **Follow up with the doctor regularly.** A pregnant woman with diabetes needs to see her doctor more often than does a pregnant woman without diabetes. Together, the woman and her doctor can work to prevent or catch problems early. Although there are no guarantees, a woman with diabetes who gets and keeps her blood sugar in control is more likely to have a healthy pregnancy and a healthy baby.

Multivitamin Supplements and Diabetes-Associated Birth Defects

It is well established that children of diabetic mothers are at increased risk for birth defects, the most common of which are heart and central nervous system defects. The prevalence of birth defects is twofold to threefold higher in children of women with diabetes than in children of women without diabetes. Studies have shown that effective control of diabetes during the periconceptional period (refers to the period of time three months before pregnancy through the first three months of pregnancy) in women with diabetes reduces the risk for birth defects in their children. However, this level of control is not always possible. Since the risk for birth defects can be reduced by the consumption of multivitamin supplements, this study examined whether the risk for birth defects among children of women with diabetes could be reduced by the consumption of multivitamin supplements during the periconceptional period.

What are the findings of this study?

This study found that children of mothers with diabetes had a fourfold increase in risk for certain birth defects, and that this excess risk was limited to the children of mothers with diabetes who did not take multivitamins. Children of mothers who had diabetes and took multivitamins during the periconceptional period did not have this excess risk for such birth defects.

What are some of the specific birth defects that can be associated with diabetes?

Birth defects associated with diabetes include those of the central nervous system, heart defects, eye defects, respiratory tract defects, cleft palate, anal atresia/stenosis, hypospadias, urinary tract defects, and positional defects of the foot.

What do the findings suggest?

Women with diabetes can reduce the risk for birth defects among their children by following good prenatal care practices, including controlling their diabetes and taking multivitamins before and early in pregnancy.

Section 9.4

Maternal High Blood Pressure

Blood pressure is the force of the blood pushing against the walls of the arteries (blood vessels that carry oxygen-rich blood to all parts of the body). When the pressure in the arteries becomes too high, it is called hypertension.

Up to 5 percent of women have hypertension before they become pregnant.[1] This is called chronic hypertension. Another 5 to 8 percent develop hypertension during pregnancy.[2] This is called gestational hypertension.

Hypertension during pregnancy can cause serious complications for mother and baby. Fortunately, serious problems usually can be prevented with proper prenatal care.

How is blood pressure measured?

At each prenatal visit, the health care provider measures blood pressure with an inflatable cuff that wraps around the woman's upper arm. The pressure in the arteries is measured as the heart contracts (systolic pressure) and when the heart is relaxed between contractions (diastolic pressure). The blood pressure reading is given as two numbers, with the top number representing the systolic pressure and the bottom number representing the diastolic pressure (for example, 110/80). A systolic reading of 140 or higher, or a diastolic reading of 90 or higher, is considered high blood pressure. Because blood pressure can go up and down during the day, health care providers often recheck a high reading to determine if a woman truly has high blood pressure.

What is chronic hypertension?

Chronic hypertension is high blood pressure that is diagnosed before pregnancy or before the twentieth week of pregnancy. This form of hypertension does not go away after delivery.

The causes of chronic hypertension are not thoroughly understood, although heredity, diet, and lifestyle may play a role. Untreated hypertension can increase the risk of serious health problems such as heart attack and stroke.

Women with chronic hypertension should see their health care provider before attempting to conceive. A pre-pregnancy visit allows the provider to ensure that the blood pressure is under control, and to evaluate any medication the woman takes to control her blood pressure. While some medications to lower blood pressure are safe during pregnancy, others—including a group of drugs called angiotensin-converting-enzyme (ACE) inhibitors—can harm the fetus. Some women with chronic hypertension may be able to stop taking their medication or reduce their dose, at least during the first half of pregnancy, as blood pressure tends to fall during this time. However, blood pressure needs to be monitored carefully during this period.

Most women with chronic hypertension have healthy pregnancies. However, about 25 percent develop a form of gestational hypertension called preeclampsia, which poses special risks.[2, 3]

What is gestational hypertension?

There are two main forms of gestational hypertension. Both occur after the twentieth week of pregnancy and go away without treatment soon after delivery. Preeclampsia is a potentially serious disorder characterized by high blood pressure and protein in the urine. When high blood pressure is not accompanied by protein in the urine, it is referred to as gestational hypertension. Gestational hypertension may progress to preeclampsia, so all women who develop high blood pressure in pregnancy are monitored closely.

Preeclampsia may be accompanied by swelling (edema) of the hands and face; sudden weight gain (five or more pounds in one week); blurred vision; severe headaches; dizziness; and intense stomach pain. A pregnant woman should contact her health care provider right away if she develops any of these symptoms.

Preeclampsia usually occurs after about thirty weeks of pregnancy. Most cases are mild, with blood pressure around 140/90. Women with mild preeclampsia often have no obvious symptoms. If left untreated, though, preeclampsia can cause serious problems.

It's important to remember that many women who develop preeclampsia or gestational hypertension do so at term (at or beyond thirty-seven weeks of gestation). These women generally have few complications.

What risks do preeclampsia and other forms of hypertension pose for a pregnant woman and her fetus?

All forms of hypertension can constrict the blood vessels in the uterus that supply the fetus with oxygen and nutrients. When this occurs before term, it can slow the fetus's growth, sometimes resulting in low birth weight. Hypertension also increases the risk of preterm delivery (before thirty-seven weeks of gestation). Premature and low-birth-weight babies face an increased risk of health problems during the newborn period and lasting disabilities, such as learning problems and cerebral palsy.

Women with hypertension also have an increased risk of placental abruption, which is separation of the placenta from the uterine wall before delivery. Severe abruption can cause heavy bleeding and shock, which are dangerous for both mother and baby. The most common symptom of abruption is vaginal bleeding after twenty weeks of pregnancy. A pregnant woman always should report any vaginal bleeding to her health care provider immediately. While all women with high blood pressure during pregnancy face some increased risk of abruption and the other complications discussed above, the risk is greatest in women who have preeclampsia along with chronic high blood pressure.[3]

Preeclampsia also can quickly progress to a rare but life-threatening condition called eclampsia, causing seizures and, sometimes, coma. Fortunately, eclampsia is rare in women who receive regular prenatal care. At each prenatal visit, blood pressure is measured and urine is checked for protein, so that preeclampsia can be diagnosed and treated before it can progress to eclampsia.

How is preeclampsia treated?

The only cure for preeclampsia is delivery. However, this is not always best for the baby. So treatment depends upon how severe the problem is and how far along a woman is in her pregnancy. If a woman is at term (thirty-seven to forty weeks), the preeclampsia is mild, and her cervix has begun to thin and dilate (signs that it's ready for delivery), her health care provider probably will recommend inducing labor. If her cervix is not yet ready for labor, her provider may recommend medication to help prepare her cervix for induction or continue to monitor her and her baby closely until labor starts on its own.

If a woman develops mild preeclampsia before her thirty-seventh week, her provider probably will recommend that she reduce her activities. In some cases, hospitalization may be recommended, though most women can be treated at home. Her baby's well-being will be closely monitored with tests such as ultrasound and fetal heart rate monitoring. Blood tests probably will be recommended for the pregnant woman to see if the preeclampsia is progressing and harming her health.

If a woman has severe preeclampsia, she should be hospitalized. Her health care provider will probably recommend inducing labor if she is beyond thirty-three to thirty-four weeks of gestation.[4] At this stage of pregnancy, the risk of prematurity is generally outweighed by the risk of progression to eclampsia. Before inducing labor, doctors generally treat women who are at less than thirty-four weeks of gestation with a drug called a corticosteroid that helps speed maturity of the fetal lungs. A woman who develops severe preeclampsia at less than thirty-two weeks of gestation sometimes may be monitored closely in the hospital.

Sometimes a woman's blood pressure continues to rise despite treatment with blood pressure medications, and her baby must be delivered early to prevent serious health problems in the mother, such as stroke, liver damage, and seizures. Babies born early may have difficulties due to prematurity, such as trouble breathing. Most of these infants will do better in an intensive care nursery than if they had stayed in the uterus.

About 10 percent of women with severe preeclampsia also develop a disorder called HELLP (an acronym for hemolysis, elevated liver enzymes, and low platelet count) syndrome, which is characterized by blood and liver abnormalities.[5] Symptoms may include nausea and vomiting, headache, upper abdominal pain, and general malaise. Women with HELLP syndrome, which also can develop in the first forty-eight hours after delivery, are treated with medications to control blood pressure and prevent seizures, and sometimes with blood transfusions. Women who develop HELLP syndrome during pregnancy almost always require early delivery to prevent serious complications.

How are women with gestational hypertension and chronic hypertension treated?

Health care providers monitor their blood pressure and urine carefully for signs of preeclampsia or worsening hypertension. Tests such as ultrasound and fetal heart rate testing may be recommended to check on fetal growth and well-being. The provider may recommend that the pregnant woman cut back on her activities and avoid aerobic exercise.

Can a woman with preeclampsia have a vaginal delivery?

A vaginal delivery is preferable to a cesarean for a woman with preeclampsia because it avoids the added stresses of surgery. It generally is appropriate for women with preeclampsia to have epidural anesthesia for pain relief during labor and delivery.

Women with severe preeclampsia or eclampsia generally are treated with a drug called magnesium sulfate to help prevent seizures during labor and delivery. It is less clear whether women with mild preeclampsia benefit from this drug.

What causes preeclampsia and who is at risk?

The causes of preeclampsia are unknown. However, women are more susceptible if they have any of these risk factors:[1, 3]

- First pregnancy
- Family history of preeclampsia
- Personal history of chronic high blood pressure, kidney disease, diabetes, systemic lupus erythematosus (a disease often characterized by a facial rash, arthritis, and other problems), and certain thrombophilias (blood-clotting disorders)
- Multiple pregnancy
- Age less than twenty years, or over thirty-five
- African-American
- Higher-than-normal weight
- Personal history of preeclampsia

Is preeclampsia likely to recur in another pregnancy?

Women who have had preeclampsia are more susceptible to developing it again in another pregnancy. The risk of recurrence appears to be highest when preeclampsia has occurred before the twenty-ninth week of gestation and, in some cases, may be as high as 65 percent in another pregnancy.[5] About 20 percent of women who have developed preeclampsia after the thirty-seventh week of pregnancy develop it again.[5]

Can preeclampsia and gestational hypertension be prevented?

Currently, there is no way to prevent preeclampsia or gestational hypertension. However, a 1999 British study suggested that some high-risk women may be able to reduce their risk of preeclampsia by taking vitamins C and E through the second half of pregnancy.[6] The researchers caution that more studies are needed before this treatment can be widely recommended.

Does the March of Dimes fund research on preeclampsia and other forms of high blood pressure in pregnancy?

Recent March of Dimes grantees have been seeking to identify genes that may play a role in preeclampsia to identify susceptible women earlier in pregnancy and, ultimately, devise ways to prevent this disorder. Another grantee has been investigating whether certain fatty acids found in fish, such as salmon and mackerel, may help reduce the risk of preeclampsia.

References

1. American College of Obstetricians and Gynecologists. Chronic Hypertension in Pregnancy. *ACOG Practice Bulletin*, number 29, July 2001.

2. American College of Obstetricians and Gynecologists. Diagnosis and Management of Preeclampsia and Eclampsia. *ACOG Practice Bulletin*, number 33, January 2002.

3. Roberts, J.M., et al. Summary of the NHLBI Working Group on Research on Hypertension During Pregnancy. *Hypertension*, volume 41, March 2003, pages 437–45.

4. Sibai, B.M. Diagnosis and Management of Gestational Hypertension and Preeclampsia. *Obstetrics and Gynecology*, volume 102, number 1, July 2003, pages 181–92.

5. Moldenhauer, J.S. and Sibai, B.M. Hypertensive Disorders of Pregnancy, in Scott, J.R. et al (eds): *Danforth's Obstetrics and Gynecology*, Ninth Edition. Philadelphia, Lippincott Williams & Wilkins, 2003, pages 257–71.

6. Chappell, L.C., et al. Effect of Antioxidants on the Occurrence of Preeclampsia in Women at Increased Risk: A Randomized Trial. *Lancet*, volume 354, September 4, 1999, pages 810–16.

Section 9.5

Maternal Obesity

"Maternal Obesity and Risk for Birth Defects" is reprinted from Centers for Disease Control and Prevention, May 5, 2003. "Body Mass Index" is reprinted from "BMI-Body Mass Index: BMI for Adults," Centers for Disease Control and Prevention, March 2006.

Maternal Obesity and Risk for Birth Defects

CDC researchers found an increased risk for certain birth defects among women who are obese or overweight when they become pregnant. This study compared characteristics of about 1,000 women who delivered an infant with and without certain birth defects in a five-county metropolitan Atlanta area between January 1993 and August 1997. The study looked at 645 infants with birth defects and 330 infants without birth defects.

What are the findings of this study?

Several studies have shown an increased risk for neural tube defects associated with prepregnancy maternal obesity. However, few recent studies have examined the risk for other birth defects among obese and overweight women. Therefore, the researchers involved in this study explored this relationship for several birth defects and compared their findings with those of previous studies.

This study had two significant findings:

- Obese women (body mass index [BMI] of 30 or more) were more likely than average-weight women to have an infant with spina bifida, omphalocele, heart defects, and multiple anomalies.

- Overweight women (BMI greater than 25, but less than 30) were more likely than average-weight women to have infants with heart defects and multiple anomalies.

What do these findings suggest?

Obese and overweight women may have a higher risk of having a child with certain birth defects. A higher risk for some birth defects is yet another adverse pregnancy outcome associated with maternal obesity. Obesity prevention efforts are needed to increase the number of women who are of healthy weight before becoming pregnant.

Body Mass Index

Body Mass Index can be calculated using pounds and inches with this equation:

$$\text{BMI} = \left(\frac{\text{Weight in Pounds}}{\text{(Height in inches)} \times \text{(Height in inches)}} \right) \times 703$$

Section 9.6

Maternal Phenylketonuria (PKU)

The information below will help you determine if having phenylketonuria (PKU) represents an increased fetal risk. With every pregnancy, all women have a 3 to 5 percent chance to have a baby with a birth defect.

What is PKU?

PKU stands for phenylketonuria, an inherited condition where the body is missing an enzyme that is needed to break down a protein called phenylalanine, or Phe for short. Since people with PKU cannot digest Phe appropriately, Phe and similar compounds build up in the body. This can lead to problems with brain development. However, treatment with a special diet can decrease the levels of Phe in the body so that this damage does not occur. Babies and children with PKU who are not on the special diet will have mental retardation.

Is there any reason to continue the diet until adulthood?

Currently, medical professionals recommend staying on the diet lifelong to ensure the healthiest development. Some people who stop the diet in early childhood have learning and behavior problems. It is particularly important for females with PKU to stay on the diet, since increased Phe levels during a pregnancy can cause problems for an unborn baby. This is referred to as Maternal PKU effects. Since half of all pregnancies are not planned, it is especially important for women with PKU to maintain the diet even if they are not actively trying to get pregnant.

What effects do high levels of Phe have on a developing baby?

Babies born to mothers with untreated PKU (women who are not on the special diet) may be born smaller, have mental retardation, a heart defect, behavior problems, and characteristic facial features.

Is there anything I can do to prevent these effects?

The same diet you were on as a child can reduce your Phe levels, which in turn reduces the chance for your baby to have any of the problems related to Maternal PKU. The goal is to get your Phe levels below 6 mg/dl. Your doctor or health care professional can measure your Phe levels with a blood test. Ideally, dietary control should start before conception, because it may take some women longer than others to get their Phe levels down.

I am eleven weeks pregnant. Will the diet help if I go on it now?

Yes. Your baby continues to grow and the brain develops throughout the pregnancy. So, it is still a good idea to go on the diet and maintain low levels of Phe. However, the first twelve weeks of pregnancy are the critical period for the organs, including the heart, to form. Therefore, starting the diet after the first trimester does not lessen the risk for birth defects.

What does the diet consist of?

Foods containing high amounts of Phe, such as meats, dairy products, and nuts need to be replaced with low-protein foods such as certain grain products, fruits, and some vegetables. There is also a special low-Phe formula to make sure that you will get the essential nutrients. A dietitian or other health care professional can provide you with more specific information on the diet.

Is there any way to know if my baby will have problems related to maternal PKU?

A detailed ultrasound after eighteen weeks of pregnancy can look for a heart defect or growth problem. Changes in intelligence, behavior, and facial features cannot, however, be determined before a baby is born.

Can I breastfeed my baby if I have PKU?

Unless the baby also has PKU, breastfeeding is not a problem for the baby, but some doctors may recommend staying on the special diet while waiting for the baby to be tested for PKU. If you stay on the diet after you deliver, the baby should not be exposed to high levels of Phe. Your doctor can also measure the Phe levels in the baby to make sure they are not elevated after breastfeeding.

Will my baby need to be on the diet?

Your baby will need to be on the diet only if he or she also has PKU. Newborns in all states are tested for PKU before they leave the hospital by testing the levels of Phe in their blood.

What if the father of the baby has PKU instead of the mother?

There have been two small studies that suggest that there is no increased risk for birth defects when the father has PKU. In some men, PKU may reduce their fertility.

What is the chance that my baby will have PKU as I do?

A baby can have PKU only if both the mother and the father carry a specific gene for PKU. A gene contains the instructions for making the proteins that our bodies need to perform their daily functions. Since you have PKU, you will always pass on one nonworking gene for PKU to your children. A person who has only one nonworking gene for PKU is called a carrier for PKU. Carriers of PKU are healthy.

If the father of the baby does not have PKU and is not a carrier, none of your children will have PKU, but they will all be carriers. However, if you have children with someone who is a carrier of PKU, then there is a 50 percent chance for each child to have PKU. Finally, if you have children with someone who also has PKU, all of your children will have PKU. Testing to find out if a partner is a carrier of PKU is possible in some families, and if the specific genetic change is found, prenatal testing may also be available. A genetic counselor or other health care professional can provide more information.

References

Burgard P, Rey F, Rupp A, Abadie V, Rey J (1997) Neuropsychologic Functions of Early Treated Patients with Phenylketonuria, On and

Off Diet: Results of a Cross-National and Cross-Sectional Study. *Ped Research*. 41(3): 368–74.

Brenton DP, Lorek A, Baudin J, Stewart A (1994) Maternal Phenylketonuria: Preconception Dietary Control and Outcome. *Int Peds*. 9(Suppl 2): 5–10.

Fisch RO, Matalon R, Weisberg S, Michals K (1991) Children of Fathers with Phenylketonuria: An International Survey. *J Peds*. 118(5): 739–41.

Fox-Bacon C, McCamman S, Therou L, Moore W, Kipp DE (1997) Maternal PKU and Breastfeeding: Case Report of Identical Twin Mothers. *Clin Peds*. 36(9): 539–42.

Gardiner RM (1990) Transport of Amino Acids across the Blood Brain Barrier: Implications for Treatment of Maternal Phenylketonuria. *J Inher Metabolic Dis*. 13:627–33.

Gottler F, Lou H, Anderson J, Kok K, Mikkelsen I, Nielsen KB, Nielsen JB (1990) Cognitive Development in Offspring of Untreated and Preconceptionally Treated Maternal Phenylketonuria. *J Inher Metabolic Dis*. 13:665–71.

Lenke RR, Levy HL (1980) Maternal Phenylketonuria and Hyperphenylalaninemia: An International Survey of the Outcome of Untreated and Treated Pregnancies. *NEJM*. 303(21): 1202–8.

Levy HL, Ghavami M (1996) Maternal Phenylketonuria: A Metabolic Teratogen. *Teratology*. 53:176–84.

Levy HL, Lobbregt D, Koch R, de la Cruz F (1991) Paternal Phenylketonuria. *Journal of Pediatrics*. 118(5): 741–43.

Levy HL, Lobbregt D, Platt LD, Benacerraf BR (1996) Fetal Ultrasonography in Maternal PKU. *Prenatal Diagnosis*. 16:599–604

Luke B, Keith LG, (1990) The Challenge of Maternal Phenylketonuria Screening and Treatment. *Journal of Reproductive Medicine*. 35(7): 667–73.

Rouse B, Azen C, Koch R, Matalon R, Hanley W, de la Cruz F, Trefz F, Friedman E, Shifrin H (1997) Maternal Phenylketonuria Collaborative Study (MPUCS) Offspring: Facial Anomalies, Malformations, and Early Neurological Sequelae. *American Journal of Medical Genetics*. 69:89–95.

Schmidt E, Rupp A, Burgard P, Pietz J, Weglage J, de Sonneville L (1994) Sustained Attention in Adult Phenylketonuria: The Influence of the Concurrent Phenylalanine-blood-level. *Journal of Clinical & Experimental Neuropsychology.* 16(5): 681–88.

Smith I, Glossop J, and Beasley M (1990) Fetal Damage Due to Maternal Phenylketonuria: Effects of Dietary Treatment and Maternal Phenylalanine Concentrations Around the Time of Conception. *Journal of Inherited Metabolic Disease.* 13:651–57.

Waisbren SE, Chang P, Levy HL, Shifrin H, Allred E, Azen C, de la Cruz F, Hanley W, Koch R, Matalon R, Rouse B (1998) Neonatal Neurological Assessment of Offspring in Maternal Phenylketonuria. *Journal of Inherited Metabolic Disease.* 21(1): 39–48.

Chapter 10

Fetal Risks Associated with Infectious Diseases

Chapter Contents

Section 10.1—Chicken Pox and Pregnancy 128
Section 10.2—Fifth Disease and Pregnancy 130
Section 10.3—Congenital Rubella 134
Section 10.4—Sexually Transmitted Infections in
                Pregnancy 137
Section 10.5—Cytomegalovirus and Pregnancy 143
Section 10.6—Listeriosis and Pregnancy: What Is Your
                Risk? 147
Section 10.7—Toxoplasmosis and Pregnancy 150

Section 10.1

Chicken Pox and Pregnancy

When you become pregnant you want to do everything you can
to stay healthy. Unfortunately it is sometimes impossible to protect
yourself from every illness out there. Chicken pox is a highly contagious viral infection that can be very serious. Fortunately there are
ways to protect you and your baby if you are threatened by chicken
pox.

What exactly is chicken pox?

Chicken pox is a viral infection also called varicella. It is accompanied by a rash, which appears as small reddish spots or pimples. A
fever and body aches usually occur before the rash appears. Chicken
pox is contracted during childhood in most cases, although there are
some instances when an adult is not immune and contracts chicken
pox. About 95 percent of women in their childbearing years are immune to chicken pox.

Who is most at risk for getting chicken pox during pregnancy?

- If you have been infected with chicken pox once before, then you
  are most likely immune to getting chicken pox again.

- If you have *not* been infected with chicken pox and are pregnant then you may be at risk of contracting the virus. You will
  want to avoid contact with anyone who has chicken pox.

- If you are not sure if you have ever been infected with chicken
  pox, your doctor can give you a blood test to determine if you
  have the chicken pox antibodies. If the test shows that you have
  antibodies than you are immune to chicken pox.

How will my baby be affected if I have chicken pox?

How your baby will be affected depends on where you are at in your pregnancy. According to the Organization for Teratology Information Service (OTIS) the following is true:

- If chicken pox occurs within the first trimester than the risk of birth defects is 0.5 to 1 percent

- If chicken pox occurs between the thirteenth and twentieth week than the risk of birth defects is 2 percent

- If chicken pox occurs within five days or less of delivery or one to two days after delivery than there is a 20 to 25 percent chance that your baby will develop chicken pox, known as congenital varicella.

- If chicken pox occurs within six to twelve days before delivery, there is a chance that the baby can still get chicken pox. In this case your baby may receive some of your newly made chicken pox antibodies, which will cause the congenital varicella to be mild.

Possible birth defects may be scars, eye problems, poor growth, small head size, delayed development, and/or mental retardation.

What can I do to protect my baby from chicken pox?

- If you have had chicken pox before, then there is nothing you need to do to protect your baby during pregnancy. Your body should have antibodies that protect you from contracting chicken pox and therefore your baby will be protected.

- If you have not had chicken pox before, you my receive the shot of zoster immune globulin (ZIG) if you are pregnant and come in contact with someone who has chicken pox. ZIG must be given within four days of first exposure. This is given only if you do not already have the antibodies against chicken pox.

- You can get a chicken pox vaccine if you do not have the chicken pox antibodies and you are not pregnant. You must wait three months before trying to conceive.

Can someone get chicken pox twice?

It is rare that a person will contract chicken pox twice, but those with immune problems are at an elevated risk of a second infection.

There are also those cases when people think they had chicken pox when they were younger, when in fact it was just a rash or something else.

Section 10.2

Fifth Disease and Pregnancy

Reprinted from "Fifth Disease (Parvovirus B19) and Pregnancy," © 2005 Organization of Teratology Information Services (OTIS). Reprinted with permission. Member programs of OTIS are located throughout the U.S. and Canada. To find the Teratogen Information Service in your area, call OTIS toll-free at 866-626-OTIS (866-626-6847), or visit their website at www.otispregnancy.org.

The information below will help you determine if your prenatal exposure to fifth disease represents an increased fetal risk. With every pregnancy, all women have a 3 to 5 percent chance to have a baby with a birth defect. The information contained in this fact sheet should not be used as a substitute for the medical care and advice of your health care provider.

What is fifth disease?

Fifth disease, also called erythema infectiosum, is a viral illness caused by human parvovirus B19. It occurs most commonly in children ages four to fourteen. The infection often starts with mild fever, sore throat, and flu-like symptoms. Children also develop a bright red rash on the face that looks like "slapped cheeks." Along with the facial rash, a lacy or bumpy rash may appear on the body, arms, and legs. Joint aches occur more commonly in adults than children. Rash and joint symptoms may develop several weeks after infection. As many as 20 to 30 percent of adults infected with parvovirus B19 have no symptoms.

Is fifth disease contagious?

Yes, fifth disease is contagious. The virus is spread through contact with secretions of the nose and lungs, and through contact with blood. The incubation period (the time between infection and the development of the illness) is between four and twenty-one days.

Individuals with fifth disease are most infectious before the onset of symptoms and are unlikely to be contagious after the development of the rash and other symptoms. This makes efforts to prevent exposure very difficult.

I don't remember ever having fifth disease. Can I develop the infection?

Because fifth disease is a mild illness, many adults may not be aware that they have had it, especially since many people do not have symptoms. About 50 percent of adults have had the infection, have antibodies to the virus, and are immune. These antibodies prevent infection for you and your unborn baby. A blood test can be done to look for the antibodies and tell if you have had a recent infection or are not immune.

I don't think I've had fifth disease and have been recently exposed at work. Should I continue to go to work?

You should ask your doctor to obtain a blood test for antibodies to parvovirus B19 to see if you are immune to fifth disease. Studies show that many women in occupations such as daycare supervision and teaching have antibodies to fifth disease and thus are not at risk for infection. However, if you are not immune to the disease, there is a 20 to 30 percent risk that you will be infected following exposure in a school or daycare setting.

You should talk to your doctor about whether you should continue working. If you continue to work, there are ways to lessen your risk of infection, including good hand washing, not sharing food or drinks, and other hygiene measures.

My children had fifth disease about three weeks ago and now my joints are sore. I am pregnant. Could I have fifth disease?

Yes, it is possible that you have fifth disease. However, there are many other causes of joint pain. Your doctor may consider ordering a blood test to check for antibodies to fifth disease. If you are not immune, you have a 50 percent risk of becoming infected from contact with an infected family member.

I am fourteen weeks pregnant and testing showed that I recently had fifth disease. Is my pregnancy at increased risk of problems because of the infection?

Many studies show that the majority of women who become infected with fifth disease deliver healthy babies, without birth defects, prematurity, or other problems. In a small number of cases, fetal loss (miscarriage or stillbirth) can occur. Infection resulting in fetal loss is more likely to occur in the first twenty weeks of pregnancy, with a risk of around 10 percent. Infections after twenty weeks gestation have a risk for fetal loss that is more in the range of 1 percent.

Fetal infection with fifth disease can lead to inflammation of the heart (myocarditis) and can damage the bone marrow so that red blood cells cannot be made. This in turn can lead to anemia. If the heart damage or anemia is severe, hydrops (excess fluid in fetal tissues) can occur and may lead to fetal death. Sometimes, the hydrops disappears and most of these babies will be normal. Rarely, a baby is born unable to make red blood cells and will need transfusions.

I had fifth disease when I was ten weeks pregnant. Are there any tests I can have done to see if my baby is ok?

An ultrasound (sound wave pictures of the fetus) can tell whether the fetus has hydrops and can look at the amount of amniotic fluid around the baby. A series of ultrasounds for several months after the maternal infection may be helpful. Other methods for detecting fetal problems are also being explored.

Are there any treatments available?

At this time there are no vaccines or medications available to prevent or treat maternal fifth disease. Frequent ultrasounds to detect hydrops are recommended when a mother tests positive to fifth disease. When a fetus develops severe anemia and hydrops in the second and third trimester, fetal blood transfusions have successfully been done. If you are in your third trimester there may be consideration of an early delivery if your baby is showing signs of hydrops.

My dog has a parvovirus infection. Can I catch it from him?

No. There are many types of parvoviruses. Each type is species-specific, meaning that dog (canine) parvoviruses infect only dogs, cat (feline) parvoviruses infect only cats, and human parvoviruses infect only humans.

References

Anderson, L.G., Human parvovirus B19. *Pediatric Annuals* 1990; 19(9): 509–13.

Committee on Infectious Disease, American Academy of Pediatrics: Parvovirus B 19, in *2003 Red Book: Report of the Committee on Infectious Disease*, 26th edition, pp 459–61.

Fairley, C.K., et al. Observational study of effect of intrauterine transfusions on outcome of fetal hydrops after parvovirus B19 infection. *Lancet* 1995; 346(8986): 1335–37.

Gillespie, S.M., et al. Occupational risk of human parvovirus B19 infection for school and daycare personnel during an outbreak of erythema infectiosum. *JAMA* 1990; 263:2061–65.

Jordan, J.A., Placental Cellular Immune Response in Women Infected with Human Parvovirus B19 during Pregnancy. *Clin. Diagno. Lab. Immunol.* 2001; 8 (2): 288–92.

Kailasam, C. Congenital parvovirus B19 infection; experience of a recent epidemic. *Fetal Diagn Ther.* 2001; 16 (1): 18–22.

Koga, M. Human parvovirus B19 in cord blood of premature infants. *Am J Perinatol.* 2001; 18 (5): 237–40.

McCarter-Spaulding, D. Parvovirus B19 in Pregnancy. *JOGNN.* 2002: 31: 107–12.

Sailer, D.N., et al. Maternal serum biochemical markers in pregnancies with fetal parvovirus B19 infection. *Prenat Diagn* 1993; 12(6): 467–71.

Soulie, J.C., Cardiac involvement in fetal parvovirus B19 infection. *Pathol Biol Paris* 1995; 43(5): 416–19.

Section 10.3

Congenital Rubella

Reprinted from "Congenital Rubella," © 2006 A.D.A.M., Inc.
Reprinted with permission.

Definition

Congenital rubella is a group of physical abnormalities that occur in an infant as a result of infection of the mother with rubella virus.

Causes, Incidence, and Risk Factors

Congenital rubella is caused by the destructive action of the rubella virus on the fetus at a critical time in development. The most critical time is the first trimester (the first three months of a pregnancy). After the fourth month, maternal rubella infection is less likely to harm the developing fetus.

The incidence of rubella syndrome has decreased dramatically since the advent of rubella vaccine.

Risk factors include lack of the recommended rubella immunization and contact with a person who has rubella. Non-immunized, non-immune pregnant women are at risk for infection and subsequent damage to the fetus.

Symptoms

- History of mother having rubella while pregnant (particularly in the first trimester)
- Skin rash at birth (purpura, petechiae)
- Low birth weight
- Small head size (microcephaly)
- Lethargy
- Irritability
- Deafness

- Seizures
- Cloudy corneas or white appearance to pupil (leukocoria)
- Developmental delay
- Mental retardation

Signs and Tests

Eye findings:

- Cataracts
- Glaucoma
- Retinitis

Congenital heart disease findings:

- Patent ductus arteriosus (PDA)
- Pulmonary artery stenosis
- Other heart defects

Central nervous system findings:

- Mental retardation
- Motor retardation
- Small head (microcephaly) from failed brain development
- Encephalitis
- Meningitis

Others associated findings:

- Deafness
- Low blood platelet count
- Enlarged liver and spleen
- Abnormal muscle tone
- Bone disease

Tests include:

- Urine tests, nasopharyngeal secretions tests, or cerebrospinal fluid tests for virus
- Antibody tests

Treatment

There is no specific treatment for rubella syndrome. Care involves appropriate treatment of affected systems in consultation with your health care providers.

Expectations (Prognosis)

The prognosis for children with congenital rubella depends on the signs and symptoms present. Some findings, such as heart defects, can be corrected. However, findings such as nervous system damage cannot.

Complications

As described above under "Signs and Tests" and "Symptoms."

Calling Your Health Care Provider

Call your health care provider if you have concerns about congenital rubella, if you are unsure of your vaccination status, or if you or your child needs rubella vaccine.

Prevention

Vaccination prior to pregnancy can prevent congenital rubella. Pregnant women who are non-immune should avoid contact with persons with rubella.

Section 10.4

Sexually Transmitted Infections in Pregnancy

Each year in the United States, about fifteen million individuals contract a sexually transmitted infection (STI). STIs are infections you can get by having sex (genital, oral, or anal) with someone who has one of these infections. Many infected individuals do not know they have an STI, because some common STIs cause no symptoms.

STIs pose special risks for pregnant women and their babies. These infections can cause miscarriage, ectopic pregnancy (when the embryo implants outside of the uterus, usually in a fallopian tube), preterm delivery (before thirty-seven weeks of pregnancy), stillbirth, birth defects, and newborn illness and death. Most frequently a baby becomes infected during delivery, as he or she passes through an infected birth canal. However, a few of these infections can cross the placenta and infect the fetus.

It's important for a pregnant woman to find out if she has an STI. During an early prenatal visit, her health care provider will probably offer screening for some of these infections, including HIV (the virus that causes AIDS) and syphilis. Some STIs can be cured with drug treatment, but others cannot. However, if a woman has an STI, steps usually can be taken to protect her baby.

What is chlamydia?

Chlamydia is a bacterial infection that can cause reproductive problems for women who contract it prior to and during pregnancy. About three million new cases occur yearly (among women and men), making this one of the most common STIs. It occurs most frequently in people under age twenty-five.

Chlamydia causes no symptoms in about 75 percent of infected women, though a minority experience burning on urination and vaginal discharge. Untreated, chlamydia can spread to the upper genital tract (uterus, fallopian tubes, and ovaries), resulting in pelvic inflammatory disease (PID). PID can damage a woman's fallopian tubes and lead to infertility or ectopic pregnancy.

About 10 percent of pregnant women have chlamydia. Untreated, they may face an increased risk of miscarriage and premature rupture of the membranes (bag of waters). A study from the National Institute of Child Health and Human Development suggested that pregnant women with chlamydia have a two- to threefold increased risk of preterm delivery. Babies of women with untreated chlamydia often become infected during vaginal delivery. Infected babies frequently develop eye infections and pneumonia, which are treated with antibiotics.

All pregnant women should be screened for chlamydia. Testing can be done on a urine sample or vaginal fluid obtained with a swab. Chlamydia can be cured with antibiotics, which can prevent complications for mother and baby. A woman's partner also should be treated, because the infection can be passed back and forth between them.

What is gonorrhea?

Gonorrhea is a common bacterial infection that causes reproductive problems much like those caused by chlamydia. About 650,000 new cases occur each year. Like chlamydia, it often causes no symptoms in infected women, though some experience vaginal discharge, burning on urination, or abdominal pain. Many develop PID.

Pregnant women with untreated gonorrhea are at increased risk of miscarriage, premature delivery, and premature rupture of the membranes. Their babies frequently contract this STI during vaginal delivery. Infected babies sometimes develop serious eye infections, joint infections, and less commonly, life-threatening blood infections, which are treated with antibiotics.

Pregnant women are routinely screened for gonorrhea, with testing done on a urine sample or vaginal fluid taken with a swab. Antibiotic treatment should cure gonorrhea and help prevent pregnancy complications and newborn infections. Both the pregnant woman and her partner should be treated. Because gonorrhea and chlamydia often occur together, providers often recommend antibiotics that can cure both.

What is syphilis?

Syphilis is a dangerous STI caused by a bacterium, which can cross the placenta and infect the fetus. Fortunately, the number of new cases in women of childbearing age has dropped to an all-time low (2,219 cases in 2000).

Syphilis begins with a hard, painless sore called a chancre in the genital or vaginal area. Without treatment, infected individuals develop a rash, fever, and other symptoms months later. If still untreated, years later some infected individuals develop devastating damage to many organs that result in heart problems, brain damage, blindness, insanity, and death.

Without treatment, syphilis during pregnancy can result in fetal or infant death in up to 40 percent of cases. Some infected infants show no symptoms at birth, but without immediate antibiotic treatment, develop brain damage, blindness, hearing loss, bone and tooth abnormalities, and other problems.

During an early prenatal visit, most pregnant women are given a blood test to screen for syphilis. A single dose of penicillin can cure syphilis if a woman has had the STI for less than a year; others will require longer periods of treatment. When a woman is treated by the fourth month of pregnancy, her baby usually will not be harmed.

What is bacterial vaginosis?

Bacterial vaginosis (BV), which affects about 16 percent of pregnant women, is caused by an overgrowth of bacteria that naturally occur in the vagina. Doctors don't know for sure how a woman gets BV, though it appears more common in women who have new sex partners or who have had multiple partners. Some women with BV experience vaginal discharge that has an unpleasant odor, burning on urination, and genital itching, while others have no symptoms.

Studies suggest that BV may double a woman's chances of preterm delivery. Women with symptoms of BV are treated with antibiotics to help reduce this risk. Because BV is often symptomless, doctors sometimes test women who are considered at high risk of preterm labor for BV. Some studies suggest that treating high-risk pregnant women with BV (even if they have no symptoms) may reduce their risk of preterm birth. However, treatment does not appear to reduce the risk in low-risk women with symptomless BV, so testing is recommended only for high-risk women.

What is trichomoniasis?

Trichomoniasis is a parasitic infection that causes yellow-green foul-smelling vaginal discharge, genital itching and redness, and pain during intercourse and urination. Each year about two million women contract this STI.

Untreated, trichomoniasis may increase the risk of premature rupture of the membranes and preterm delivery. Rarely, an infant can contract the infection during delivery and develop a fever after birth.

Trichomoniasis is diagnosed by testing vaginal fluid obtained with a swab. It usually can be cured with a drug called metronidazole. Both partners should be treated.

What is genital herpes?

Genital herpes is a common STI that is caused by a group of viruses. About 25 percent of American women are infected, but most do not know it because the majority of infected individuals have no symptoms.

A minority of infected individuals develop blisters in the genital area that itch and become painful. Someone who contracts genital herpes for the first time also may develop fever, fatigue, swollen glands, and body aches. The virus remains in the body forever and can cause repeated outbreaks of blisters. Doctors usually diagnose herpes by looking at the sores; however, in some cases, they may take a swab of the blisters for testing.

A small minority of women with herpes pass it on to their infants during vaginal delivery. The risk is highest (30 to 50 percent) when the pregnant woman contracts herpes (whether or not she has symptoms) for the first time late in pregnancy. Some infected infants develop skin or mouth sores, which usually can be effectively treated with anti-viral drugs. However, in spite of treatment, the infection sometimes spreads to the brain and internal organs, resulting in brain damage, blindness, mental retardation, and even death. If a woman has symptoms of herpes at the time of delivery, a cesarean delivery will probably be recommended to protect her baby.

What are genital warts?

Genital warts are pink, white, or gray swellings in the genital area that are caused by a large group of viruses called human papillomaviruses. Some of the viruses also increase the risk of cervical cancer. The warts often appear in small cauliflower-shaped clusters, which may itch or burn. About 1 percent of all sexually active adults have genital warts.

Sometimes pregnancy-related hormones cause genital warts to grow. Occasionally, they may grow so large that they block the birth canal, making a cesarean delivery necessary. Rarely, an infected mother can pass the virus on to her baby, causing warts to grow on the vocal cords in childhood. A cesarean delivery usually is not recommended to protect the baby because this complication is rare and it is not known whether a cesarean will prevent it.

If the warts grow large or become uncomfortable, they can be safely removed during pregnancy with laser surgery or cryotherapy (freezing).

What is human immunodeficiency virus (HIV)?

HIV (human immunodeficiency virus) is the virus that causes AIDS (acquired immune deficiency syndrome), which can damage the immune system and threaten the lives of mothers and babies. An estimated 120,000 to 160,000 women in the United States are living with HIV. The majority were infected sexually, although intravenous drug use is another common source of the infection.

The Centers for Disease Control and Prevention (CDC) and the March of Dimes recommend that all pregnant women be offered counseling and voluntary testing for HIV. Women who learn they carry the virus can get treatment to help protect their babies. New drug treatments can now reduce to 2 percent or less the risk of a treated mother's passing HIV on to her baby, compared to about 25 percent of untreated mothers.

How can a pregnant woman protect her baby from STIs?

A pregnant woman can help protect her baby from STIs by making sure she doesn't contract one of them during pregnancy. She should have sex with only one partner who does not use drugs (a common source of HIV) or have symptoms of an STI. If her partner has a history of herpes, she should avoid intercourse when he has symptoms, and use a condom even when he has no sores, since there's no way to tell if he's having a symptomless outbreak. Condoms also help to protect against HIV and other STIs.

A woman should contact her provider right away if she suspects she has an STI, or if she has had sex with a partner who may have an STI. This way she can be treated promptly, to protect her health and that of her baby.

Does the March of Dimes support research on STIs in pregnancy?

The March of Dimes supports research grants aimed at improving understanding of how STIs adversely affect pregnancy, and improving the outcome for infected newborns. For example, two grantees are studying how a gene from the herpes virus allows the virus to evade the newborn's immature immune system and spread to numerous organs, with the goal of developing drugs that can prevent or treat these dangerous infections. A grantee also is studying how the viruses that cause genital warts (human papillomaviruses [HPVs]) may affect the developing placenta and contribute to miscarriages.

References

Andrews, W.W., et al. The preterm prediction study: association of second-trimester genitourinary chlamydia infection with subsequent spontaneous preterm birth. *American Journal of Obstetrics and Gynecology*, volume 183, number 3, September 2000, pages 662–68.

Carey, J.C., et al. Metronidazole to prevent preterm delivery in pregnant women with asymptomatic bacterial vaginosis. *New England Journal of Medicine*, volume 342, number 8, February 24, 2000, pages 534–40.

Centers for Disease Control and Prevention (CDC). Tracking the hidden epidemics: trends in STDs in the United States 2000. Atlanta, GA, 2001.

Centers for Disease Control and Prevention (CDC). Bacterial vaginosis, chlamydia, genital herpes, genital HPV infection, gonorrhea, syphilis, trichomoniasis. Atlanta, GA, March 12, 2002.

Section 10.5

Cytomegalovirus and Pregnancy

© 2001 Organization of Teratology Information Services (OTIS). Reprinted with permission. Member programs of OTIS are located throughout the U.S. and Canada. To find the Teratogen Information Service in your area, call OTIS toll-free at 866-626-OTIS (866-626-6847), or visit their website at www.otispregnancy.com.

The information below will determine if your prenatal exposure to cytomegalovirus represents an increased fetal risk. With every pregnancy, any woman has a 3 to 5 percent chance to have a baby with a birth defect.

What is cytomegalovirus (CMV)?

CMV is a member of the herpes family of viruses and is primarily a sexually transmitted disease, but it can also be transmitted from mother-to-child (congenitally), through blood transfusions, by close personal contact, and via organ transplantation. CMV spreads from one person to another through contact with saliva, semen, cervical and vaginal secretions, blood, urine, tears, feces, or breast milk. In the United States, the rate of CMV infection in women varies from 50 to 80 percent. A healthy immune system keeps this virus in check. There are two different types of infection: primary CMV infections and recurrent CMV infections.

Who is at increased risk for CMV?

Women who work in daycare centers or women who are exposed to toddlers and young children have an increased risk of CMV infection. Women who work in the healthcare profession may also be at an increased risk, although the transmission to a health professional from an infected patient has never been documented.

How can I find out if I am infected with CMV?

A blood test can determine if you have a nonactive (latent) CMV infection. Ideally, testing should be done prior to conception. If an infection is identified during pregnancy, several tests may need to be performed to determine whether the infection is new (primary) or old (recurrent). You should discuss whether you should be tested with your healthcare provider. Because testing for CMV infection can be difficult to interpret, your test may need to be performed at a special laboratory.

What precautions can I take to avoid CMV infection?

Women of childbearing age should practice good hygiene, especially if they are routinely exposed to young children. Good hand washing after changing diapers and after any contact with any of the bodily fluids mentioned above is encouraged. Mouth-to-mouth kissing with children attending daycare is discouraged. Pregnant women should refrain from sharing food, eating utensils, and drinking utensils. All women with non-monogamous relationships are strongly encouraged to use latex condoms during intercourse.

I am pregnant and have just found out that I have recently been infected (primary infection) with the CMV virus. Is my fetus at risk?

Primary maternal infection occurs in 0.7 to 4.0 percent of pregnancies. The reported transmission rates to the fetus are between 24 and 75 percent, with an average transmission rate of about 40 percent. Fetuses that become infected during pregnancy are said to have "congenital CMV infection." Of the approximately 40 percent of fetuses that become infected, 10 percent of neonates show symptoms of congenital CMV infections after primary maternal infection at birth. The brain, eyes, liver, spleen, blood, and skin are at risk for problems. Long-term effects may include sensorineural hearing loss, mental retardation, developmental delay, and visual impairment. Of the remaining 90 percent with asymptomatic (no evidence of disease at birth) congenital infection, 5 to 15 percent are at risk to develop some of the long-term effects. Discuss with your healthcare provider whether you should see a specialist for further information.

I had a CMV infection a year ago and I was recently diagnosed with a recurrent infection. I am pregnant. Is my fetus at risk?

Recurrent maternal CMV infection occurs (1 to 14 percent) in women more commonly than primary CMV infection, but only 0.2 to

2 percent of recurrent infections produce congenital infection. The incidence of symptomatic neonatal disease after recurrent maternal CMV infection is quite low, less than 1 percent, but long-term effects may still occur in 5 to 10 percent of congenital CMV infections, with sensorineural hearing loss being the most common effect. Discuss with your healthcare provider whether you should see a specialist for further information.

Does it matter when in my pregnancy I am diagnosed with a primary or recurrent CMV infection?

Gestational age has no influence on the risk of transmission to the fetus. However, the severity of the disease tends to be worse when the infection takes place before twenty weeks of gestation. This is true for primary maternal infections more so than recurrent maternal infections. Recurrent maternal CMV infections typically cause no effects that are clinically apparent in the neonatal period regardless of timing of the infection; however there are a few reports of recurrent maternal CMV infections in which the neonate showed clinical signs of infection.

How can I find out if my fetus has been infected with CMV?

Once you have been shown to be infected, there are several ways to check if your fetus has been infected. Amniocentesis can be performed to check the fluid around the fetus or fetal blood can be examined to determine the presence of infection. Testing the fluid around the fetus has been determined to be more accurate than fetal blood testing. However, if the fetus is infected, these tests cannot tell you the severity of the infection in the fetus. In some cases, infected fetuses may have visible signs of problems on ultrasound such as a decreased amount of amniotic fluid (oligohydramnios), smallness in size for the fetus's age (intrauterine growth retardation), and enlarged tissues in the brain (cerebral ventriculomegaly) to name a few. After birth, a saliva, urine, or blood test can be performed on the baby. You should discuss these tests with your healthcare provider.

Is there treatment for CMV during pregnancy?

Maternal CMV infections may be treated with one of two drugs: ganciclovir or foscarnet. Unfortunately, there is no accepted prenatal or postnatal therapy for congenital CMV infections. The use of ganciclovir during pregnancy to prevent or reduce the effects of congenital CMV infection has been considered. Current recommendations limit the use of ganciclovir in pregnancy to severe (life-threatening or sight-threatening) maternal CMV infections. Your healthcare provider can discuss specific treatment options with you.

References

Adler S, et al. Prevention of child-to-mother transmission of cytomegalovirus by changing behaviors: a randomized controlled trial. *Pediatr Infect Dis J* 15: 240–46, 1996.

Ahlfors K. Harris S. Ivarsson S. Svanberg L. Secondary maternal cytomegalovirus infection causing symptomatic congenital infection. *N Engl J Med.* 305: 284, 1981.

Azam A, et al. Prenatal diagnosis of congenital cytomegalovirus infection. *Obstet Gynecol* 97: 443–48, 2001.

Boppana S, et al. Symptomatic congenital cytomegalovirus infection in infants born to mothers with pre-existing immunity to cytomegalovirus. *Pediatrics.* 104: 55–60, 1999.

Demmler G. Acquired cytomegalovirus infections. In Feigin RD, Cherry JD (eds.), *Textbook of Pediatric Infectious Diseases*. Philadelphia: W.B. Saunders Co., pp. 1532–47, 1992.

Ho M. *Cytomegalovirus: Biology and Infection*. New York: Plenum Medical Book Co., 1991.

Nelson C, Demmler G. Cytomegalovirus infection in the pregnant mother, fetus, and newborn infant. *Clinic in Perinatology* 24: 151–60, 1997.

Piper J, Wen T. Perinatal cytomegalovirus and toxoplasmosis: challenges of antepartum therapy. *Clinical Obstetrics and Gynecology* 42: 81–96, 1999.

Section 10.6

Listeriosis and Pregnancy: What Is Your Risk?

Reprinted from "Listeriosis and Pregnancy: What Is Your Risk? Safe Food Handling for a Healthy Pregnancy," United States Department of Agriculture (USDA), September 2001.

When you're expecting, it's natural to be concerned about your health and that of your unborn baby. Maintaining a healthful diet, drinking plenty of liquids, and taking prenatal vitamins are all important for the health of the expectant mother and her baby. Food safety is also very important. This information will help you make safe decisions when selecting and preparing food for yourself and your family.

Sometimes, what we eat can make us sick. Food contaminated by harmful bacteria can cause serious illness. One type of bacteria, *Listeria monocytogenes* (pronounced lis-TIR-ee-ya mon-o-si-TAH-gin-eez), can cause an illness called listeriosis. The Centers for Disease Control and Prevention (CDC) estimates that 2,500 people become seriously ill with listeriosis each year in the United States. Of these, one in five die from the disease. Listeriosis can be particularly dangerous for pregnant women and their unborn babies. Food-borne illness caused by *Listeria* in pregnant women can result in premature delivery, miscarriage, fetal death, and severe illness or death of a newborn from the infection.

What is **Listeria?**

Listeria is a type of bacteria found everywhere in soil and groundwater and on plants. Animals and people can carry *Listeria* in their bodies without becoming sick. Despite being so widespread, most infections in humans result from eating contaminated foods.

Most people are not at increased risk for listeriosis. However, there are some people who are considered at risk because they are more susceptible to listeriosis. In addition to pregnant women and their unborn babies and newborns, other at-risk groups include older adults and people with weakened immune systems caused by cancer treatments,

147

AIDS, diabetes, kidney disease, and so on. By carefully following food safety precautions, persons at risk for listeriosis can substantially reduce their chances of becoming ill.

Why is listeriosis especially dangerous for me and my child?

Hormonal changes during pregnancy have an effect on the mother's immune system that lead to an increased susceptibility to listeriosis in the mother. According to the CDC, pregnant women are about twenty times more likely than other healthy adults to get listeriosis. In fact, about one-third of listeriosis cases happen during pregnancy. Listeriosis can be transmitted to the fetus through the placenta even if the mother is not showing signs of illness. This can lead to premature delivery, miscarriage, stillbirth, or serious health problems for her newborn.

Is Listeria transmitted from the mother to the baby through breast milk?

While there is a theoretical possibility that *Listeria monocytogenes* could be transmitted via mother's milk, this has never been proven.

How will I know if I have listeriosis?

Because the symptoms of listeriosis can take a few days or even weeks to appear and can be mild, you may not even know you have it. This is why it's very important to take appropriate food safety precautions during pregnancy.

In pregnant women, listeriosis may cause flu-like symptoms with the sudden onset of fever, chills, muscle aches, and sometimes diarrhea or upset stomach. The severity of the symptoms may vary. If the infection spreads to the nervous system, the symptoms may include headache, stiff neck, confusion, loss of balance, or convulsions. Consult your doctor or healthcare provider if you have these symptoms. A blood test can be performed to find out if your symptoms are caused by listeriosis.

What is the treatment for listeriosis?

During pregnancy, antibiotics are given to treat listeriosis in the mother. In most cases, the antibiotics also prevent infection of the fetus or newborn. Antibiotics are also given to babies who are born with listeriosis.

What steps can I take to prevent listeriosis?

The U.S. Department of Agriculture's Food Safety and Inspection Service (FSIS) and the U.S. Food and Drug Administration (FDA) provide the following advice for pregnant women and all at-risk consumers:

- Do not eat hot dogs, luncheon meats, or deli meats unless they are reheated until steaming hot.

- Do not eat soft cheeses such as feta, Brie, Camembert, blue-veined cheeses, and Mexican-style cheeses such as "queso blanco fresco." Hard cheeses, semi-soft cheeses such as mozzarella, pasteurized processed cheese slices and spreads, cream cheese, and cottage cheese can be safely consumed.

- Do not eat refrigerated pâté or meat spreads. Canned or shelf-stable pâté and meat spreads can be eaten.

- Do not eat refrigerated smoked seafood unless it is an ingredient in a cooked dish such as a casserole. Examples of refrigerated smoked seafood include salmon, trout, whitefish, cod, tuna, and mackerel which are most often labeled as "nova-style," "lox," "kippered," "smoked," or "jerky." This fish is found in the refrigerated section or sold at deli counters of grocery stores and delicatessens. Canned fish such as salmon and tuna or shelf-stable smoked seafood may be safely eaten.

- Do not drink raw (unpasteurized) milk or eat foods that contain unpasteurized milk.

What can all consumers do to prevent listeriosis and keep their food safe?

Because *Listeria* can grow at refrigeration temperatures of 40° F or below, FSIS and FDA advise all consumers to:

- Use all perishable items that are precooked or ready-to-eat as soon as possible.

- Clean their refrigerators regularly.

- Use a refrigerator thermometer to make sure that the refrigerator always stays at 40° F or below.

What should I do if I've eaten a food that has been recalled because of Listeria contamination?

If you have eaten a contaminated product and do not have any symptoms, most experts believe you don t need any tests or treatment, even if you are pregnant. However, you should inform your physician or healthcare provider if you are pregnant and have eaten the contaminated product and within two months experience flu-like symptoms.

It's important to learn how to protect yourself and your unborn baby from food-borne illnesses. Getting in the habit of eating a safe and nutritious diet not only benefits your baby, but will also give you peace of mind.

Remember—new information on food safety is constantly emerging. Recommendations and precautions are updated as scientists learn more about preventing food-borne illness. You need to be aware of and follow the most current information on food safety. Consult your healthcare provider if you have questions.

Section 10.7

Toxoplasmosis and Pregnancy

Reprinted from "Toxoplasmosis," Center for the Evaluation of Risks to Human Reproduction, National Institute of Environmental Health Sciences, December 21, 2005.

Overview

Toxoplasmosis is an infection caused by a parasite. If a pregnant woman contracts toxoplasmosis, there is a 40 percent chance that her unborn child will also become infected. However, such infections are not common in the United Sates. One to two per one thousand babies that are born each year have toxoplasmosis. The toxoplasmosis parasite may be found in cat feces, soils, and undercooked infected meat. Cats may contract toxoplasmosis after eating infected birds or rodents, and the infection can spread to persons only through direct contact with the cat's feces or soils in contact with the feces. Unborn children infected in early pregnancy are most likely to suffer severe health effects, which may include blindness, deafness, seizures, and mental retardation. Often, infected infants appear normal at birth, but develop symptoms months or years later. Toxoplasmosis is easily prevented by taking some simple precautions such as having someone else clean cat litter boxes, keeping cats indoors, thoroughly cooking meats and washing fruits and vegetables before eating, wearing gloves while gardening, and washing hands after handling raw meats. If toxoplasmosis is suspected in a pregnant woman, tests can be done to determine if the unborn child is also infected. Medications can prevent or reduce severity of health effects in unborn children.

Description of Toxoplasmosis

According to the Organization of Teratology Information Services (OTIS, 2002), "Toxoplasmosis is an infection caused by the parasite *Toxoplasma gondii*. You can get it by eating undercooked, infected meat, or handling soil or cat feces that contain the parasite. Swelling of the lymph nodes or a mononucleosis-type (fever, fatigue, and sore throat) illness may be seen. Most adults have no symptoms. In most cases, once you have gotten toxoplasmosis, you cannot get it again."

The March of Dimes (MOD, 2001) has stated that, "Cats often become infected when they eat an infected rodent or bird. The parasite reproduces in the cat's intestine, and a form of the parasite ends up in the cat's litter box, sand or soil. This form of the parasite becomes infectious within days, and is resistant to most disinfectants. Under certain temperature and humidity conditions, the parasite may live in soil for more than a year. Infected cats usually appear healthy."

Toxoplasmosis and Pregnancy

If a woman contracts toxoplasmosis during pregnancy, there is a possibility that her unborn child will be infected. Unborn children of women who have contracted toxoplasmosis prior to pregnancy are usually not at risk. According to OTIS (OTIS, 2002), "Congenital toxoplasmosis only occurs when the mother has an active infection during pregnancy. In general, there is no increased risk to the fetus when toxoplasmosis occurs more than six months prior to conception. If you had toxoplasmosis in the past, you are usually immune, and the fetus is not at risk."

The Organization of Teratology Information Services (OTIS, 2002) has stated, "In about 40 percent of the cases in which a pregnant woman has toxoplasmosis, the baby is also infected. Infants who become infected during pregnancy are said to have 'congenital toxoplasmosis' infection. In the United Sates, one to two per one thousand babies that are born each year have toxoplasmosis." According to the March of Dimes (MOD, 2001), about one in ten infected babies has a severe Toxoplasma infection evident at birth. These newborns often have eye infections, an enlarged liver and spleen, jaundice (yellowing of the skin and eyes), and pneumonia. Some die within a few days of birth. Those who survive can have mental retardation, severely impaired eyesight, cerebral palsy, seizures, and other problems. Although up to 90 percent of infected babies appear normal at birth, between 55 and 85 percent of them develop problems months to years later, including eye infections that may affect sight, hearing loss, and learning disabilities. Toxoplasmosis during pregnancy also can result in miscarriage or stillbirth.

Toxoplasmosis Prevention

To prevent toxoplasmosis, the March of Dimes (MOD, 2001) suggests that pregnant woman take the following precautions:

- Don't empty the cat's litter box. Have someone else do this.

- Don't feed the cat raw or undercooked meats.

- Keep the cat indoors to prevent it from hunting birds or rodents.

- Don't eat raw or undercooked meat, especially lamb or pork. Meat should be cooked to an internal temperature of 160° F throughout.

- If you handle raw meat, wash your hands immediately with soap. Never touch your eyes, nose, or mouth with potentially contaminated hands.

- Wash all raw fruits and vegetables before you eat them.

- Wear gloves when gardening, since outdoor soil may contain the parasite from cats. Keep your hands away from your mouth and eyes, and wash your hands thoroughly when finished. Keep gloves away from food products.

- Avoid children's sandboxes. Cats may use them as a litter box.

Diagnosis and Treatment

According to the March of Dimes (MOD, 2001), "If a health care provider suspects that a pregnant woman has an active Toxoplasma infection, he or she may recommend one or more of several available blood tests. These tests require expert interpretation and, therefore, the Centers for Disease Control and Prevention recommends that all positive test results be confirmed by a Toxoplasma reference laboratory (one with special expertise in diagnosing this disorder)."

If the reference laboratory confirms that a pregnant woman has an active infection, the next step is to determine whether the fetus is infected. Prenatal tests including amniocentesis and ultrasound may help to determine whether the fetus is infected. Fetuses suspected of being infected are treated by giving the mother pyrimethamine and sulfadiazine. This approach appears to reduce the frequency and severity of the newborn's symptoms. Time is of the essence and the earlier the treatment of the mother, the less likely her baby is to have symptoms.

If tests show that the fetus is not yet infected, the mother may be given an antibiotic called spiramycin. Some studies suggest that spiramycin can reduce by about 50 percent the likelihood of the fetus becoming infected. Although spiramycin has not yet been approved for use in this country by the Food and Drug Administration (FDA), and is therefore considered an experimental drug, it can be obtained from the FDA.

Chapter 11

Rh Incompatibility

If you just found out you're pregnant, one of the first—and most important—tests you should expect is a blood-type test. This basic test determines your blood type and Rh factor. Your Rh factor may play a role in your baby's health, so it's important to know this information early in your pregnancy.

What is the Rh factor?

People with different blood types have proteins specific to that blood type on the surfaces of their red blood cells. There are four blood types—A, B, AB, and O.

Each of the four blood types is additionally classified according to the presence of another protein on the surface of red blood cells that indicates the Rh factor. If you carry this protein, you are Rh positive. If you don't carry the protein, you are Rh negative.

Most people—about 85 percent—are Rh positive. But if a woman who is Rh negative and a man who is Rh positive conceive a baby, there is the potential for a baby to have a health problem. The baby growing inside the Rh-negative mother may have Rh-positive blood, inherited from the father. Approximately half of the children born to an Rh-negative mother and Rh-positive father will be Rh positive.

Reprinted from "What Is Rh Incompatibility?" This information was provided by KidsHealth, one of the largest resources online for medically reviewed health information written for parents, kids, and teens. For more articles like this one, visit www.KidsHealth.org, or www.TeensHealth.org. © 2005 The Nemours Center for Children's Health Media, a division of The Nemours Foundation.

Rh incompatibility usually isn't a problem if it's the mother's first pregnancy because, unless there's some sort of abnormality, the fetus's blood does not normally enter the mother's circulatory system during the course of the pregnancy.

However, during delivery, the mother's and baby's blood can intermingle. If this happens, the mother's body recognizes the Rh protein as a foreign substance and can begin producing antibodies (protein molecules in the immune system that recognize, and later work to destroy, foreign substances) against the Rh proteins introduced into her blood.

Other ways Rh-negative pregnant women can be exposed to the Rh protein that might cause antibody production include blood transfusions with Rh-positive blood, miscarriage, and ectopic pregnancy.

Rh antibodies are harmless until the mother's second or later pregnancies. If she is ever carrying another Rh-positive child, her Rh antibodies will recognize the Rh proteins on the surface of the baby's blood cells as foreign, and pass into the baby's bloodstream and attack those cells. This can lead to swelling and rupture of the baby's red blood cells. A baby's blood count can get dangerously low when this condition, known as hemolytic or Rh disease of the newborn, occurs.

How is Rh disease of the newborn prevented and treated?

In generations past, Rh incompatibility was a very serious problem. Fortunately, significant medical advances have been made to help prevent complications from Rh incompatibility and to treat any newborn affected by Rh disease.

Today, when a woman with the potential to develop Rh incompatibility is pregnant, doctors administer a series of two Rh immune-globulin shots during her first pregnancy. The first shot is given around the twenty-eighth week of pregnancy and the second within seventy-two hours after giving birth. Rh immune-globulin acts like a vaccine, preventing the mother's body from producing any potentially dangerous Rh antibodies that can cause serious complications in the newborn or complicate any future pregnancies.

A dose of Rh immune-globulin may also be given if a woman has a miscarriage, an amniocentesis, or any bleeding during pregnancy.

If a doctor determines that a woman has already developed Rh antibodies, then the pregnancy will be closely monitored to make sure that those levels are not too high. In rare cases, if the incompatibility is severe and the baby is in danger, a series of special blood transfusions (called exchange transfusions) can be performed either while the baby is still in the uterus or after delivery.

Exchange transfusions replace the baby's blood with red blood cells that have the Rh-negative factor. This procedure stabilizes the baby's level of red blood cells and minimizes further damage caused by circulating Rh antibodies already present in the baby's bloodstream.

Because of the success rate of the Rh immune-globulin shots, exchange transfusions are needed in fewer than 1 percent of Rh-incompatible pregnancies in the United States today.

What can happen if Rh disease is not prevented?

Rh incompatibility rarely causes complications in a first pregnancy and does not affect the health of the mother. But Rh antibodies that develop during subsequent pregnancies can be potentially dangerous to mother and child. Rh disease can result in severe anemia, jaundice, brain damage, and heart failure in a newborn. In extreme cases, it can cause the death of the fetus because too many red blood cells have been depleted.

If you're not sure what your Rh factor is and think you're pregnant, it's important to start regular prenatal care as soon as possible—including blood type testing. With early detection and treatment of Rh incompatibility, you can focus on more important things—like welcoming a new, healthy baby into your household.

Chapter 12

Gestational Concerns

Chapter Contents

Section 12.1—Fetal Growth Restriction 160
Section 12.2—Amniotic Fluid Abnormalities 163
Section 12.3—Placental Conditions 171
Section 12.4—Umbilical Cord Abnormalities 177

Section 12.1

Fetal Growth Restriction

The most common definition of fetal growth restriction is a fetal weight that is below the tenth percentile for gestational age as determined through an ultrasound. This can also be called small for gestational age (SGA) or intrauterine growth restriction (IUGR).

Are there different types of fetal growth restriction?

There are basically two different types of fetal growth restriction:

- **Symmetric or primary growth restriction** is characterized by all internal organs being reduced in size. Symmetric growth restriction accounts for 20 to 25 percent of all cases of growth restriction.

- **Asymmetric or secondary growth restriction** is characterized by the head and brain being normal in size, but the abdomen is smaller. Typically this is not evident until the third trimester.

What are the risk factors for developing fetal growth restriction?

Pregnancies that have any of the following conditions may be at a greater risk for developing fetal growth restriction:

- Maternal weight of less than one hundred pounds
- Poor nutrition during pregnancy
- Birth defects or chromosomal abnormalities
- Use of drugs, cigarettes, and/or alcohol
- Pregnancy-induced hypertension (PIH)

- Placental abnormalities
- Umbilical cord abnormalities
- Multiple pregnancy
- Gestational diabetes in the mother
- Low levels of amniotic fluid or oligohydramnios

How is fetal growth restriction diagnosed?

One of the most important things when diagnosing fetal growth restriction is to ensure accurate dating of the pregnancy. Gestational age can be calculated by using the first day of your last menstrual period (LMP) and also by early ultrasound calculations.

Once gestational age has been established the following methods can be used to diagnose fetal growth restriction:

- Fundal height that does not coincide with gestational age
- Measurements calculated in an ultrasound that are smaller than would be expected for the gestational age
- Abnormal findings discovered by a Doppler ultrasound

How is fetal growth restriction treated?

Despite new research, the optimal treatment for fetal growth restriction remains problematic. Most likely the treatment will depend on how far along you are in your pregnancy.

If gestational age is thirty-four weeks or greater, healthcare providers may recommend being induced for an early delivery.

If gestational age is less than thirty-four weeks, healthcare providers will continue monitoring until thirty-four weeks or beyond. Fetal well-being and the amount of amniotic fluid will be monitored during this time. If either of these becomes a concern, then immediate delivery may be recommended.

Depending on your healthcare provider, you will likely have appointments every two to six weeks until you deliver. If delivery is suggested prior to thirty-four weeks, your healthcare provider may perform an amniocentesis to help evaluate fetal lung maturity.

What risks are associated with a baby born with fetal growth restriction?

- Increased risk for cesarean delivery

- Increased risk for hypoxia (lack of oxygen when the baby is born)

- Increased risk for meconium aspiration, which is when the baby swallows part of the first bowel movement. This can cause the alveoli to be overdistended, a pneumothorax to occur, and/or the development of bacterial pneumonia.

- Hypoglycemia (low blood sugar)

- Polycythemia (increased number of red blood cells)

- Hyperviscosity (decreased blood flow due to an increased number of red blood cells)

- Increased risk for motor and neurological disabilities

References

Cunningham, F. Gary, Kenneth J Leveno, Steven L. Bloom, John C. Hauth, Larry Gilstrap III, and Katharine D. Wenstrom ed. *Williams Obstetrics* 22nd ed. (New York: McGraw-Hill Publishers), 2005.

Scott, James R., Ronald S. Gibbins, Beth Y. Karlan, Arthur F. Haney ed. *Danforth's Obstetrics and Gynecology* 9th ed. (Philadelphia: Lippincott Williams & Wilkins), 2003.

Olds, Sally B, Marcia L. London, and Patricia Wieland Ladewig, eds. *Maternal-Newborn Nursing: A Family-Centered Approach* 5th ed. (New York: Addison-Wesley Nursing), 1996.

Section 12.2

Amniotic Fluid Abnormalities

Abnormalities in the Amniotic Fluid

The amniotic fluid that surrounds a developing baby plays a crucial role in normal development. This clear-colored liquid cushions and protects the baby and provides it with fluids. By the second trimester, the baby is able to breathe the fluid into his lungs and to swallow it, promoting normal growth and development of the lungs and gastrointestinal system. Amniotic fluid also allows the baby to move around, which aids in normal development of muscle and bone.

The amniotic sac that contains the embryo forms about twelve days after conception. Amniotic fluid immediately begins to fill the sac. In the early weeks of pregnancy, amniotic fluid consists mainly of water supplied by the mother. After about twelve weeks, fetal urine makes up most of the fluid.

The amount of amniotic fluid increases until about twenty-eight to thirty-two weeks of pregnancy, when it measures a little less than one quart. After that time, the level of fluid generally stays about the same until the baby is full term (about thirty-seven to forty weeks), when the level begins to decline.

In some pregnancies, however, there may be too little or too much amniotic fluid. These conditions are referred to as oligohydramnios and polyhydramnios, respectively. Both can sometimes cause problems for mother and baby or be a sign of other problems. However, in the majority of cases, the baby is born healthy. Here's what expectant parents should know about these disorders.

How are oligohydramnios and polyhydramnios diagnosed?

An ultrasound examination can diagnose either too little or too much amniotic fluid. Doctors commonly measure the depth of the fluid in four quadrants in the uterus and add them up. This method of measuring amniotic fluid is referred to as the amniotic fluid index (AFI). If the amniotic fluid depth measures less than 5 centimeters, the pregnant woman has oligohydramnios. If fluid levels add up to more than 25 centimeters, she has polyhydramnios.

How common is oligohydramnios?

About 8 percent of pregnant women have too little amniotic fluid. Oligohydramnios can develop at any time during pregnancy, though it is most common in the last trimester. About 12 percent of women whose pregnancies last about two weeks beyond their due dates (about forty-two weeks gestation) develop oligohydramnios, because the level of amniotic fluid decreases by about half by forty-two weeks gestation.

What fetal problems and pregnancy complications are associated with oligohydramnios?

The problems associated with too little amniotic fluid differ depending on the stage of pregnancy. Oligohydramnios that occurs in the first half of pregnancy is more likely to have serious consequences than if it occurs in the last trimester. Too little amniotic fluid early in pregnancy can compress fetal organs and cause birth defects, such as lung and limb defects. Oligohydramnios that develops in the first half of pregnancy also increases the risk of miscarriage, preterm birth, and stillbirth.

When oligohydramnios occurs in the second half of pregnancy, it may be associated with poor fetal growth. Near term, oligohydramnios may increase the risk of complications of labor and delivery, including potentially dangerous umbilical cord accidents that can deprive the baby of oxygen, and stillbirth. Women with oligohydramnios are more likely than unaffected women to need a cesarean delivery.

What causes too little amniotic fluid?

The causes of oligohydramnios are not completely understood. The majority of pregnant women who develop oligohydramnios have no identifiable cause.

The most important known causes of early oligohydramnios are certain birth defects and ruptured membranes (a rupture in the bag of waters that surrounds the baby). About 7 percent of babies of women with oligohydramnios have birth defects. Birth defects involving the kidneys and urinary tract are the most likely causes because affected fetuses produce less urine (which makes up most of the amniotic fluid).

Certain maternal health problems also have been associated with oligohydramnios. These include high blood pressure, diabetes, systemic lupus erythematosus (SLE) (an autoimmune condition), and placental problems. A group of medications used to treat high blood pressure, called angiotensin-converting enzyme inhibitors (like captopril), can damage the fetal kidneys and cause severe oligohydramnios and fetal death. Women who have chronic high blood pressure should consult their health care provider prior to pregnancy to make sure their blood pressure is under control and that any medications they take are safe during pregnancy.

How is oligohydramnios treated?

Recent studies suggest that women with otherwise normal pregnancies who develop oligohydramnios near term probably need no treatment, and their babies are likely to be born healthy. They do, however, require close surveillance. Their health care provider will probably recommend weekly or more frequent ultrasound examinations to see if the level of amniotic fluid is decreasing. If the level of amniotic fluid does drop, he or she may recommend inducing labor early to help prevent complications during labor and delivery. About 40 to 50 percent of cases of oligohydramnios resolve themselves without treatment in as little as a few days.

Besides ultrasound examinations, providers will likely recommend tests of fetal well-being, such as the nonstress and contraction stress tests, both of which measure fetal heart rate. These tests can alert the provider that the baby is having difficulties. In such cases, the provider is likely to recommend early delivery to help prevent serious problems.

Developing babies with poor growth whose mothers have oligohydramnios are at high risk of complications, such as asphyxia (lack of oxygen), both before and during birth. Mothers of these babies are monitored very closely, and they sometimes need to be hospitalized.

If a woman has severe oligohydramnios near the time of delivery, her provider may suggest inserting salty water (saline solution) through the cervix into the uterus. This may help reduce complications during labor and delivery and reduce the need for cesarean delivery.

Studies suggest that this approach is especially beneficial when fetal heart rate monitoring shows that the baby may be having difficulties. Some studies also suggest that women with oligohydramnios can help increase their levels of amniotic fluid by drinking extra water. Also, many doctors suggest decreasing physical activity or even bed rest. A pregnant woman with oligohydramnios should discuss with her healthcare provider which, if any, treatment may be best for her.

How common is polyhydramnios?

About 2 percent of pregnant women have too much amniotic fluid. Most cases are mild and result from a gradual buildup of excess fluid in the second half of pregnancy. However, a small number have a rapid buildup of fluid occurring as early as sixteen weeks of pregnancy that usually results in very early delivery.

What complications does polyhydramnios cause for mother and baby?

While women with mild polyhydramnios may experience few symptoms, those who are more severely affected may have abdominal discomfort and breathing difficulties as a result of the uterus crowding the abdominal organs and lungs. Polyhydramnios also may increase the risk of pregnancy complications including preterm rupture of the membranes, preterm delivery, umbilical cord accidents, placental abruption (when the placenta partially or completely peels away from the uterine wall before delivery), poor fetal growth, stillbirth, and cesarean delivery. Women with polyhydramnios may be more likely to have severe bleeding after delivery.

What causes polyhydramnios?

In about two-thirds of cases, the cause of polyhydramnios is unknown. The most common known cause of polyhydramnios is birth defects in the fetus, especially birth defects that hinder fetal swallowing (such as birth defects involving the esophagus or gastrointestinal tract and central nervous system). Normally, swallowing by the fetus helps reduce the level of amniotic fluid, helping to balance out the input caused by fetal urination. Heart defects in the baby also can contribute to polyhydramnios.

Other fetal problems that can cause polyhydramnios include maternal-fetal blood incompatibilities (such as Rh disease) and twin-twin transfusion syndrome (a complication affecting identical twin pregnancies, in which one baby gets too much blood flow and the other too little due to connections between blood vessels in their shared placenta). Women with chronic diabetes are at increased risk of polyhydramnios, though they have fewer complications from it than women without diabetes.

How is polyhydramnios treated?

When an ultrasound examination shows that a woman has polyhydramnios, she will probably need additional tests. Her health care provider will most likely suggest a detailed ultrasound examination to diagnose or, more likely, rule out birth defects and twin-twin transfusion syndrome. Her provider also may recommend amniocentesis (a small amount of amniotic fluid is removed through a needle inserted into the mother's abdomen to test for certain birth defects) and a blood test for diabetes.

About half the time, polyhydramnios goes away without treatment. In other cases, it may resolve when the problem causing it is corrected. For example, treating high blood sugar levels in women with diabetes or treating certain fetal heart rhythm disturbances (by medicating the mother) often reduces amniotic fluid levels.

Healthcare providers usually closely monitor women with polyhydramnios with weekly (or more frequent) ultrasound examinations to check amniotic fluid levels. Tests of fetal well-being are also usually recommended to check for signs of fetal difficulties. If the pregnant woman becomes too uncomfortable, her provider may recommend a drug called indomethacin. This drug helps reduce fetal urine production and reduce amniotic fluid levels. Amniocentesis also can be used to drain off excess fluid. This procedure, which may be repeated a number of times, can reduce symptoms and may prolong pregnancy.

If tests show that mother and baby appear healthy, a woman with mild polyhydramnios near term usually does not need any treatment. While she may have an increased risk of cesarean delivery, she appears to be at low risk of other complications, and her baby is likely to be healthy.

Does discolored amniotic fluid pose a risk to the baby?

Normal amniotic fluid is clear or tinted yellow. Abnormal coloring seen at amniocentesis or at birth can sometimes suggest problems. Green or brown-tinged fluid usually indicates that the baby has passed stool. This can be a sign of fetal stress. Pink-tinged fluid suggests bleeding, while wine-colored amniotic fluid suggests bleeding in the past. These conditions may be of little or no consequence, but tests may be suggested to find possible causes.

Does the March of Dimes support research on amniotic fluid disorders?

A March of Dimes grantee is currently evaluating the safety of a new drug treatment developed for oligohydramnios that aims to increase the levels of amniotic fluid by increasing urination in the baby. The treatment could play a major role in preventing umbilical cord accidents, stillbirths, and preterm delivery associated with too little amniotic fluid.

References

Biggio, J.R., et al. Hydramnios prediction of adverse outcome. *Obstetrics and Gynecology*, volume 94, number 5, November 1999, pages 773–77.

Casey, B.M. Pregnancy outcomes after antepartum diagnosis of oligohydramnios at or beyond 34 weeks gestation. *American Journal of Obstetrics and Gynecology*, volume 184, number 4, April 2000, pages 909–12.

Cunningham, F.G., et al. Abnormalities of the fetal membranes and amniotic fluid, in *Williams Obstetrics*, 21st edition, New York, McGraw/Hill Medical Publishing Division, 2001, pages 813–25.

Lembet, A., and Berkowitz, R.L. Polyhydramnios. *Contemporary Ob / Gyn*, September 1999, pages 67–80.

Panting-Kemp, A., et al. Idiopathic polyhydramnios and perinatal outcome. *American Journal of Obstetrics and Gynecology*, volume 181, number 5, November 1999, pages 1079–82.

Ross, M.G., Brace, R.A., and NIH Workshop Participants. National Institute of Child Health and Development conference summary: amniotic fluid biology—basic and clinical aspects. *Journal of Maternal-Fetal Medicine*, volume 10, February 2001, pages 2–19.

Amniotic Band Syndrome

In amniotic band syndrome, strands of the amniotic sac ensnare parts of the developing body, causing a variety of problems. These may include syndactyly (joined fingers or toes), bands or constriction rings, amputations, swelling, or other deformities. There are several different names for this condition.

Does amniotic band syndrome cause my baby any pain?

No, typically there is no pain associated with this condition. However, occasionally, if there is a very tight band associated with some skin breakdown or infection, there may be minor discomfort.

What are the different types of amniotic band syndrome?

Amniotic band syndrome may present in many different forms. For example, it may cause only a minor groove or indentation in one of the limbs; or it may cause syndactyly of multiple digits on the hand or foot with multiple bands or constriction rings on multiple digits; or amputations of digits or larger parts of the limbs. Each case is unique.

Who gets amniotic band syndrome?

Amniotic band syndrome can occur in any newborn infant. There is no pattern of inheritance. This condition occurs in approximately one in fifteen thousand newborns.

What causes amniotic band syndrome?

Although there are many theories, the cause of amniotic band syndrome has not been determined.

What are the main issues related to amniotic band syndrome?

The primary issue in most types of amniotic band syndrome is function of the hand and digits; appearance of the hand is also an issue, but is secondary to function. When there is syndactyly of the digits (fingers or toes joined together), independent function of the digits is limited. When the digits are short because of growth arrest or intrauterine amputations, function may also be limited.

Are there other problems that occur commonly with amniotic band syndrome?

The most common problems that are associated with amniotic band syndrome are cleft lip/palate and clubfoot. Associated anomalies may occur in approximately 40 to 60 percent of cases. Usually, there are no abnormalities of the internal organs.

What is the treatment for babies with amniotic band syndrome?

While every patient is treated individually, with treatment plans made specifically for him or her, some generalizations are possible. Amniotic band syndrome is treated surgically. The exact type, number, timing, and sequence of operations depends upon the specific deformity present in each case. When the fingertips are joined together (acrosyndactyly), the first operation usually is done to release the fingertips so that the fingers may move more independently. This procedure is done in the first three to six months of life. After that, procedures may be done to deepen the web spaces between digits to increase their effective length; these operations may involve the use of skin grafts from the abdomen. Constriction bands are "contoured" by excising them and rearranging the skin and soft tissues on either side of the band to create a smooth, cylindrical shape to the digit or limb. Occasionally, even more complicated procedures may be done to lengthen digits, such as using distraction osteogenesis to stretch the bones or using microsurgery to transfer toes to the hand.

Section 12.3

Placental Conditions

The placenta is an unborn baby's lifeline. It forms from the same cells as the embryo, and attaches to the inner wall of the uterus. The placenta forms connections with the mother's blood supply, from which it transfers oxygen and nutrients to the baby. It also connects with the baby's blood supply, from which it removes wastes and transfers them to the mother's blood (her kidneys then dispose of the waste).

The placenta has other functions that also are crucial for normal pregnancy. These include production of hormones that play a role in triggering labor and delivery. The placenta also helps to protect the unborn baby from infections and potentially harmful substances. After the baby is delivered, the placenta's job is done and it is delivered as the afterbirth.

The mature placenta is flat and circular, and weighs about one pound. But sometimes the placenta is structured abnormally, is poorly positioned in the uterus, or does not function properly. Placental problems are among the most common complications of the second half of pregnancy. Here are some of the most frequent placental problems and how they can affect mother and baby.

What is placental abruption?

Placental abruption (sometimes written abruptio placentae) is a condition in which the placenta peels away from the uterine wall, partially or almost completely, before delivery. It can deprive the baby of oxygen and nutrients and cause bleeding in the mother that, in severe cases, can endanger both her and the baby.

Placental abruption also increases the risk of preterm delivery (before thirty-seven completed weeks of gestation). Although the outlook for premature babies has greatly improved, they still face an

171

increased risk of newborn complications, lasting disabilities, and even death. A 1999 study at Mount Sinai School of Medicine in New York City found that women with abruptions were about four times more likely than women without abruptions to deliver prematurely (40 percent vs. 9 percent). Abruption also increases the risk of stillbirth.

How common is placental abruption?

Abruption occurs in about one in one hundred pregnancies. It occurs most often in the third trimester, but it can happen any time after about twenty weeks of pregnancy.

What are the symptoms of abruption?

The main sign of placental abruption is vaginal bleeding. Bleeding sometimes is accompanied by uterine discomfort and tenderness, or sudden, continuous abdominal pain. A pregnant woman always should contact her health care provider if she is bleeding vaginally.

If the health care provider suspects an abruption, she probably will recommend going to the hospital for a complete evaluation. An ultrasound examination often is used to help diagnose placental abruption.

How is placental abruption treated?

A mild abruption usually is not dangerous unless it progresses. If a woman has a mild abruption at term, her health care provider may recommend prompt delivery (either by inducing labor or by c-section) to avoid any risks associated with a worsening abruption.

If a woman has a mild abruption and her baby would be very premature if delivered immediately, her health care provider will probably admit her to the hospital for careful monitoring. If tests show that neither mother nor baby is having difficulties, the provider may try to prolong the pregnancy to avoid prematurity-related complications for the baby. If the provider suspects that the abruption is likely to result in preterm delivery before thirty-four weeks of pregnancy, he or she will probably recommend the mother be given a drug (corticosteroid) to help speed maturation of the unborn baby's lungs and decrease the risk of certain other complications of preterm birth.

If an abruption progresses, a woman is bleeding heavily, or the baby is having difficulties, then prompt delivery, usually by cesarean section, probably will be necessary.

What causes placental abruption?

The cause of abruption is unknown, but high blood pressure, cocaine use, and cigarette smoking during pregnancy greatly increase the risk. Pregnant women with high blood pressure should do their best to keep it under control by seeing their health care provider regularly and taking medication, if recommended. All pregnant women should avoid cigarettes and cocaine, which contribute to abruption and certain other pregnancy complications.

Other factors that increase the risk of abruption include abdominal trauma (such as may be caused by an automobile accident or abuse); abnormalities of the uterus or umbilical cord; being over thirty-five years of age; twin or higher multiple pregnancy; premature rupture of the membranes (water breaking before labor); and having too little amniotic fluid. A recent study in Israel found that women with genetic changes that make them more prone to blood clotting disorders may be at increased risk of abruption. Although this study is preliminary, it may eventually be possible to screen for these genetic changes in women who have had an abruption, and then treat them in future pregnancies with medications that may help prevent abruptions. Currently, a woman who has had an abruption has about a 10 percent chance of it happening again in any later pregnancy.

What is placenta previa?

Placenta previa, which occurs in about one in two hundred pregnancies, is a low-lying placenta that covers part or all of the inner opening of the cervix. This placement of the placenta can block the baby's exit from the uterus. And, as the cervix begins to thin and dilate in preparation for labor, blood vessels that connect the abnormally placed placenta to the uterus may tear, resulting in bleeding. During labor and delivery, bleeding can be severe, endangering mother and baby. As with placental abruption, placenta previa can result in the birth of a premature baby.

What are the symptoms of placenta previa?

The most common symptom of placenta previa is painless uterine bleeding during the second half of pregnancy. When this occurs, a health care provider generally will recommend going to the hospital for an evaluation, which will probably include an ultrasound examination to pinpoint the placenta's location. When placenta previa is suspected, a vaginal examination usually is avoided because it may trigger heavy bleeding.

Some women who have not experienced vaginal bleeding learn during a routine ultrasound examination that they have a low-lying placenta. A pregnant woman should not be too worried if this happens to her, especially if she is in the first half of pregnancy. More than 90 percent of the time, apparent placenta previa diagnosed in the second trimester corrects itself by term.

How is placenta previa treated?

A woman who has been diagnosed with placenta previa may need to stay in the hospital until delivery. If the bleeding stops, as it often does, her physician will continue to monitor her and her baby. The pregnant woman will probably be treated with a corticosteroid drug if she is likely to deliver before thirty-four weeks. At thirty-six weeks, if she hasn't delivered, the provider may suggest a test of the amniotic fluid (obtained by amniocentesis) to see if the baby's lungs are mature. If they are, the provider will likely recommend a c-section at that time to prevent risks associated with any future bleeding episodes.

If the bleeding does not stop, or if the woman goes into labor, her health care provider will probably recommend a prompt c-section. Cesarean delivery is recommended for nearly all women with placenta previa because c-sections usually can prevent severe bleeding.

What causes placenta previa?

The cause of placenta previa is unknown, but like placental abruption, it's more common among women who smoke, use cocaine, or are over thirty-five. It occurs far more frequently in women having their second or later babies than in first pregnancies. Women also are at increased risk if they've had previous uterine surgery, including a c-section; a D&C (dilation and curettage, in which the lining of the uterus is scraped), which is often done just after a miscarriage; an abortion; or if they are carrying twins (or higher multiples). Women who've had a placenta previa in a previous pregnancy have a 4 to 8 percent chance of a recurrence.

What is placenta accreta?

Placenta accreta is a placenta that implants too deeply and too firmly into the uterine wall. Similarly, placenta increta and percreta are placentas that imbed themselves even more deeply, into uterine muscle or through the entire thickness of the uterine wall, sometimes extending into nearby structures such as the bladder. These disorders, which occur in about 1 in 2,500 deliveries, are most common in women with placenta previa and in those who have had a previous c-section or other uterine surgery. Like placenta previa, these disorders often cause vaginal bleeding in the third trimester and frequently result in the birth of a premature baby.

How are placenta accreta and related disorders treated?

In these disorders, the placenta does not completely separate from the uterus as it should after delivery of the baby. This can lead to dangerous bleeding after vaginal delivery. The placenta usually must be surgically removed to stop the bleeding, and often a hysterectomy (removal of the uterus) is necessary. When placenta accreta is diagnosed by ultrasound before birth, a cesarean delivery immediately followed by a hysterectomy often is planned in order to reduce blood loss and other complications in the mother. In some cases, other surgical procedures can be used to save the uterus.

What are some other placental problems?

In some cases, the placenta may not develop correctly or function as well as it should. It may be too thin, too thick, have an extra lobe, connect abnormally to the umbilical cord, or attach abnormally to the fetal membranes. And problems can occur during pregnancy that damage the placenta, including infections, blood clots, and areas of tissue destruction (infarcts). These placental abnormalities can contribute to various complications, including miscarriage, poor fetal growth, prematurity, excessive maternal bleeding at delivery, and possibly certain birth defects. A doctor will examine the placenta after delivery and perhaps send it to the laboratory, especially if the newborn has certain complications such as poor growth, to help identify the cause of the problem.

Does the March of Dimes support research on placental conditions?

March of Dimes grantees are studying how certain infections, such as papilloma viruses (which cause genital warts) and cytomegalovirus (CMV) may damage the placenta, possibly contributing to miscarriage, poor fetal growth, and birth defects such as cerebral palsy.

Others are exploring how certain genes regulate the development and function of the placenta, in order to develop ways to prevent miscarriages and growth problems that may result from placental abnormalities.

References

ACOG Committee on Obstetric Practice. Placenta Accreta. *ACOG Committee Opinion*, Number 266, January 2002.

Anath, C.V., et al. Placental abruption and adverse perinatal outcomes. *Journal of the American Medical Association*, volume 282, number 17, November 3, 1999, pages 1646–51.

Craven, C., and Ward, K. Embryo, Fetus, and Placenta: Normal and Abnormal, in Scott, J., et al. (eds.): *Danforth's Obstetrics and Gynecology*, Eighth Edition, Philadelphia, Lippincott Williams & Wilkins, 1999, pages 29–45.

Kupferminc, M.J., et al. Increased frequency of genetic thrombophilia in women with complications of pregnancy. *New England Journal of Medicine*, volume 340, number 1, January 7, 1999, pages 9–13.

Yetter, J.F. Examination of the placenta. *American Family Physician*, March 1, 1998.

Section 12.4

Umbilical Cord Abnormalities

The umbilical cord is a narrow, tube-like structure that connects the developing baby (also referred to, in medical terms, as the fetus) to the placenta. The cord is sometimes called the baby's "supply line" because it delivers the nutrients and oxygen the baby needs for normal growth and development and removes waste products.

The umbilical cord begins to form about five weeks after conception. It becomes progressively longer until about twenty-eight weeks of pregnancy, reaching an average length of twenty-two inches. As it gets longer, the cord generally twists around itself and becomes coiled.

There are three blood vessels inside the umbilical cord—two arteries and one vein. The vein carries oxygen-rich blood and nutrients from the placenta to the baby, while the two arteries transport waste from the baby back to the placenta (where waste is transferred to the mother's blood and disposed of by her kidneys). A gelatin-like tissue called Wharton's jelly cushions and protects these blood vessels.

A number of abnormalities can affect the umbilical cord. Sometimes the cord is too long, too short, connects improperly to the placenta, or becomes knotted or compressed. Cord abnormalities can lead to problems during pregnancy or during labor and delivery. In some cases, cord abnormalities are discovered after delivery when a doctor examines the cord and the placenta. Here are some of the most frequent cord problems and how they can affect mother and baby.

What is single umbilical artery?

About 1 percent of singleton and about 5 percent of multiple pregnancies have an umbilical cord that contains only two blood vessels, instead of the normal three, as one artery is missing. The cause of this abnormality is unknown. If an ultrasound examination shows that the

177

baby appears to have no other abnormalities, the baby is likely to be born healthy.

However, studies suggest that about 25 percent of babies with single umbilical artery have birth defects, including chromosomal and/or other abnormalities. A woman whose baby is diagnosed with single umbilical artery during an ultrasound examination may be offered prenatal testing using ultrasound evaluation of the fetal heart and amniocentesis to diagnose or rule out chromosomal abnormalities. Even if the baby does not appear to have birth defects, the pregnant woman will probably be monitored carefully for the remainder of the pregnancy because of a somewhat increased risk of poor fetal growth, preterm delivery, and stillbirth.

What is umbilical cord prolapse?

Umbilical cord prolapse occurs when the cord slips into the vagina after the membranes have ruptured, before the baby descends into the birth canal. This complication affects about one in three hundred births. The baby can then put pressure on the cord as he or she passes through the cervix and vagina during labor and delivery, reducing or cutting off his or her oxygen supply. Umbilical cord prolapse can result in stillbirth unless the baby is delivered promptly, usually by cesarean section. Babies who are delivered promptly are usually unharmed.

If a pregnant woman's membranes rupture outside of the hospital, and she feels something in her vagina, she should have someone take her to the hospital immediately or call 911. A health care provider may suspect that a woman in labor in the hospital has umbilical cord prolapse if her unborn baby develops heart rate abnormalities after the membranes have ruptured. The provider can confirm that the cord has prolapsed by doing a pelvic examination. This is an emergency situation, and the provider will take steps to relieve pressure on the umbilical cord by lifting the presenting fetal part away from the cord while preparing the woman for prompt cesarean delivery. Occasionally, if a woman's cervix is fully dilated, she may be able to deliver vaginally.

The risk of umbilical cord prolapse is increased if the baby is in a breech (foot-first) position or if the baby is premature. In these cases, the baby's presenting part (the foot or a smaller than-normal head) does not fill the pelvis and allows the cord to slip. Prolapse is more common when the umbilical cord is too long, when there is too much amniotic fluid, or when the membranes are ruptured artificially to start or speed up labor. Umbilical cord prolapse also is frequent in vaginal twin deliveries, with the second twin most commonly affected.

What is vasa previa?

Vasa previa is an uncommon cord abnormality (occurring in about one in three thousand births) that can be life-threatening for the unborn baby. This complication occurs when the umbilical cord inserts abnormally in the fetal membranes of the placenta, instead of in the center of the placenta (which may be abnormally shaped or positioned). The abnormal cord placement results, in a minority of cases, in fetal blood vessels that run through the membranes being unprotected by the umbilical cord. Vasa previa occurs when these unprotected fetal blood vessels cross the cervix, sometimes rupturing when the membranes do, causing life-threatening bleeding in the baby. Even if the fetal blood vessels don't rupture, the baby may suffer from lack of oxygen due to pressure on the blood vessels.

When vasa previa occurs unexpectedly at delivery, more than half of affected babies are stillborn. However, recent studies show that vasa previa can be diagnosed with ultrasound by mid-pregnancy. Fetal deaths generally can be prevented when the baby is delivered somewhat early by cesarean section, prior to the onset of labor, once the lungs are mature. Pregnant women with vasa previa may have painless vaginal bleeding in the second or third trimester. A pregnant woman who experiences vaginal bleeding should always report it to her health care provider so that the cause can be determined, and her provider can take any necessary steps to protect her baby.

A pregnant woman may be at increased risk of vasa previa if she has certain placental abnormalities (such as a low-lying placenta that covers part or all of the cervix [placenta previa] or an abnormally shaped placenta) or if she is expecting more than one baby. Studies also suggest that women whose pregnancies result from in vitro fertilization may also be at increased risk.

What are nuchal loops?

Up to 25 percent of babies are born with their umbilical cords wrapped one or more times around their necks. This rarely causes any problems, and babies with nuchal loops, also called "nuchal cords," are generally healthy.

Sometimes fetal monitoring shows heart rate abnormalities during labor and delivery in babies with nuchal loops. This may reflect pressure on the cord. However, the pressure is rarely serious enough to cause death or any lasting problems, though occasionally a cesarean delivery may be needed.

Less frequently, the umbilical cord becomes wrapped around other parts of the baby's body, such as a foot or hand. Generally, this doesn't harm the baby.

What are umbilical cord knots?

About 1 percent of babies are born with one or more knots in the umbilical cord. Some knots form during delivery when a baby with a nuchal loop is pulled through the loop. Others form during pregnancy when the baby moves around. Knots occur most often when the umbilical cord is too long, and in identical-twin pregnancies that share a single amniotic sac, when the babies' cords become entangled.

As long as the knot remains loose, it generally does not harm the baby. However, sometimes the knot or knots can be pulled tight, cutting off the baby's oxygen supply. Cord knots result in miscarriage or stillbirth in 5 percent to 10 percent of cases. During labor and delivery, a tightening knot can cause the baby to have heart rate abnormalities that are detected by fetal monitoring. In some cases, a cesarean delivery may be necessary.

Are there other umbilical cord abnormalities?

Occasionally, the baby moves around in a way that causes the cord to become too tightly coiled, reducing blood flow. This is sometimes referred to as a "cord accident." Sometimes babies with tightly coiled cords begin to move less. Pregnant women should report decreased fetal movement to their health care provider immediately.

Pregnancies with too little amniotic fluid, called oligohydramnios, can experience umbilical cord compression leading to decreased oxygen supply, poor growth, or fetal death. This condition can be followed with ultrasound and fetal testing.

An extremely short cord can make a safe vaginal delivery impossible and can contribute to placental abruption, in which the placenta peels away (partially or completely) from the uterine wall prior to delivery, endangering mother and baby.

Sometimes an ultrasound examination will show bulging in a cord blood vessel. This may be a "false cyst," which is actually a varicose vein, or a "true cyst," a fluid-filled sac. Neither form of cyst is proven to pose a risk to the pregnancy. However, some studies suggest true cysts may be associated with birth defects, including chromosomal abnormalities, so the health care provider may recommend some additional tests to diagnose or rule out these problems.

Does the March of Dimes support research on umbilical cord abnormalities?

March of Dimes grantees are seeking ways to prevent umbilical cord abnormalities and the complications they cause. One grantee is studying the role of a gene in causing single umbilical artery to prevent it and the birth defects that sometimes accompany it. Another is developing drug treatment that can boost amniotic fluid levels in women who have too little fluid to help prevent the umbilical cord compression (sometimes resulting in fetal death) that sometimes goes along with this condition.

References

Catanzarite, V.A., et al. The two-vessel cord: how concerned should we be? *Contemporary Ob/Gyn*, April 1997, pages 43–54.

Collins, J.H., et al. *Silent Risk: Issues about the Human Umbilical Cord*. 6/14/02.

Cunningham, F.G., et al. Abnormalities of the umbilical cord, in *Williams Obstetrics*, 21st edition, New York, McGraw-Hill Medical Publishing Division, 2001, pages 831–35.

Dildy, G.A., and Clark, S.L. Umbilical cord prolapse. *Contemporary Ob/Gyn*, November 1993, pages 23–31.

International Vasa Previa Foundation. *Vasa previa*. Moline, IL, 6/20/02.

Lee, W., et al. Vasa previa: prenatal diagnosis, natural evolution, and clinical outcome. *Obstetrics and Gynecology*, volume 95, number 4, April 2000, pages 572–76.

Chapter 13

Fetal Surgery and
Other Treatment Techniques

What is fetal intervention?

Fetal intervention is reaching inside the uterus to help a fetus who
has a problem. It is surprisingly new because our ability to detect fetal problems has advanced so rapidly over the last few decades. While
many diseases can now be accurately diagnosed before birth by genetic and imaging techniques, only a few require intervention before
birth. These are generally simple anatomic problems that cause ongoing damage to the developing fetus and can be corrected using the
techniques described in the following.

All fetal intervention is really maternal-fetal intervention, and the
most important consideration in all fetal intervention is the safety of
the mother and her reproductive potential. The intervention is designed to benefit the fetus who has a problem, but the mother is an
innocent bystander who assumes some risk for the sake of her unborn fetus. In weighing the risks versus the benefits of an intervention, the most important consideration is the mother, her health, her
family, and her ability to have other children.

What are the techniques of fetal intervention?

There are three general approaches to fetal intervention, all of
which have been developed in the last few decades. The most definitive and most invasive is open fetal surgery.

Excerpted from "Techniques of Fetal Intervention," © 2006 Fetal Treatment
Center, University of California, San Francisco. All rights reserved. Reprinted with
permission. For additional information, see http://fetus.ucsfmedicalcenter.org.

Open Fetal Surgery. In open fetal surgery, the mother is anesthetized, an incision is made in the lower abdomen to expose the uterus, the uterus is opened using a special stapling device to prevent bleeding, the surgical repair of the fetus is completed, the uterus followed by the maternal abdominal wall are closed, and the mother is awakened. The magnitude of the surgery is about the same as any intra-abdominal operation like removal of the gall bladder or cesarean section, except that at the end of the operation the mother is still pregnant. The anesthetic and surgical techniques were worked out in the 1980s and have proven quite safe for mother and fetus. However, this is major surgery which requires hospitalization for three to seven days, requires Cesarean delivery of this and future pregnancies, and often causes preterm labor and preterm delivery. The pregnancy must be closely monitored for preterm labor, and drugs to control preterm labor are required.

Fetendo Fetal Surgery. "Fetendo" is the name we apply to fetoscopic intervention that was developed in the 1990s to avoid making an incision in the uterus and, hopefully, to minimize preterm labor. The ability to see the fetus through very small endoscopes, which have been available for several decades, was refined to allow surgical manipulation of the fetus with very small instruments guided by direct fetoscopic view on a television monitor. We called it "Fetendo" because the actual manipulation is much like younger people playing video games. As we developed these techniques, we learned that visualization of the fetus in real time is both endoscopic, that is, looking through the telescope, and sonographic, that is, looking at a cross-sectional image of the fetus in real time on a separate screen. The combination of image-guided manipulation and sonographically guided manipulation has proved to be quite powerful in solving a number of fetal problems. Fetendo intervention can be done either through the mother's skin (percutaneous) or, in some circumstances, requires a small opening in the mother's abdomen (mini-laparotomy). See Figure 13.1 for an illustration of this procedure.

The good part of Fetendo intervention is that it is less invasive than open surgery. It is easier on the mother in terms of postoperative recovery, and causes less trouble with preterm labor. Unfortunately, it has not eliminated the problem of preterm labor and, so, monitoring and drugs are usually still necessary. Fetendo is technically difficult and required the development of many new devices and techniques to allow us to see through the amniotic fluid, maintain the fetal position, and do delicate work within the fetus.

Fetendo has replaced open fetal surgery for some fetal problems but not all. It has proven particularly useful for treating problems with the placenta, like twin-twin transfusion syndrome, and for looking inside the fetus, for example, to place a balloon in the fetal trachea or deal with obstruction of the fetal bladder.

Fetal Image-Guided Surgery (FIGS-IT). FIGS-IT is a term we coined for fetal image-guided surgery for intervention or therapy, and describes the method of manipulating the fetus without either an incision in the uterus or an endoscopic view inside the uterus. The manipulation is done entirely under real-time cross-sectional view provided by the sonogram. This is the same sonogram as is used for diagnostic purposes, but in this case it is used to guide instruments. Like Fetendo, it can be done either through the mother's skin or, in

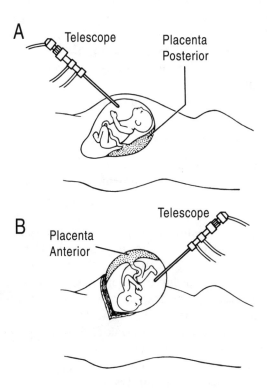

Figure 13.1. These pictures demonstrate the position of the telescope with respect to placental position. An anterior placenta necessitates forward displacement of the uterus.

some cases, with a small opening in the mother's abdomen. It can often be done under a regional anesthesia like an epidural or a spinal, or even under local anesthesia. This is the least invasive of the fetal access techniques and, thus, causes the least problem for mother in terms of hospitalization and discomfort. It also causes the least problem with preterm labor. Disappointingly, it has not completely eliminated the problem of preterm labor, and so monitoring and drugs are often still necessary. Image-guided intervention was first used for amniocentesis and fetal blood sampling, but now can be used for a variety of fetal manipulations, including placement of catheter-shunts in the bladder, abdomen, or chest; radiofrequency ablation to solve problems with anomalous twins; and even for some cardiac manipulation. It is generally not useful for serious structural problems that require surgery.

It is easiest to think of fetal intervention in terms of invasiveness—open surgery being most invasive; FIGS-IT least invasive; and Fetendo in between. It is important to remember that the fetus can be accessed non-invasively through the mother's circulation. For some problems such as fetal cardiac arrhythmias, medicines and nutrients can be delivered to the fetus by giving them to the mother and letting them cross the placenta naturally.

Table 13.1 provides examples of each type of fetal intervention.

What is the risk to the mother?

The most important consideration in all fetal intervention is the affect on the mother. She is, in general, an innocent bystander who chooses to accept some risk to help her fetus. The risk varies with the invasiveness of the procedure. For open surgery, the risk is of general anesthesia and of the abdominal incision, but most important is the consequence of the incision in the uterus itself. The immediate consequence is preterm labor and the need for monitoring and drugs to control preterm labor. The longer-term consequence is cesarean delivery in this and subsequent pregnancies. This is because the incision in the uterus in mid-gestation is not the same as that used for elective cesarean section at term. The risk of Fetendo procedures is less because the procedure is less invasive. Anesthesia may be regional or local, and an incision in the mother's abdomen may not be necessary. However, the risk of piercing the uterine muscle and, more importantly, the membranes lining the inside of the uterus, remains a problem. There is still the risk of amniotic fluid leaking through the membranes and contributing to preterm labor. Unfortunately, this remains a significant risk and requires monitoring of the amniotic fluid volume, the membranes, and preterm labor.

The risk of fetal image guided surgery is less than either Fetendo or open fetal surgery. FIGS-IT can usually be done under local or regional anesthesia and usually without the incision in the maternal abdomen. However, the problem with membrane puncture, subsequent leakage, separation of membranes, and preterm labor persists. The problem of sealing the membranes remains one of the unsolved problems of fetal intervention.

Table 13.1. Fetal Intervention

Type of Intervention	Description	Examples
Open Surgery	Hysterotomy	• Congenital Cystic Adenomatoid Malformation (CCAM)–Lobectomy • Sacrococcygeal Teratoma (SCT)–Resection • Myelomeningocele (MMC)–Repair • Cervical Teratoma–Resection • Ex-utero Intrapartum Treatment (EXIT) • Tracheal occlusion • Neck tumors • Congenital Diaphragmatic Hernia (CDH) (EXIT to Extracorporeal Membrane Oxygenation [ECMO]) • CCAM (EXIT lobectomy)
Fetendo	Fetoscopic Surgery	• Balloon Occlusion of Trachea • Laser Ablation of Vessels (Twin-to-Twin Transfusion Syndrome [TTTS]) • Cord Ligation/Division • Cystoscopic Ablation Valves • Amniotic Bands Division
FIGS	Fetal Image Guided Surgery	• Amnioreduction/Infusion • Fetal Blood Sampling • Radio Frequency Ablation (RFA) Anomalous Twins • Vesico/Pleuro Amniotic Shunts • Cord Monopolar Cautery • Balloon Dilation Aortic Stenosis

Part Two

Prematurity and
Other Birth Complications

Chapter 14

Premature Labor and Delivery

Chapter Contents

Section 14.1—Premature Labor 192
Section 14.2—Premature Birth Complications 196
Section 14.3—What to Expect in the Neonatal Intensive
                     Care Unit 200

Section 14.1

Premature Labor

Pregnancy is normally a time of happiness and anticipation, but it can also be a time of unknowns. Many women have concerns about what is happening with their baby. Is everything okay? Some women wonder about going into labor early. Premature labor occurs in about 12 percent of all pregnancies. However, knowing the symptoms and avoiding particular risk factors can lower a woman's chance of premature labor.

What is premature labor?

A normal pregnancy should last about forty weeks. Occasionally, labor may begin prematurely before the thirty-seventh week of pregnancy because uterine contractions cause the cervix to open earlier than normal. When this happens, the baby is born premature and can be at risk for health problems. Fortunately, due to research, technology, and medicine along with dedicated professionals in Neonatal Intensive Care Units, the health of premature babies is improving.

What risk factors place me at a high risk for premature labor?

Certain factors may increase a woman's risk of having premature labor, although the specific causes of premature labor are not known. However, having a specific risk factor does not mean a woman is predetermined to have premature labor. A woman may have premature labor for no apparent reason. If you have any of these risk factors, it's important to know the symptoms of premature labor and what you should do if they occur.

Women are at greatest risk for premature labor if:

- They are pregnant with twins, triplets, or more;
- They have had a previous premature birth;

- They have certain uterine or cervical abnormalities.

Medical risk factors include:

- Recurring bladder and/or kidney infections;

- Urinary tract infections, vaginal infections, and sexually transmitted infections;

- Infection with fever (greater than 101 degrees Fahrenheit) during pregnancy;

- Unexplained vaginal bleeding after twenty weeks of pregnancy;

- Chronic illness such as high blood pressure, kidney disease, or diabetes;

- Multiple first trimester abortions or one or more second trimester abortions;

- Underweight or overweight before pregnancy;

- Clotting Disorder (thrombophilia);

- Being Pregnant with a single fetus after in vitro fertilization (IVF);

- Short time between pregnancies (less than six to nine months between birth and beginning of the next pregnancy).

Lifestyle risks for premature labor include:

- Little or no prenatal care;

- Smoking;

- Drinking alcohol;

- Using illegal drugs;

- Domestic violence, including physical, sexual, or emotional abuse;

- Lack of social support;

- High levels of stress;

- Low income;

- Long working hours with long periods of standing.

What are warning signs of premature labor?

It may be possible to prevent a premature birth by knowing the warning signs and calling your healthcare provider if you suspect you are having premature labor. Warning signs and symptoms of premature labor include:

- A contraction every ten minutes, or more frequently within one hour (five or more uterine contractions in an hour);

- Watery fluid leaking from your vagina (this could indicate that your bag of water is broken);

- Menstrual-like cramps felt in the lower abdomen that may come and go or be constant;

- Low dull backache felt below the waistline that may come and go or be constant;

- Pelvic pressure that feels like your baby is pushing down;

- Abdominal cramps that may occur with or without diarrhea;

- Increase or change in vaginal discharge.

What does a contraction feel like?

As the muscles of your uterus contract, you will feel your abdomen harden. As the contraction goes away, your uterus becomes soft. Throughout pregnancy, the layers of your uterus will tighten irregularly, which is usually not painful. These are known as Braxton-Hicks contractions and are usually irregular and do not open the cervix. If these contractions become regular or more frequent (one every ten to twelve minutes for at least an hour) they may be premature labor contractions, which can cause the cervix to open. It is important to contact your healthcare provider immediately.

How can I check for contractions?

While lying down, use your fingertips to feel your uterus tighten and soften. This is called "palpation." During a contraction your abdomen will feel hard all over, not just in one area. However, as your baby grows you may feel your abdomen become firmer in one area and then become soft again.

What should I do if I think I am experiencing premature labor?

If you suspect you are having signs and symptoms of premature labor call your healthcare provider immediately. This can be a scary time for you but there are some ways you can help to prevent premature labor by becoming aware of the symptoms and following these directions:

- Empty your bladder.
- Lie down tilted toward your left side; this may slow down or stop signs and symptoms.
- Avoid lying flat on your back. This may cause the contractions to increase.
- Drink several glasses of water because dehydration can cause contractions.
- Monitor contractions for one hour by counting the minutes that elapse from the beginning of one contraction to the beginning of the next.

If symptoms get worse, or don't go away after one hour, call your healthcare provider again or go to the hospital. When you call your doctor, be sure to mention that you are worried about premature labor. The only sure way to know if you are in premature labor is by having a doctor do an examination of your cervix. If your cervix is opening up, premature labor could be starting.

What is the treatment to prevent premature labor from starting or continuing?

- Magnesium sulfate is a medication given through an intravenous line (IV), which may cause nausea temporarily. A large dose is given initially and then a smaller continuous dose is given for twelve to twenty-four hours or more.
- Corticosteroid is a medication given twenty-four hours before birth to help accelerate the baby's lung and brain maturity.
- Oral medications are sometimes used to decrease the frequency of contractions, and may make women feel better.

What impact does premature labor have on my pregnancy?

The longer your baby is in the womb, the better the chance he or she will be healthy. Babies who are born prematurely are at higher risks for brain and other neurological complications as well as breathing and digestive problems. Some premature babies grow up with a developmental delay or have learning difficulties in school. The earlier in pregnancy a baby is born, the more health problems are likely to develop.

Premature labor does not always result in premature delivery. Some women with premature labor and early dilation of the cervix are put on bed rest until the pregnancy progresses further.

Most babies born prior to twenty-four weeks have little chance of survival. Only about 50 percent will survive and the other 50 percent may die or have permanent problems due to being born too early. However, babies born after thirty-two weeks have a very high survival rate, and usually do not have long-term complications.

Babies born at hospitals with neonatal intensive care units (NICU) do best. If you deliver at a hospital that does not have a NICU, you may be transferred to one that does.

Section 14.2

Premature Birth Complications

Babies born before the thirty-seventh week of gestation are considered to be born prematurely. Premature newborns are sometimes given the nickname "preemies." Mothers who have their baby prematurely are often scared and nervous. It is true that premature newborns face an increased chance of having one or more complications. The earlier the baby is born, the higher the risk of complications. Any complications that a premature newborn experiences will be cared for in the neonatal intensive care unit (NICU). Following is a list of the most common complications that a premature newborn may face.

Immature lungs. On average most babies have mature lungs by thirty-six weeks of gestation. However, this may not be true for all babies, since every baby develops at a different rate. If a mother and her doctor know that she may be delivering early, an amniocentesis may be performed to check the maturity level of the lungs. In some cases, an injection of steroids can be given to the baby before delivery occurs. This can help speed up the development of the lungs. The biggest concern when it comes to premature labor is the development of the newborn's lungs. Here are a few complications that can occur with immature lungs:

- Respiratory distress syndrome (RDS) causes harsh, irregular breathing and difficulties due to the lack of a certain agent in the lungs called surfactants, which helps prevent the lungs from collapsing. Treatment involves one or more of the following: supplemental oxygen (through an oxygen hood), use of a respirator (ventilator), continuous positive airway pressure, endotracheal intubation, and in severe cases, doses of surfactant.

- Transient tachypnea is rapid shallow breathing. This can occur in both premature babies and full-term babies. Recovery usually occurs within three days. Before recovery, the newborns' feedings are postponed and in some cases intravenous feedings are done. There is usually no other treatment necessary.

- Bronchopulmonary dysplasia (BPD) occurs when a baby's lungs have shown evidence of deterioration. Unfortunately, when preemies are put on a ventilator (also known as a respirator) their lungs are still immature and sometimes cannot withstand the constant pressure of the respirator. Preemies that have been on a respirator for more than twenty-eight days are at risk for developing BPD. Preemies do recover from this; however, it may take some longer than others.

Pneumonia. Due to all of the complications with premature-related respiratory problems, pneumonia can occur. Pneumonia is an infection in the area of the lung involved in the exchange of carbon dioxide and oxygen and causes inflammation that reduces the amount of space available for the exchange of air. This results in inadequate amounts of oxygen to the body. Treatment involves antibiotics as well as the possibility of supplemental oxygen and intubation. If this is left untreated, it can evolve into a deadly infection or lead to sepsis or meningitis.

Apnea and bradycardia. Apnea is the absence of breathing. In the NICU an alarm will sound if your newborn has an irregular breathing pattern that consists of intervals of pauses longer than ten to fifteen seconds. Bradycardia is the reduction of heart rate. In the

NICU an alarm will sound if your newborn's heart rate falls below one hundred beats per minute. Usually a little tap or simple rub on the back helps remind the preemie to breathe or brings the heart rate up.

Infection. A premature baby may not be ready to fight off certain infections, and for his own protection he is placed in an incubator to provide protection against potential infections.

Jaundice. A yellowish skin color caused by the buildup of substances in the blood called bilirubin. Treatment involves being placed under a bilirubin light called phototherapy. This may last about a week to ten days.

Intraventricular hemorrhage (IVH). Babies born at less than thirty-four weeks have an increased risk of bleeding in their brain. This happens because immature blood vessels may not tolerate the changes in circulation that take place during labor. This can lead to future complications such as cerebral palsy, mental retardation, and learning difficulties. Intracranial hemorrhage occurs in about one-third of babies born at twenty-four to twenty-six weeks of gestation. If preterm labor is identified and is inevitable, there are medications that can be given to the mother to help lessen the chances of severe intracranial hemorrhage in the newborn.

Inability to maintain body heat. Premature babies are born with little body fat and immature skin that does not allow them to maintain body heat. Treatment involves warmers or incubators to help them keep warm.

Immature gastrointestinal and digestive system. Premature newborns are born with gastrointestinal systems that are too immature to absorb nutrients safely. Therefore they receive their initial nutrients through intravenous (IV) feeding, which is called total parenteral nutrition (TPN). After a few days, newborns may be fed through a tube with breast milk or formula because the newborn may still not be mature enough to swallow or suck on his or her own.

Anemia. This is a medical condition caused by abnormally low concentrations of red blood cells. Red blood cells are important because they carry a substance called hemoglobin, which carries oxygen. Most newborns should have levels higher than 15 grams. However, preemies are at a high risk of having low levels and are at risk for anemia. If the anemia is severe, treatment involves transfusion of red blood cells to the newborn.

Patent ductus arteriosus (PDA). This is a cardiac disorder that causes breathing difficulties after delivery due to an open blood vessel, called the ductus arteriosus. During fetal development the ductus arteriosus is open to allow blood to be diverted from the lungs into the aorta since the baby does not breathe until after delivery. A fetus makes a chemical compound called prostaglandin E that circulates his or her blood, keeping the ductus arteriosus open. At a full term birth levels of prostaglandin E fall, causing the ductus arteriosus to close and allowing a baby's lungs to receive the blood they need to function properly once they have entered the world. With preterm labor, the prostaglandin E level may stay the same, causing an open ductus arteriosus, which causes breathing complications. Treatment involves a medication that stops or slows the production of prostaglandin E.

Retinopathy of prematurity (ROP). This is a potentially blinding eye disorder. It affects most preemies between twenty-four and twenty-six weeks of gestation and rarely affects preemies beyond thirty-three to thirty-four weeks of gestation. There are many different stages, and treatment depends on severity and may include laser surgery or cryosurgery.

Necrotizing enterocolitis (NEC). This condition occurs when a portion of the newborn's intestine develops poor blood flow that can lead to infection in the bowel wall. Treatment includes intravenous feeding and antibiotics. Only in severe cases is an operation necessary.

Sepsis. This is a medical condition in which bacteria enters the blood stream. Sepsis often brings infection to the lungs, and therefore can lead to pneumonia. Treatment involves antibiotics.

Section 14.3

What to Expect in the Neonatal Intensive Care Unit

Reprinted from "Care for the Premature Baby."
Reprinted with permission from the American Pregnancy Association,
http://www.americanpregnancy.org, © 2006. All rights reserved.

Babies born before the thirty-seventh week of gestation are born prematurely. Premature newborns are sometimes given the nickname "preemies." Mothers who have their baby prematurely are often scared and nervous. It is true that premature newborns face an increased risk of having one or more complications. The earlier the baby is born, the greater the risk of complications. Any complications that a premature newborn experiences will be cared for in the neonatal intensive care unit (NICU). Following is a brief description of what to expect when it comes to the care for your newborn preemie.

Why Do Premature Newborns Need Special Care?

A premature newborn is not fully equipped to deal with our world. Their little bodies still have areas that need to mature and fully develop. Some of these areas include the lungs, digestive system, immune system, and skin. Thankfully, medical technology has made it possible for preemies to get through the first few days, weeks, or months of life until they are able to make it on their own.

A First Glance at the Neonatal Intensive Care Unit (NICU)

The NICU is your newborn's protected environment. It may also be his or her home for a while. Therefore it is a good idea to get acquainted and know as much as you can about it. You should know that it is equipped with a caring staff, monitoring and alarm systems, respiratory and resuscitation equipment, access to physicians in every pediatric specialty, twenty-four-hour laboratory service, and you!

When it comes to all of the equipment in the NICU, it can be over-whelming and sometimes scary. Knowing what everything does can help you relax and prevent you from being distracted.

Monitoring and Alarm Systems

Monitoring machines vary depending on the hospital you are in. Different hospitals use different equipment. However, all monitors monitor the heart rate, respiratory rate, blood pressure, and temperature. A pulse oximeter is an instrument that may be used to measure the amount of oxygen in the blood. You may notice that your newborn has various sticky pads or cuffs on his chest, legs, arms, or other body parts. These sticky pads and cuffs have wires that connect to the monitor, which often looks like a television screen that displays lots of numbers.

Alarm systems go off periodically in the NICU and it does not always indicate an emergency. In fact, more often than not it is nothing to worry about. Therefore do not panic when you experience this and do not be surprised when everyone else does not panic.

Methods of Respiratory Assistance

These depends on the premature newborn's individual needs.

Endotracheal tube. This is a tube that is placed down the newborn's windpipe. It delivers warm humidified air and oxygen.

Ventilator. This is also sometimes referred to as a respirator. This is the breathing machine that the endotracheal tube is connected to. It can monitor the amount of oxygen, air pressure, and number of breaths.

Continuous positive airway pressure (C-PAP). This method is used for preemies who can breathe on their own but just need some help getting air to their lungs.

Oxygen hood. This is an actual clear plastic box that is placed over the preemie's head and is attached to a tube that pumps oxygen to the preemie.

Methods of Feeding

These depends on the premature newborn's individual needs.

Intravenous lines. This method carries nutrition directly into the bloodstream. This method is used for premature babies who have immature digestive systems and are not able to suck, swallow, and breathe in a coordinated manner. This method may also be used when treatment for other health complications is being implemented. An intravenous line (IV) may be placed in the scalp, arm, or leg.

Umbilical catheter. This method involves a tube that is surgically placed into a vessel of the umbilical cord. Don't worry, it is not painful. This method can carry potential risks (infection or blood clots) and therefore is used for only the most critical infants and with those who may need this type of feeding for several weeks. For these critical preemies, it is the safest and most appropriate way to supply nutrients.

Oral and nasal feeding. This method involves a narrow flexible tube threaded through the nose (nasogastric tube) or mouth (orogastric tube). This method is provided for preemies who are ready to digest breast milk or formula but still not able to suck, swallow, and breathe in a coordinated manner.

Central line (sometimes referred to as a PICC line). This is an intravenous line that is inserted into a vein, often in the arm, since this allows use of a larger vein. This is normally used to deliver nutrients and medicines that would otherwise irritate smaller veins.

Other Equipment

Incubator. A clear plastic crib that keeps babies warm and help protect them from germs and noise.

Bili light. This is a bright blue fluorescent light that is located over your baby's incubator. This light is used to treat jaundice (yellowing of skin and eyes).

The Staff

The staff is made up of respiratory therapists, occupational therapists, dietitians, lactation consultants, pharmacists, social workers, hospital chaplains, and a neonatologist. A neonatologist is a pediatrician with additional training in the care of sick and premature babies. Get to know the staff. They are very informative and encourage parental involvement.

Knowing that your newborn is receiving the best care can provide comfort and reassurance.

What Is Kangaroo Care?

Kangaroo care consists of placing a diaper-clad premature baby in an upright position on a mother's bare chest, allowing tummies to touch and placing the premature baby in between the mother's breasts. The baby's head is turned so that the ear is above the parent's heart. Many studies have shown significant benefits. According to Krisanne Larimer, author of "Kangarooing Our Little Miracles," kangaroo care has been shown to help premature newborns with:

- Body temperature: Studies have shown that mothers have thermal synchrony with their babies. The study also concluded that when the baby was cold, the mother's body temperature would increase to warm the baby up and vice versa.

- Breastfeeding: Kangaroo care allows easy access to the breast, and skin-to-skin contact increases milk let-down.

- Weight gain: Kangaroo care allows the baby to fall into a deep sleep, which allows the baby to conserve energy for more important things. Increase in weight gain means shorter hospital stay.

- Increased intimacy and attachment

Breastfeeding

We have all heard how breastfeeding strengthens a baby's immune defenses and provides emotional connections between a mother and her baby. However, when a newborn is born prematurely a mother may not be allowed to breastfeed her baby. Most premature newborns between twenty-five and twenty-nine weeks gestational age are feed intravenously or through a tube. If you are planning to breastfeed you should tell your doctor and nurses immediately after labor. Then you can begin expressing and storing your breast milk for when your baby is ready for it. Your baby's digestive system and control of electrolytes will determine when he or she will be able to handle breast milk through a tube. This is when you can use the milk you have stored. Once your baby's respiratory system is stabilized he or she can begin breastfeeding. Most babies born at thirty-five to thirty-seven weeks can go straight to breastfeeding.

How You Can Participate in the Neonatal Intensive Care Unit (NICU)

There are other ways besides breastfeeding and kangaroo care in which mothers and fathers can help care for their baby in NICU. Both the mother and father are encouraged by the NICU staff to interact with their baby. As a mother or father you may not see how it is possible to interact with your baby with the wires, machines, and incubator in the way. Surprisingly, there are quite a few ways you can accomplish this:

- Touch your baby as much as possible. You can do this through gentle touch or even stroking motions.

- Talk to your baby. Your baby is used to your voice(s) and it could be comforting to hear you. Along with talking you can read or sing to your baby.

- Change your baby's diaper.

- Participate in your baby's first bath. Depending on your baby's progress, you may use washcloths, sponges, or Q-tips to do this.

- Take your baby's temperature.

Chapter 15

Medical Complications of Prematurity

Chapter Contents

Section 15.1—Apnea of Prematurity.. 206
Section 15.2—Bronchopulmonary Dysplasia 210
Section 15.3—Retinopathy of Prematurity 215

Section 15.1

Apnea of Prematurity

This information was provided by KidsHealth, one of the largest resources online for medically reviewed health information written for parents, kids, and teens. For more articles like this one, visit www.KidsHealth.org, or www.TeensHealth.org. © 2005 The Nemours Center for Children's Health Media, a division of The Nemours Foundation.

Once a baby is born, he or she needs to breathe continuously to get oxygen. In a premature baby, the part of the central nervous system (brain and spinal cord) that controls breathing is not yet mature enough to allow nonstop breathing. This causes large bursts of breath followed by periods of shallow breathing or stopped breathing. The medical term for this condition is apnea of prematurity, or AOP.

Apnea of prematurity is fairly common in preemies. Doctors usually diagnose the condition before the mother and baby are discharged from the hospital, and the apnea usually goes away on its own as the infant matures. Once apnea of prematurity goes away, it does not come back. But there's no doubt about it—it's frightening while it's happening.

What Is Apnea of Prematurity?

Apnea is a medical term that means a baby has stopped breathing. Most experts define apnea of prematurity as a condition in which premature infants stop breathing for fifteen to twenty seconds during sleep.

Generally, babies who are born at less than thirty-five weeks' gestation have periods when they stop breathing or their heart rates drop. (The medical name for a slowed heart rate is bradycardia). These breathing abnormalities may begin after two days of life and last for up to two to three months after these premature infants are born. The lower the infant's weight and level of prematurity at birth, the more likely it is that the infant will have AOP spells.

Although it's normal for all infants to have pauses in breathing and heart rates, those with AOP have drops in heart rate below eighty beats per minute, which causes them to become pale or bluish. They may also appear limp, and their breathing may be noisy. They then either start breathing again by themselves or require help to resume breathing.

AOP may happen once a day or many times a day. Doctors will closely evaluate your infant to make sure the apnea isn't due to another condition, such as infection or internal bleeding.

Apnea of prematurity should not be confused with periodic breathing, which is also common in premature newborns. Periodic breathing is marked by a pause in breathing that lasts just a few seconds and is followed by several rapid and shallow breaths. Periodic breathing is not accompanied by a change in facial color (such as blueness around the mouth) or a drop in heart rate. A baby who has periodic breathing resumes regular breathing on his or her own.

Although it can be frightening, periodic breathing typically causes no other problems in newborns.

How Is Apnea of Prematurity Treated?

Most of the time, premature infants (especially those less than thirty-four weeks' gestation at birth) will receive medical care for apnea of prematurity in the hospital's neonatal intensive care unit (NICU). When they are first born, many of these premature infants must get help breathing from a ventilator because their lungs are too immature to allow them to breathe on their own.

During mechanical ventilation, a tube is placed into the baby's trachea (windpipe) and breaths of air are blown through the tube into the baby's lungs. These breaths are given at a set pressure. The ventilator is also programmed to give a certain number of breaths per minute, and the baby's breathing, heart rate, and oxygen levels are continuously monitored.

Sometimes babies with apnea of prematurity are given medications to help mature their lungs and allow the preemies to come off mechanical ventilation within a few weeks and breathe on their own.

When infants are disconnected from a mechanical ventilator, often they require a form of assisted breathing called nasal continuous positive airway pressure (CPAP). A nasal CPAP device consists of a large tube with tiny prongs that fit into the baby's nose, which is hooked to a machine that provides oxygenated air into the baby's air passages and lungs. The pressure from the CPAP machine helps keep a preemie's lungs open so he or she can breathe. However, the machine does not provide breaths for the baby, so the baby breathes on his or her own.

Once preemies are off a mechanical ventilator and breathing on their own—with or without nasal CPAP—they are monitored continuously for any evidence of apnea. The cardiorespiratory monitor (also known as an apnea and bradycardia, or A/B, monitor) also tracks the infant's heart rate. An alarm on the monitor sounds if there's no breath for a set number of seconds. When the monitor sounds, a nurse immediately checks the baby for signs of distress. False alarms are not uncommon.

If a baby doesn't begin to breathe again within fifteen seconds, a nurse will rub the baby's back, arms, or legs to stimulate the breathing. Most of the time, babies with apnea of prematurity spells will begin breathing again on their own with this kind of stimulation.

However, if the nurse handles the baby, and the baby still hasn't begun breathing on his or her own and becomes pale or bluish in color, oxygen may be administered with a handheld bag and mask. The nurse or doctor will place the mask over the infant's face and use the bag to slowly pump a few breaths into the baby's lungs. Usually only a few breaths are needed before the baby begins to breathe again on his or her own.

If a baby begins to have many such apnea spells, medication is sometimes given intravenously or by mouth to stimulate the part of the brain that controls breathing. This often reduces the apnea spells.

When Your Baby Is on a Home Apnea Monitor

Although apnea spells are usually resolved by the time most preemies go home, a few will continue to have apnea spells. In these cases, if the doctor thinks it's necessary, the baby will be discharged from the NICU with an apnea monitor.

An apnea monitor consists of two main parts: a belt with sensory wires that your child wears around his or her chest and a monitoring unit with an alarm. The sensors measure the baby's chest movement and breathing rate while the monitor continuously records these rates. Before the baby leaves the hospital, the NICU staff will thoroughly review the monitor with you and give you detailed instructions on how and when to use it, as well as how to respond to an alarm. Parents and caregivers will also be trained in infant CPR, even though it's unlikely they'll ever have to use it.

If the baby isn't breathing when you check him or her or your baby's face seems pale or bluish, follow the instructions given to you by the NICU staff. Usually, your response will involve some gentle stimulation techniques and, if these don't work, starting CPR and calling 911. Remember, never shake your baby to wake him or her.

It can be very stressful to have a baby at home on an apnea monitor. Some parents find themselves watching the monitor, afraid even to take a shower or run to the mailbox. This usually becomes easier with time. If you're feeling this way, it may help to share your feelings with the NICU staff. They may be able to reassure you and even put you in touch with other parents of preemies who have gone through the same thing.

Your child's doctor will determine how long your baby wears the monitor, so be sure to talk to him or her if you have any questions or concerns.

Caring for Your Child

Apnea of prematurity usually resolves on its own with time. For most preemies, this means AOP stops around forty-four weeks of postconceptional age. Postconceptional age is defined as the gestational age (how many weeks of pregnancy at the time of birth) plus the postnatal age (weeks of age since birth). In rare cases, AOP continues for a few weeks longer.

Healthy infants who have had AOP usually do not go on to have more health or developmental problems than other babies. The apnea of prematurity does not cause brain damage. If a healthy baby is apnea free for a week, he or she will probably never have apnea again.

Although sudden infant death syndrome (SIDS) does occur more often in premature infants, no relationship between AOP and SIDS has ever been proven.

Aside from AOP, there may be other complications with your premature baby that may limit the time and interaction that you can have with your child. Nevertheless, you can bond with your baby in the NICU. It's a good idea to talk to the NICU staff about what type of interaction would be best for your baby, whether it's holding, feeding, caressing, or just speaking softly. The NICU staff is trained not only to care for premature babies, but also to reassure and support the parents of preemies.

Section 15.2

Bronchopulmonary Dysplasia

This information was provided by KidsHealth, one of the largest resources online for medically reviewed health information written for parents, kids, and teens. For more articles like this one, visit www.KidsHealth.org, or www.TeensHealth.org. © 2005 The Nemours Center for Children's Health Media, a division of The Nemours Foundation.

Babies who are born prematurely or who experience respiratory problems shortly after birth are at risk for bronchopulmonary dysplasia (BPD), sometimes called chronic lung disease. Although most infants fully recover from BPD and have few long-term health problems as a result, BPD can be a serious condition requiring intensive medical care.

A child is not born with BPD. It is something that develops as a consequence of prematurity and progressive lung inflammation.

What Is BPD?

Bronchopulmonary dysplasia involves abnormal development of lung tissue. It is characterized by inflammation and scarring in the lungs. It develops most often in premature babies, who are born with underdeveloped lungs.

"Broncho" refers to the airways (the bronchial tubes) through which the oxygen we breathe travels into the lungs. "Pulmonary" refers to the lungs' tiny air sacs (alveoli), where oxygen and carbon dioxide are exchanged. "Dysplasia" means abnormal changes in the structure or organization of a group of cells. The cell changes in BPD take place in the smaller airways and lung alveoli, making breathing difficult and causing problems with lung function.

Along with asthma and cystic fibrosis, BPD is one of the most common chronic lung diseases in children. According to the National Heart, Lung, and Blood Institute (NHLBI) of the National Institutes of Health (NIH), between five thousand and ten thousand cases of BPD occur every year in the United States. Children with extremely low birth weight (less than 2.2 pounds or 1,000 grams) are most at risk for developing BPD. Although most of these infants eventually outgrow the more serious symptoms, in rare cases BPD—in combination with other complications of prematurity—can be fatal.

What Causes BPD?

The majority of BPD cases occur in premature infants, usually those who are born at thirty-four weeks' gestation or before and weigh less than 4.5 pounds (2,000 grams). These babies are more likely to be affected by a condition known as infant respiratory distress syndrome (RDS) or hyaline membrane disease, which occurs as a result of tissue damage to the lungs from being on a mechanical ventilator for a significant amount of time.

Mechanical ventilators do the breathing for babies whose lungs are too immature to allow them to breathe on their own. The ventilators also supply necessary oxygen to the lungs of these premature infants. Oxygen is delivered through a tube that has been inserted into the baby's trachea (windpipe) and is given under pressure from the machine to properly move air into stiff, underdeveloped lungs. Sometimes, for these babies to survive, the amount of oxygen given must be higher than the oxygen concentration in the air we commonly breathe.

Although mechanical ventilation is essential to their survival, over time the pressure from the ventilation and excess oxygen intake can injure a newborn's delicate lungs, leading to RDS. Almost half of all extremely low birth weight infants will develop some form of RDS. If symptoms of RDS persist, then the condition will be considered BPD if a baby is oxygen dependent at thirty-six weeks' postconceptional age.

BPD also can arise from other adverse conditions that a newborn's fragile lungs have difficulty coping with, such as trauma, pneumonia, and other infections. All of these can cause the inflammation and scarring associated with BPD, even in a full-term newborn or, very rarely, in older infants and children.

Among babies who are premature and have a low birth weight, white male infants seem to be at greater risk for developing BPD, for reasons unknown to doctors. Genetics may contribute to some cases of BPD as well.

Diagnosis and Treatment of BPD

Important factors in diagnosing BPD are prematurity, infection, mechanical ventilator dependence, and oxygen exposure.

BPD is typically diagnosed if an infant still requires additional oxygen and continues to show signs of respiratory problems after twenty-eight days of age (or past thirty-six weeks' postconceptional age). Chest x-rays may be helpful in making the diagnosis. In babies with RDS, the x-rays may show lungs that look like ground glass. In babies with BPD, the x-rays may show lungs that appear spongy.

No available medical treatment can immediately cure bronchopulmonary dysplasia. Treatment is geared to support the breathing and oxygen needs of infants with BPD and to enable them to grow and thrive. Babies first diagnosed with BPD receive intense supportive care in the hospital, usually in a newborn intensive care unit (NICU) until they are able to breathe well enough on their own without the support of a mechanical ventilator. Some babies also may receive jet ventilation, a continuous low-pressure ventilation that is used to minimize the lung damage from ventilation that contributes to BPD. Not all hospitals use this procedure to treat BPD, but some hospitals with large NICUs do.

Infants with BPD are also treated with different kinds of medications that help to support lung function. These include bronchodilators (such as albuterol) to help keep the airways open and diuretics (such as furosemide) to reduce the buildup of fluid in the lungs.

Antibiotics are sometimes needed to fight bacterial infections because babies with BPD are more likely to develop pneumonia. Part of a baby's treatment may involve the administration of surfactant, a natural lubricant that improves breathing function. Babies with RDS who have not yet been diagnosed with BPD may have disrupted surfactant production, so administering natural or synthetic surfactant may reduce the chance that BPD develops.

In addition, babies sick enough to be hospitalized with BPD may need feedings of high-calorie formulas through a gastric tube inserted into the stomach to ensure they get enough calories and nutrients and start to grow.

In severe cases, babies with BPD cannot use their gastrointestinal systems to digest food. These babies require intravenous (IV) feedings—called TPN, or total parenteral nutrition—made up of fats, proteins, sugars, and nutrients. These are given through a small tube that is inserted into a large vein through the baby's skin.

The time spent in the NICU for infants with BPD can range from several weeks to a few months. The NIH estimates that the average length of intensive in-hospital care for babies with BPD is 120 days. Even after a baby leaves the hospital, he or she may require continued medication, breathing treatments, or even oxygen at home. Although most children are weaned from supplemental oxygen by the end of their first year, a few with serious cases may need a ventilator for several years or even their entire lives (although this is rare).

Improvement for any baby with BPD is gradual. Some infants will be slow to improve; others may not recover from the condition if their lung disease is very severe. Lungs continue to grow for five to seven years, and there can be subtle abnormal lung function even at school age, although the majority of children function well. Many babies diagnosed with BPD will recover close to normal lung function, but this takes time. Scarred, stiffened lung tissue will always have poor function. However, as infants with BPD grow, new healthy lung tissue can form and grow, and may eventually take over much of the work of breathing for diseased lung tissue.

Complications of BPD

After coming through the more critical stages of BPD, some infants still have longer-term complications. They are often more susceptible to respiratory infections such as influenza, respiratory syncytial virus (RSV), and pneumonia. When they come down with an infection, they tend to get sicker than most children do.

Another respiratory complication of BPD includes excess fluid buildup in the lungs, known as pulmonary edema, which makes it more difficult for air to travel through the airways.

Occasionally, kids with a history of BPD may also develop complications of the circulatory system, such as pulmonary hypertension in which the pulmonary arteries—the vessels that carry blood from the heart to the lungs—become narrowed and cause high blood pressure. However, this is relatively uncommon and a late complication.

Effects of the medications they may need to take include dehydration and low sodium levels from diuretics. Kidney stones, hearing problems, and low potassium and calcium levels can result from long-term furosemide use.

Infants with BPD often grow more slowly than other babies and have difficulty gaining weight. They tend to lose weight when they are sick. Premature infants with severe BPD also have a higher incidence of cerebral palsy.

Overall, though, the risk of serious permanent complications from BPD is fairly small.

Caring for Your Child

As with any child, parents have a critical role in the care of an infant with BPD. One important precaution you can take is to reduce your child's exposure to potential respiratory infections. Limit visits from people who are sick, and if your child needs day care, pick a small center, where there will be less exposure to infectious agents. Ensuring that your child receives all the recommended vaccinations can help ward off problems as well. And keep your child away from tobacco smoke, particularly in your home, as it is a serious respiratory irritant.

If your baby requires oxygen at home, your baby's health care providers will show you how to work the tube and check oxygen levels.

Children with asthma-type symptoms may need bronchodilators to relieve asthma-like attacks. You can give this medication to your child with a puffer or nebulizer, which produces a fine spray of medicine that your child then breathes in.

Because infants with BPD sometimes have trouble growing due to breathing problems, you may also need to feed your baby a high-calorie formula. Sometimes, babies with BPD who are slower to gain weight will go home from the intensive care nursery on gastric tube feedings. Formula feedings may be given alone or as a supplement to breastfeeding.

When to Call Your Child's Doctor

Once a baby comes home from the hospital, parents still need to watch for signs of respiratory distress or BPD emergencies, instances in which a child has serious trouble breathing. Signs that an infant might need immediate care include:

- shallow breathing
- faster breathing than normal
- working much harder than usual to breathe
  - belly sinking in with breathing
  - pulling in of the skin between the ribs with each breath
  - bobbing of the head with each breath
- growing tired or lethargic from working to breathe
- more coughing than usual
- panting or grunting
- wheezing
- a bluish tinge to the skin
- trouble feeding or excess spitting up or vomiting of feedings

If you notice any of these symptoms in your child, call your child's doctor or seek emergency medical attention.

Section 15.3

Retinopathy of Prematurity

Reprinted from the National Eye Institute,
National Institutes of Health, April 2005.

What is retinopathy of prematurity?

Retinopathy of prematurity (ROP) is a potentially blinding eye disorder that primarily affects premature infants weighing about 2.75 pounds (1,250 grams) or less that are born before thirty-one weeks of gestation (A full-term pregnancy has a gestation of thirty-eight to forty-two weeks). The smaller a baby is at birth, the more likely that baby is to develop ROP. This disorder—which usually develops in both eyes—is one of the most common causes of visual loss in childhood and can lead to lifelong vision impairment and blindness. ROP was first diagnosed in 1942.

How many infants have ROP?

Today, with advances in neonatal care, smaller and more premature infants are being saved. These infants are at a much higher risk for ROP. Not all babies who are premature develop ROP. There are approximately 3.9 million infants born in the United States each year; of those, about 28,000 weigh 2.75 pounds or less. About 14,000 to 16,000 of these infants are affected by some degree of ROP. The disease improves and leaves no permanent damage in milder cases of ROP. About 90 percent of all infants with ROP are in the milder category and do not need treatment. However, infants with more severe disease can develop impaired vision or even blindness. About 1,100 to 1,500 infants annually develop ROP that is severe enough to require medical treatment. About 400 to 600 infants each year in the United States become legally blind from ROP.

What causes ROP?

ROP occurs when abnormal blood vessels grow and spread throughout the retina, the tissue that lines the back of the eye. These abnormal

215

blood vessels are fragile and can leak, scarring the retina and pulling it out of position. This causes a retinal detachment. Retinal detachment is the main cause of visual impairment and blindness in ROP.

Several complex factors may be responsible for the development of ROP. The eye starts to develop at about sixteen weeks of pregnancy, when the blood vessels of the retina begin to form at the optic nerve in the back of the eye. The blood vessels grow gradually toward the edges of the developing retina, supplying oxygen and nutrients. During the last twelve weeks of a pregnancy, the eye develops rapidly. When a baby is born full-term, the retinal blood vessel growth is mostly complete (The retina usually finishes growing a few weeks to a month after birth). But if a baby is born prematurely, before these blood vessels have reached the edges of the retina, normal vessel growth may stop. The edges of the retina—the periphery—may not get enough oxygen and nutrients.

Scientists believe that the periphery of the retina then sends out signals to other areas of the retina for nourishment. As a result, new abnormal vessels begin to grow. These new blood vessels are fragile and weak and can bleed, leading to retinal scarring. When these scars shrink, they pull on the retina, causing it to detach from the back of the eye.

Are there different stages of ROP?

Yes. ROP is classified in five stages, ranging from mild (stage I) to severe (stage V):

Stage I. Mildly abnormal blood vessel growth. Many children who develop stage I improve with no treatment and eventually develop normal vision. The disease resolves on its own without further progression.

Stage II. Moderately abnormal blood vessel growth. Many children who develop stage II improve with no treatment and eventually develop normal vision. The disease resolves on its own without further progression.

Stage III. Severely abnormal blood vessel growth. The abnormal blood vessels grow toward the center of the eye instead of following their normal growth pattern along the surface of the retina. Some infants who develop stage III improve with no treatment and eventually develop normal vision. However, when infants have a certain

216

degree of Stage III and "plus disease" develops, treatment is considered. "Plus disease" means that the blood vessels of the retina have become enlarged and twisted, indicating a worsening of the disease. Treatment at this point has a good chance of preventing retinal detachment.

Stage IV. Partially detached retina. Traction from the scar produced by bleeding, abnormal vessels pulls the retina away from the wall of the eye.

Stage V. Completely detached retina and the end stage of the disease. If the eye is left alone at this stage, the baby can have severe visual impairment and even blindness.

Most babies who develop ROP have stages I or II. However, in a small number of babies, ROP worsens, sometimes very rapidly. Untreated ROP threatens to destroy vision.

How is ROP treated?

The most effective proven treatments for ROP are laser therapy or cryotherapy. Laser therapy "burns away" the periphery of the retina, which has no normal blood vessels. With cryotherapy, physicians use an instrument that generates freezing temperatures to briefly touch spots on the surface of the eye that overlie the periphery of the retina. Both laser treatment and cryotherapy destroy the peripheral areas of the retina, slowing or reversing the abnormal growth of blood vessels. Unfortunately, the treatments also destroy some side vision. This is done to save the most important part of our sight—the sharp, central vision we need for "straight ahead" activities such as reading, sewing, and driving.

Both laser treatments and cryotherapy are performed only on infants with advanced ROP, particularly stage III with "plus disease." Both treatments are considered invasive surgeries on the eye, and doctors don't know the long-term side effects of each.

In the later stages of ROP, other treatment options include:

- **Scleral buckle:** This involves placing a silicone band around the eye and tightening it. This keeps the vitreous gel from pulling on the scar tissue and allows the retina to flatten back down onto the wall of the eye. Infants who have had a scleral buckle need to have the band removed months or years later, since the eye continues to grow; otherwise they will become nearsighted. Scleral buckles are usually performed on infants with stage IV or V.

- **Vitrectomy:** Vitrectomy involves removing the vitreous and replacing it with a saline solution. After the vitreous has been removed, the scar tissue on the retina can be peeled back or cut away, allowing the retina to relax and lay back down against the eye wall. Vitrectomy is performed only at stage V.

What happens if treatment does not work?

While ROP treatment decreases the chances for vision loss, it does not always prevent it. Not all babies respond to ROP treatment, and the disease may get worse. If treatment for ROP does not work, a retinal detachment may develop. Often, only part of the retina detaches (stage IV). When this happens, no further treatments may be needed, since a partial detachment may remain the same or go away without treatment. However, in some instances, physicians may recommend treatment to try to prevent further advancement of the retinal detachment (stage V). If the center of the retina or the entire retina detaches, central vision is threatened, and surgery may be recommended to reattach the retina.

Are there other risk factors for ROP?

In addition to birth weight and how early a baby is born, other factors contributing to the risk of ROP include anemia, blood transfusions, respiratory distress, breathing difficulties, and the overall health of the infant.

An ROP epidemic occurred in the 1940s and early 1950s when hospital nurseries began using excessively high levels of oxygen in incubators to save the lives of premature infants. During this time, ROP was the leading cause of blindness in children in the United States. In 1954, scientists funded by the National Institutes of Health determined that the relatively high levels of oxygen routinely given to premature infants at that time were an important risk factor, and that reducing the level of oxygen given to premature babies reduced the incidence of ROP. With newer technology and methods to monitor the oxygen levels of infants, oxygen use as a risk factor has diminished in importance.

Although it had been suggested as a factor in the development of ROP, researchers supported by the National Eye Institute determined that lighting levels in hospital nurseries has no effect on the development of ROP.

Can ROP cause other complications?

Yes. Infants with ROP are considered to be at higher risk for developing certain eye problems later in life, such as retinal detachment, myopia (nearsightedness), strabismus (crossed eyes), amblyopia (lazy eye), and glaucoma. In many cases, these eye problems can be treated or controlled.

What research is the National Eye Institute supporting?

The National Eye Institute (NEI)-supported clinical studies on ROP include:

- The Cryotherapy for Retinopathy of Prematurity (CRYO-ROP) outcome study examined the safety and effectiveness of cryotherapy (freezing treatment) of the peripheral retina in reducing the risk of blindness in certain low-birth-weight infants with ROP. Follow-up results confirm that applying a freezing treatment to the eyes of premature babies with ROP helps save their sight. The follow-up results also give researchers more information about how well the babies can see in the years after cryotherapy.

- The Effects of Light Reduction on Retinopathy of Prematurity (Light-ROP) study evaluated the effect of ambient light reduction on the incidence of ROP. The study determined that light reduction has no effect on the development of a potentially blinding eye disorder in low-birth-weight infants. The study determined that light reduction in hospital nurseries has no effect on the development of ROP.

- The Supplemental Therapeutic Oxygen for Prethreshold Retinopathy of Prematurity (STOP-ROP) multicenter trial tested the efficacy, safety, and costs of providing supplemental oxygen in moderately severe retinopathy of prematurity (prethreshold ROP). Results showed that modest supplemental oxygen given to premature infants with moderate cases of ROP may not significantly improve ROP, but definitely does not make it worse.

- The Early Treatment for Retinopathy of Prematurity (ETROP) study is designed to determine whether earlier treatment in carefully selected cases of ROP will result in an overall better visual outcome than treatment at the conventional disease threshold point used in the CRYO-ROP study.

Chapter 16

Multiple Births

Chapter Contents

Section 16.1—Preparing for Twins, Triplets, and More 222
Section 16.2—Twin Pregnancy Complications 228
Section 16.3—Fetal Surgery for Twin-Twin Transfusion
           Syndrome 232
Section 16.4—High Order Multiples: Special Concerns 236

Section 16.1

Preparing for Twins, Triplets, and More

A multiple gestation is a pregnancy in which a woman is carrying two or more babies (fetuses). In the past two decades, the number of multiple births in the United States has jumped dramatically. Between 1980 and 2000, the number of twin births has increased 74 percent, and the number of higher order multiples (triplets or more) has increased fivefold, according to the National Center for Health Statistics. Today, about 3 percent of babies in this country are born in sets of two, three, or more, and about 95 percent of these multiple births are twins.

The rising number of multiple gestations is a concern because women who are expecting more than one baby are at increased risk of certain pregnancy complications, including preterm delivery (before thirty-seven completed weeks of pregnancy). Babies who are born preterm are at risk of serious health problems during the newborn period, as well as lasting disabilities and death.

Some of the complications associated with multiple gestation can be minimized or prevented when they are diagnosed early. There are a number of steps a pregnant woman and her health care provider can take to help improve the chances that her babies will be born healthy.

Why are multiple gestations increasing?

About one-third of the increase in multiple gestations is due to the fact that more women over age thirty (who are more likely to conceive multiples) are having babies. The remainder of the increase is due to the use of fertility-stimulating drugs and assisted reproductive techniques (ART) such as in vitro fertilization (IVF)(in which eggs are removed from the mother, fertilized in a laboratory dish, and then transferred to the uterus). According to the most recent survey of ART programs in the United States, 56 percent of births resulting from these procedures were multiples.

Doctors now realize that it is crucial to monitor fertility treatments so that women will have fewer, but healthier, babies. This involves limiting the number of embryos transferred during IVF, or halting treatment with fertility drugs during a cycle if ultrasound shows that a large number of eggs could be released. In fact, the rate of higher-order multiple births has declined slightly in the past two years.

A woman also has a higher-than-average chance of conceiving twins if she has a personal or family history of fraternal (non-identical) twins or if she is obese.

How are multiple gestations diagnosed?

Although previous generations often were surprised by the delivery of twins (or other multiples), today most parents to-be learn the news fairly early. An ultrasound examination can detect more than 95 percent of multiples by the beginning of the second trimester. (Sometimes a seemingly normal twin gestation that is identified very early is later found to have only one fetus. These so-called vanishing twin events are not well understood.)

An abnormal result on the triple or quadruple screen—blood tests done around the sixteenth week of pregnancy to identify babies at increased risk of certain birth defects—also alerts a health care provider to the possibility of multiples, as does hearing more than one fetal heartbeat during a routine examination. A provider also may suspect that a woman is carrying more than one baby if she puts on weight more rapidly than anticipated in the first trimester, if her uterus is larger than expected, or if she has severe pregnancy-related nausea and vomiting (morning sickness). Some women also may notice more fetal movement than in a previous singleton pregnancy. Whenever a multiple gestation is suspected, the health care provider will most likely recommend an ultrasound examination to find out for sure.

What complications occur more frequently in a multiple gestation?

Twins generally face the fewest medical complications and are usually born healthy. The more babies a woman carries at once, the greater her risk of complications.

Close to 60 percent of twins, over 90 percent of triplets, and virtually all quadruplets and higher multiples are born preterm. The length of gestation decreases with each additional baby. On average, most singleton pregnancies last thirty-nine weeks; for twins, thirty-six weeks; for triplets, thirty-two weeks; for quadruplets, thirty weeks; and for quintuplets, twenty-nine weeks.

Most preterm multiples weigh less than 5.5 pounds (2,500 grams), which is considered low birth weight. Low-birth-weight babies, especially those born before thirty-two weeks of gestation and/or weighing less than 3.3 pounds (1,500 grams), are at increased risk of health complications in the newborn period as well as lasting disabilities, such as mental retardation, cerebral palsy, and vision and hearing loss. While advances in caring for very small infants has brightened the outlook for these tiny babies, chances remain slim that all infants in a set of sextuplets or more will survive and thrive.

Before birth, identical twins face an additional risk. One-third of all twin pairs are identical—they begin as one fertilized egg that subsequently divides in half. The remaining two-thirds of twins are fraternal, resulting from two different eggs fertilized by two different sperm. Fraternal twins are no more similar genetically than are any other siblings. They may not be the same sex; they may not even look alike. Higher-order multiples can result from three (or more) eggs being fertilized, one egg splitting twice (or more), or a combination of both.

Identical twin fetuses have a 15 percent chance of developing a serious complication called twin-to-twin transfusion syndrome. This condition, which occurs when there is a connection between the two babies' blood vessels in their shared placenta, can result in one baby getting too much blood flow and the other too little. Until recently, severe cases often resulted in the loss of both babies. Recent studies, though, suggest that the use of amniocentesis to drain off excess fluid can save about 60 percent of affected babies. Removing the excess fluid appears to improve blood flow in the placenta and reduces the risk of preterm labor. Recent studies also suggest that using laser surgery to seal off the connection between the blood vessels may save a similar number of babies. An advantage of laser surgery is that only one treatment is needed, while amniocentesis generally must be repeated more than once.

Women who are pregnant with multiples also face an increased risk of pregnancy-related forms of high blood pressure (preeclampsia) and diabetes. More than half of triplet pregnancies are complicated by preeclampsia. With proper treatment, these disorders usually do not pose a major risk to mother or baby.

Should a woman expecting multiples gain extra weight?

Eating right and gaining the recommended amount of weight reduces the risk of having a low-birth-weight baby in singleton, as well as multiple, gestations. A healthy weight gain is especially important if a woman is pregnant with twins or more, as multiples have a higher risk of preterm birth and low birth weight than do singletons.

Women who begin pregnancy at a normal weight and who are expecting one baby usually are advised to gain twenty-five to thirty-five pounds over nine months. Women of normal weight who are expecting twins are usually advised to gain thirty-five to forty-five pounds. Women pregnant with triplets should probably aim for a gain of fifty to sixty pounds.

Studies show that gaining enough weight in the first twenty to twenty-four weeks of pregnancy is especially important for women carrying multiples. In a twin pregnancy, a gain of at least twenty-four pounds by the twenty-fourth week of pregnancy helps reduce the risk of having preterm and low-birth-weight babies. A good early weight gain may be especially important in multiple gestations because these pregnancies tend to be shorter than singleton pregnancies. Studies also suggest that a good early weight gain aids in development of the placenta, possibly improving its ability to pass along nutrients to the babies.

The American College of Obstetricians and Gynecologists recommends that women with multiple pregnancies consume about 300 more calories a day than women carrying one baby (a total of about 2,700 to 2,800 calories a day). However, women pregnant with multiples should discuss the number of extra calories they should eat with their health care providers. They also should take a prenatal vitamin that is recommended by their health care provider and that contains at least 30 milligrams of iron. Iron-deficiency anemia is common in multiple gestations, and it can increase the risk of preterm delivery.

What special care is needed in a multiple gestation?

Women who are expecting multiples generally need to visit their health care providers more frequently than women expecting one baby to help prevent, detect, and treat the complications that develop more often in a multiple gestation. Health care providers usually recommend twice-monthly visits during the second trimester and weekly (or more frequent) visits during the third trimester.

Starting around the twentieth week of pregnancy, a health care provider will monitor the pregnant woman carefully for signs of preterm labor. She may do an internal exam or recommend a vaginal ultrasound examination to see if the woman's cervix is shortening (a possible sign that labor may begin soon). Some providers also do electronic uterine monitoring. Home uterine monitoring was once recommended for women at especially high risk of preterm labor, but studies of women expecting twins did not find it useful.

When a woman develops preterm labor, her provider may recommend bed rest in the hospital and, possibly, treatment with drugs that may postpone labor. If the provider does not believe labor will stop and if the babies are likely to be born before thirty-four weeks gestation, she will probably recommend that the pregnant woman be treated with drugs called corticosteroids. These drugs help speed fetal lung development and reduce the likelihood and severity of breathing and other problems during the newborn period.

Even if a woman pregnant with twins has no signs of preterm labor, her provider may recommend cutting back on activities sometime between the twentieth and thirtieth weeks of pregnancy. She may be advised to cut back on activities even sooner and to rest several times a day if she is expecting more than two babies.

As a multiple gestation progresses, the health care provider will regularly check the pregnant woman's blood pressure for preeclampsia. Regular ultrasound examinations often are recommended to check on the babies' rates of growth—including growth differences among them, which can be signs of serious problems. During the third trimester, the provider may recommend tests of fetal well-being (such as the nonstress test, which measures fetal heart rate when the baby is moving).

Can a woman expecting multiples deliver vaginally?

While the chance of a cesarean delivery is higher in twin than in singleton births, about half of women expecting twins can have a normal vaginal delivery. Chances are good if both babies are in a normal, head-down position. However, when a woman is carrying three or more babies, a cesarean delivery is usually recommended because it is safer for the babies.

Does the March of Dimes support research relevant to multiple gestation?

The March of Dimes supports a number of grants aimed at improving understanding of the causes of preterm delivery. Although these studies generally focus on singleton pregnancies, the largely unknown mechanisms leading to preterm delivery of singletons and of multiples may be much the same.

References

American College of Obstetricians and Gynecologists (ACOG). Special problems of multiple gestation. *ACOG Educational Bulletin*, number 253, November 1998.

Centers for Disease Control and Prevention. Use of assisted reproductive technology—United States 1996 and 1998. *Morbidity and Mortality Weekly Report*, volume 51, number 2, February 8, 2002.

Mari, G., et al. Perinatal morbidity and mortality rates in severe twin-twin transfusion syndrome. *American Journal of Obstetrics and Gynecology*, volume 185, 2001, pages 708–15.

Martin, J., et al. Births: final data for 2000. *National Vital Statistics Reports*, volume 50, number 5, February 12, 2002.

Newman, R.B., and Luke, B. *Multifetal Pregnancy: A Handbook for Care of the Pregnant Patient*, Philadelphia, Lippincott, Williams and Wilkins, 2000.

Section 16.2

Twin Pregnancy Complications

Twin to Twin Transfusion Syndrome

What is twin to twin transfusion syndrome(TTTS)?

TTTS and other complications of monochorionic (MC; shared placenta) twin pregnancies are generally diagnosed by ultrasound. These problems do not occur in twins who have two placentas (dichorionic, DC), and therefore it is important to distinguish between MC and DC twins at an ultrasound examination. The earlier in pregnancy, the easier this can be achieved.

TTTS is a serious, progressive disorder that affects up to 15 percent of MC twins. The twins do not have malformations, but one transfuses the other through a particular blood vessel connection. In this situation, an artery from the donor twin enters the placental substance to exchange oxygen and nutrients. Unfortunately, the corresponding vein returns "by mistake" to the other twin (the recipient) via this arteriovenous connection.

What is the outcome for a fetus with TTTS?

In TTTS the donor twin responds by partially shutting down blood supply to many of its internal organs, especially the kidneys, and has reduced urine output and therefore a small amniotic fluid volume (oligohydramnios) in its amniotic cavity. The recipient responds to the blood transfusion by producing excessive amounts of urine, and is surrounded by a large volume of amniotic fluid (polyhydramnios). It is the combination of oligohydramnios and polyhydramnios that suggests the diagnosis of TTTS. The twins are often discrepant in size, as well, with significant discordance in estimated fetal weights. The recipient's blood becomes thick and difficult to pump around the body, and this can result in heart failure, generalized soft tissue swelling (hydrops), and fetal death. Because of the blood vessel connections across the placenta, if one twin dies, the co-twin faces significant risk for death or damage to vital organs. If a co-twin survives, there is a high risk of brain injury. Without treatment, about 70 to 80 percent of twins with TTTS will die. Survivors may have injuries to their brains, hearts, and kidneys.

How serious is my fetus's TTTS?

The severity of the problem is based on the stage in pregnancy during which it becomes evident (the earlier, the more serious it is). In addition the degree of fluid imbalance is important in grading or staging the problem. A serious situation is associated with a deepest pocket of ultrasound measurable fluid in the sac of the donor of less than 2 cm, and greater than 8 cm in the recipient. A bladder that is unfilled in the donor and evidence of heart failure in the recipient are also very serious signs. The most serious situation is when in addition to this there is abnormal blood flow in the umbilical cords of the twins, measured with ultrasound. Finally evidence of heart failure (hydrops) in the recipient is the gravest situation.

What options do I have?

Because twin-twin transfusion syndrome is a progressive disorder, early treatment may prevent complications, including preterm labor and premature rupture of membranes secondary to polyhydramnios. The most commonly used treatment is amnioreduction (serial large-volume amniocenteses), in which large volumes of amniotic fluid are drained with a needle placed through the abdomen of the mother into the sac of the recipient twin. This procedure may be repeated, if necessary. Survival rates with this treatment reach about 60 percent. Although it is not known exactly how amnioreduction improves the state of both twins, it is effective in many cases.

However, some cases of TTTS do not respond to amnioreduction, and one or both fetuses may die if other methods are not tried. These cases are appropriately treated with a direct approach to try to stop transfusion in the abnormal arteriovenous connection. This can be achieved by introducing a thin fiberoptic scope through the mother's abdomen, through the wall of the uterus and into the amniotic cavity of the recipient. By examining the surface placental vessels directly, the abnormal vascular connections can be found and eliminated by directing a laser beam at them. The procedure should be as selective as possible, and detailed ultrasound examination prior to the procedure may help locate the abnormal connection, making it quicker and easier to locate with the fetoscope.

Unequal Placental Sharing

What is unequal placental sharing?

Not all MC twin pregnancies in which there is a difference in size of the twins and different levels of amniotic fluid have TTTS as the cause. These findings are also seen in unequal placental sharing. In this case the twins do not have equal access to the placenta. This leads to the smaller one having slower growth and lower amounts of amniotic fluid. This usually gets progressively worse and can lead to stillbirth of the smaller twin. As discussed previously, death of one of the twins will also place the survivor at risk because of the blood vessel connections in the placenta. In unequal placental sharing the larger, normally growing twin does not have increased amniotic fluid, in contrast to TTTS. Unequal placental sharing and TTTS can coexist to varying degrees.

How serious is my fetus's condition?

Ultrasound evaluations provide us with the information to determine the severity of the situation. The greater the degree of size and weight difference between the twin fetuses the more serious the problem is. Also the less fluid present in the sac of the smaller twin, the more serious the situation. We also monitor the blood flow in the umbilical cords of the fetuses using Doppler ultrasound. A high resistance pattern is characteristic in the smaller, sicker one, and a normal one in the larger.

What options do I have?

There are no treatments that can be performed to improve the situation in this case. Amnioreduction and laser treatment are not appropriate, and could make things worse. Management is based on keeping a very close watch on the smaller twin. This may allow us to see when the smaller one is getting sick. Depending on the stage of the pregnancy, this may lead to hospitalization for closer follow-up or delivery. It is very important to keep such a close eye on the smaller one because stillbirth will possibly lead to serious problems even in the survivor.

Acardiac Twin (TRAP Sequence)

What is an acardiac twin or the TRAP sequence?

This is a very rare problem, happening on average once in every thirty-five thousand pregnancies. One twin is usually completely normal. The other is body-like tissue, often with legs and a lower body, but no upper body or heart. Abnormal blood vessels on the placental surface allow the normal twin to (or pump twin) to pump blood though the tissue of the abnormal one. Because the pump twin heart has to pump for two, there is a high risk of going into heart failure. This would then lead to death of the normal twin, unless it is delivered if it is far enough along in pregnancy.

How serious is my fetus's condition?

The risk of the normal or pump twin going into heart failure and dying seems to depend on the size of the acardiac. The larger the acardiac compared to the pump twin, the greater the risk. The amount of blood flow into the acardiac also seems to play a role. The more blood flow, the higher the risk. The harder the pump twin's heart is working, the greater the risk of heart failure also. All of these things can be looked for with ultrasound tests. In critical cases these tests may have to be repeated frequently.

What options do I have?

One option in this case is simply watching for the earliest signs of heart failure in the pump twin, with frequent ultrasounds. If heart failure is identified, and the pregnancy is far enough along, then the pump twin would simply be delivered. The other option, if the acardiac twin is large enough and we are worried about the amount of blood flow to it causing heart failure in the healthy twin, is to stop the blood flow with surgery. We currently do this using a thin needle, which we guide into the place where the blood vessels feed into the acardiac twin, using ultrasound. Once in place, this instrument, called a radio-frequency ablation (RFA) device, produces a very high local heat, to burn the tissue and destroy the blood vessels, to stop the blood flow. The needle is so thin that no incision is necessary and the pain and recovery are similar to those after an amniocentesis.

Section 16.3

Fetal Surgery for
Twin-Twin Transfusion Syndrome

Excerpted from "Twin to Twin Transfusion Syndrome," © 2005–2006 The Fetal Treatment Program. All rights reserved. Reprinted with permission. For additional information, visit http://bms.brown.edu/pedisurg/ FetalTreatment.html.

What Are the Treatment Options?

Observation and Bed rest

If twin-to-twin transfusion syndrome occurs after twenty-five to twenty-eight weeks, conservative measures (bed rest, single amnioreduction) and early delivery are usually recommended. Amnioreduction means the removal, through a fine needle, of the excess amniotic fluid from the recipient twin with polyhydramnios. As the pregnancy comes closer to term, it may be best to "wait and see," and to plan early delivery if either twin shows signs of distress. In this situation, the risks associated with (mild to moderate) prematurity may be smaller than the risk of an intervention in the womb (such as the ones described in the following).

Amnioreduction

Removal of excess amniotic fluid from the recipient twin has been, until recently, the best available treatment for twin-to-twin transfusion syndrome. The reason for its effectiveness is not completely clear, but removing the excess amniotic fluid may help decrease the risk of preterm, premature rupture of the membranes (PPROM) and premature labor. It may also be beneficial by relieving the pressure on the umbilical cord of the twin with excess fluid, and thus improving blood flow between the fetus and the placenta.

Amnioreduction does not, however, treat the cause of twin-to-twin transfusion syndrome, only one of its effects. Since the fluid is likely to accumulate again (usually within a few days to a week or two), the procedure will have to be repeated. With each amnioreduction, the risk of bleeding or infection increases, as does the risk of injury to the membranes.

The results of repeated amnioreduction depend on how often this has to be done and how rapidly fluid accumulates again. In general, the earlier in gestation the syndrome develops and the quicker poly-hydramnios recurs after amnioreduction, the worse the outcome. Whereas survival of either twin in twin-to-twin transfusion syndrome is very low if the condition develops early (before twenty weeks of gestation), repeated amnioreduction can improve survival of at least one twin to 50 to 60 percent of cases. Unfortunately, the risk of se-vere complications in the surviving twins may be as high as 20 to 35 percent, and includes severe heart or brain anomalies.

Laser Coagulation of the Communicating Placental Vessels

This technique, a form of fetal surgery, was originally described in 1995 by Dr. Julian DeLia, and is now being performed in several cen-ters worldwide. This is the only known form of treatment for twin-to-twin transfusion syndrome where the likely cause of the condition is addressed. In essence, a laser fiber is used, through a very small en-doscope (a long telescopic lens) inserted into the uterus, to block all vessels that run from one twin to the other (see Figure 16.1)

Fetal surgery is done under epidural or general anesthesia. A small incision is made on the mother's abdomen and, under ultrasound guid-ance, a long and thin instrument (less than one-eighth inch in diam-eter) is introduced into the amniotic cavity. This instrument contains an endoscope, which allows the surgeon to directly look into the uterus, and a laser fiber to coagulate, or block, the blood vessels that are seen to cross from one twin to the other. All blood vessels that connect the fetus to its own side of the placenta are left alone.

The procedure has been performed hundreds of times since it was first described. It was initially developed in the United States, but the majority of cases have been performed in Europe. Today, several cen-ters in the United States are offering this technique.

The results of laser fetal surgery appear to be better than those of other techniques, when patients are properly selected. Survival of at least one twin has been reported to be 70 to 80 percent, and survival of both twins is seen in 30 to 40 percent of the pregnancies. Also, the complication rate appears to be much lower. There are many fewer cases of severe heart and brain damage, and the overall complication rate (including a few instances of infection and damage to the membranes) is less than 10 percent, not including PPROM.

Preterm, premature rupture of the membranes (PPROM) usually leads to premature delivery; it is common in twin gestations (5 to 15 percent), particularly if TTTS is present. While decreasing the polyhydramnios reduces that risk, it may still occur as a result of the invasive procedure itself. After laser coagulation, the incidence of PPROM may be as high as 15 percent, particularly if multiple procedures (such as repeated amnioreductions) preceded the endoscopic operation.

Since its first description, the technique has undergone many improvements. For example, the use of special endoscopes that can be custom-curved now allows the treatment of patients with an anterior placenta. The use of magnetic resonance imaging (MRI) and computerized three-dimensional reconstruction allows the surgeons to plan the procedures on a virtual reality model, before the uterus is even entered.

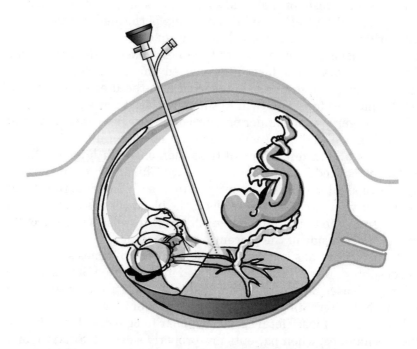

Figure 16.1. *The blood vessels that allow transfusion from one twin to the other are closed off by laser. The laser is introduced through a very thin endoscope into the uterus. As a result, each twin gets a separate portion of the placenta, and the twins are now completely separated.*

It is important to note that this is a form of fetal surgery and the most aggressive of the treatment options for TTTS, and that risks, although reduced to a minimum, exist for the mother and the fetuses. While the procedure aims at separating the two blood circulations, communications may still persist after the operation. As a result, one fetus's demise could theoretically still affect the other (although that risk is clearly much reduced compared with any of the other treatment options). Complications of TTTS, such as fetal death, brain damage, limb necrosis, and others, have been reported even when laser therapy was performed. It is our belief that most of these represented previously undiagnosed abnormalities (undiagnosed, perhaps, because of limitations on the ability of ultrasound to detect evolving problems in their early stages); nevertheless, the possibility also exists that the treatment may not be successful and the TTTS may progress.

Until recently, it had not yet been demonstrated in a scientific way that endoscopic laser ablation of placental vessels was clearly superior to amnioreduction. Therefore, our center participated in a randomized, controlled trial involving many institutions throughout several continents, and administered by Eurofoetus. Patients who qualified were offered the chance to enroll in the study, which aimed to compare serial amnioreduction with endoscopic laser surgery. The study was completed last year, and showed that laser ablation was

Table 16.1 Outcome of Severe TTTS With and Without Treatment

Outcome	Untreated	Amnioreduction	Laser
Survival of both twins	0–10%	26%	35%
Survival of at least one twin	0–30%	51%	76%
Maternal complications			
	PPROM (5–15%)	PPROM (5–15%)[a] Infection[a] Bleeding	PPROM (5–15%) Infection Bleeding
Fetal complications			
Neurologic/Cardiac damage	20–35%	20–35%	less than 5%
Limb necrosis	described	described	described
Organ damage/absence	described	described	described

[a]Risk increases with increasing number of amnioreductions.

superior to amnioreduction for advanced-stage TTTS. This is the first time a randomized controlled study has been performed for fetal treatment of TTTS. It is also the first study to demonstrate that laser surgery is superior to amnioreduction; it is not the only study on the subject, however: The National Institute of Child Health and Human Development (NICHD), part of the National Institutes of Health (NIH), is currently sponsoring a similar study.

Amniotic Septostomy

A few centers have, in the past, offered an alternative procedure, whereby one or more small holes are created between the two amniotic cavities, in the hope that fluid from the recipient twin (with polyhydramnios) will flow toward the donor twin (who has oligohydramnios). The reasoning is that this way, both twins will have a normal amount of amniotic fluid. Some early results appeared promising, but this technique has since been abandoned.

Section 16.4

High-Order Multiples: Special Concerns

Introduction

Infertility treatments are expensive, are often not covered by health insurance plans, and can be emotionally and physically draining. As a result, many infertility patients feel that a multiple pregnancy—twins, triplets, quadruplets, or more—would be a good outcome. Many wonder, "If I want to have more than one child, shouldn't I try to have twins so I don't have to undergo infertility treatment again?" According to a

2004 study,[1] a multiple birth would be the most desired outcome of infertility treatment for one in five women surveyed. A minority (46%) of the women in this study was well informed about the possible complications and risks associated with a twin pregnancy; awareness of risks associated with triplets was higher (76%).[2]

While there are many grateful parents of families built through multiple births, you should know that multiple-gestation pregnancy and birth, even of twins, are associated with a greater chance of pregnancy-related problems as well as risks to the infants.

Types of Multiples

There are two types of twins: monozygotic (identical) and dizygotic (fraternal). Identical twins occur when one fertilized egg divides into two embryos. They may share the same placenta but have different gestational sacs. Identical twins have identical genes, are the same sex, and are identical in appearance (at birth). Fraternal twins occur when two eggs are fertilized by two separate sperm. These twins have a different genetic makeup, can be different genders, and do not generally look alike.

"High order multiples" is a term used to describe triplets or three fetuses or babies; quadruplets ("quads"), four; quintuplets ("quints"), five; sextuplets, six; and septuplets, seven. High order multiples are usually the result of treatment with injectable fertility drugs combined with insemination or intercourse, or in vitro fertilization (IVF). High-order-multiple pregnancy rates due to IVF have been declining as IVF technology has improved, resulting in higher pregnancy rates with lower numbers of embryos transferred.

Who Is at Risk for Having Multiples?

Those at the greatest risk for having multiples are as follows:

- Women under thirty undergoing intrauterine insemination (IUI) with ovulation-stimulating drugs, known commonly as fertility drugs (e.g., Clomiphene, Pergonal, Repronex, Gonal-F, Bravelle and Follistim). IUI is a procedure in which sperm is placed directly in the uterus within hours of ovulation. When fertility drugs are used, multiple eggs may be produced. Because more mature eggs are generally released in women using fertility drugs, more eggs can be fertilized and thus, the multiple pregnancy rate is increased. While the eggs can be monitored, their fertilization cannot be controlled in this procedure. The twin pregnancy rate from cycles using timed IUI in combination with fertility drugs is 15 to 20 percent and the triplet and greater (quads, quints, etc.) pregnancy rate is 5 percent. High order births are usually the result of a cycle that used injectable ovulatory-stimulating drugs combined with IUI or intercourse.

* Women undergoing assisted reproductive technologies (ART) such as in vitro fertilization (IVF). With IVF, a woman uses fertility drugs to produce multiple eggs that are fertilized in a lab, and the resulting embryos are transferred back to her uterus. The multiple pregnancy rate for ART depends upon the number of embryos transferred, the age of the woman, the quality of the embryos, and many other factors. According to the Centers for Disease Control and Prevention (CDC)'s 2002 *Assisted Reproductive Technology Success Rates Report* the multiple pregnancy rate for women using ART is 36.2 percent: 29.4 percent were twins and 6.8 percent were triplets or more. Because miscarriage is common in woman with multiples, the multiple infant live birth rate for these same women was 35.4 percent; 31.6 percent were twins and 3.8 percent were triplets or more.

* Women using donated eggs from a woman less than thirty years old, regardless of the age of the recipient.

* Women who use Clomiphene, an oral drug used to stimulate ovulation. Clomiphene can increase the twin rate from 1 to 2 percent to 5 to 10 percent; but triplets and other high order multiples are rare using this drug.

* Women with a body mass index of at least 30 may be at a higher risk for having fraternal twins.[3]

* Women with polycystic ovarian syndrome (PCOS), a hormonal imbalance that results in the ovaries creating many immature follicles. PCOS patients tend to be at above average risk for high order multiples because they tend to over respond to fertility drugs. For this reason, it may make sense for some patients with PCOS to avoid stimulated cycles using injectable medications combined with IUI or intercourse and consider IVF because doctors can control the number of embryos transferred using IVF.

What Are the Risks During Pregnancy?

A woman with a multiple gestation pregnancy may experience complications during her pregnancy and at delivery including:

- Severe nausea and vomiting, particularly in the first trimester.

- Toxemia or preeclampsia, which occurs when the woman develops high blood pressure and protein is passed into her urine. If severe and untreated, it can result in stroke, seizure, or kidney failure.

- Gestational diabetes, which can result in premature babies who may have high birth weight and who may have respiratory problems at birth.

- Maternal anemia, a condition that causes weakness and tiredness due to low levels of iron in the blood.

- Premature aging of the placenta, which may result in a slow flow of nutrients to the fetus. This can occur during the third trimester and may delay fetal growth.

- Maternal hemorrhage or severe bleeding during labor, delivery, or after delivery.

- Cesarean delivery, which can result in bleeding, infection, and scarring in the pelvic area.

Multiple gestation pregnancy and multiple births can put a family at financial risk, as well. Obstetricians often order women carrying multiple fetuses to remain in bed and to restrict their physical activity during the last trimester of pregnancy, which can impact the family's income.

While many new parents of multiples adjust well, the stress of parenting, feeding, and caring for several infants can lead to anxiety, marital difficulties, depression, and social isolation. Furthermore, multiple births create abrupt lifestyle changes that may be difficult for some parents to adjust to.

What Are the Risks to Babies?

Premature labor and delivery is a serious risk if a woman is pregnant with multiples. The average length of pregnancy for a singleton (one child) is thirty-nine to forty weeks. A multiple gestation pregnancy is usually much shorter: thirty-six weeks for twins; thirty-three weeks for triplets; and thirty-one weeks for quadruplets.[4]

Babies born prematurely may have the following complications:

- Low birth weight;

- Underdeveloped lungs;
- Brain damage resulting in cerebral palsy;
- Vision problems or blindness.

Studies report that twins are four times more likely to die in the first month of life than a singleton, and that triplets are ten times as likely to die in the first month as a singleton.[5] Other studies have shown that triplets may have up to a 30 percent higher risk than singletons of neurological problems.[6]

How Is Multiple Gestation Pregnancy Controlled?

Careful monitoring of the ovarian response is the most effective method of preventing a multiple gestation pregnancy in cycles where fertility drugs are used in combination with intercourse or IUI. Monitoring includes frequent vaginal ultrasounds of the ovaries to determine how many follicles and eggs are developing, and blood tests to measure estrogen levels.

If the physician determines that too many follicles are developing during the cycle, he or she may offer the patient several options:

- Stop taking the follicle-stimulating medications.

- Stop taking the hCG shot (Novarel, Pregnyl, Ovidrel), which triggers the release of eggs from the follicles; with this option the cycle will be canceled. It is important to know that a woman may still ovulate and conceive without taking the hCG shot, so the only safe way to avoid multiple gestation is to not have intercourse during that cycle.

- The physician may recommend a "coasting" treatment in which the patient discontinues the stimulating drugs until her estrogen levels drop, after which she resumes medications.

- The physician may suggest that the patient switch the IUI cycle to an IVF cycle to control the number of embryos transferred into the uterus; extra embryos may be frozen for use in future cycles.

- The patient stops taking the medications and the IVF or IUI is canceled.

The best way to prevent multiple gestation pregnancies in patients undergoing IVF treatment is to limit the number of embryos that are transferred. In September 2004 the American Society for Reproductive

Medicine (ASRM) and the Society for Assisted Reproductive Technology (SART) issued revised "Practice Guidelines" to assist clinics and their patients in determining the appropriate number of embryos to transfer during an IVF cycle. The guidelines recommend the following:

- Women under the age of thirty-five should consider using only two embryos for transfer.

- Women ages thirty-five to thirty-seven with a favorable prognosis (a sufficient number of embryos that result in extra embryos available to freeze for future cycles, or previous success with IVF) should transfer no more than two embryos. If they do not have a favorable prognosis, no more than three embryos should be transferred.

- Women ages thirty-eight to forty with a favorable prognosis should have no more than three embryos transferred. Women in this age group with an unfavorable prognosis should have only four embryos transferred.

ASRM guidelines also recommend that the number of embryos to transfer should be agreed upon by the physician and the patient and included in the informed consent document and clinical record. (The informed consent is a document outlining the procedure and any associated risks, and is signed by the patient and the clinic or doctor.)

Other factors that may impact the decision regarding how many embryos to transfer include:

- The IVF clinic's success rates;

- The patient's previous clinical pregnancy rate;

- The quality of the embryos;

- The individual's or couple's feelings about multifetal reduction, an outpatient procedure used to reduce the number of embryos in the uterus.

Clinics may use several techniques, described in the following, to improve embryo quality or implantation success, so that fewer embryos can be transferred during IVF (note that not all fertility clinics offer all of these techniques):

- **Blastocyst transfer to increase implantation rates.** Blastocysts are embryos that are cultured for five to six days rather

than the usual three days. By culturing embryos to the blastocyst stage, implantation rates improve thereby allowing the doctor to put fewer embryos back during the embryo transfer
procedure.

- **Fragment removal to increase embryo quality.** Before
  transfer, microscopic cellular fragments are removed from the
  embryos that if left in place could decrease the quality of the
  embryo and possibly impact implantation and development of
  the embryos.

- **Embryos can be grown in a variety of co-culture medi-
  ums** that contain cells from fallopian tubes, maternal blood cells,
  or special products that are thought to help embryo growth.

- **Assisted hatching** is a technique in which the embryologist
  makes a small opening in the embryo wall to allow it to attach
  better to the uterine wall.. This technique has been shown to
  improve embryo implantation.

- **Preimplantation genetic diagnosis (PGD)** is a procedure in
  which each embryo is biopsied and only those that are chromo-
  somally normal are transferred. PGD has been shown to increase
  embryo implantation rates, allowing for transfer of fewer embryos,
  which can lower the risk for multiples.

- **Single embryo transfer,** in which only the best quality embryo
  is transferred, dramatically lowers multiple pregnancy rates.

Miscarriage

The miscarriage rate for women pregnant with multiples is higher
than with a singleton. Miscarriage occurs in up to 20 percent of twin
pregnancies and up to 40 percent of pregnancies with triplets or more.
In some cases a twin pregnancy becomes a singleton due to a syndrome called "The Vanishing Twin," in which one of the fetal sacs is
reabsorbed before twelve weeks.

Multifetal Reduction

If three or more embryos implant, the patient and physician will
have to make some difficult choices. One choice to consider is multifetal
pregnancy reduction, an outpatient procedure that involves reducing
the number of embryos that have become implanted to improve the
chance of having a healthy pregnancy and a positive outcome.

Patients should ask the physician or nurse about this procedure before taking fertility drugs prior to being faced with this difficult decision. The assistance of an infertility counselor or therapist can be extremely helpful in making this decision, as well as connecting with others who have faced this dilemma.

Questions to Ask Your Medical Team

If you are considering taking ovulation-stimulating medications, either oral or injectable, and attempting pregnancy through intercourse, IUI, or ART, ask your medical team to answer these questions:

- How will the clinic monitor your response to fertility medications? What procedures are involved?

- How long does a monitoring appointment take?

- What time of day are appointments scheduled?

- How will the clinic manage your care if your ovaries produce too many follicles or your estrogen levels increase too much? At what points might the clinic recommend cycle cancellation? Will the clinic switch the IUI to an IVF cycle? If so, is that noted in your medical chart in case your doctor is not available when a decision has to be made?

- How many embryos would the clinic recommend be transferred during an IVF cycle based on your age and past pregnancy and medical history? What number is recommended if you use donor eggs?

- If you have at least three good quality embryos, will the clinic culture your embryos to the blastocyst stage?

- Does the clinic offer PGD?

- Does the clinic do assisted hatching on embryos before transfer?

- Does the clinic have facilities for freezing embryos that are not transferred during a "fresh" cycle?

- If more than three embryos implant, what is the clinic's protocol? Does it offer multifetal reduction?

Information and Support

The course of infertility treatment is filled with excitement and hope but also emotional strain, as patients have to face decisions that will impact their family building experience. It is essential to become well informed about options before beginning treatment.

References

1. Ryan, G.L., S.H. Zhang, A. Dokras, C. Syrop, B. Van Voorhis. The desire of infertile patients for multiple births. *Fertility and Sterility*, March 2004, vol. 81, no. 3, p. 500–505.

2. Ibid

3. Reddy, U. Relationship of maternal body mass index and height to twinning. *Obstetrics & Gynecology*, March 2005, vol. 105, no. 5, p. 593–97.

4. March of Dimes Updates, *Contemporary OB/GYN*, July 2003, p. 67.

5. Ryan G.L., S.H. Zhang, A. Dokras, C. Syrop & B. Van Voorhis. The desire of infertile patients for multiple births. *Fertility and Sterility* vol. 81, no. 3, March 2004, p. 504.

6. Chen, S. Multiple births: Risks and rewards. *Family Building* vol. 2, issue 3, Spring 2003, p 8.

Chapter 17

Birth Complications Associated with Birth Defects

Chapter Contents

Section 17.1—Cesarean Childbirth: Why and How It Is
        Performed 246
Section 17.2—What to Expect in Labor and Delivery When
        Your Baby Has a Health Problem 249

Section 17.1

Cesarean Childbirth:
Why and How It Is Performed

This text is from *About Cesarean Childbirth*; it is reprinted by permission of the American College of Surgeons. © 2002 American College of Surgeons.

Cesarean section refers to the delivery of a baby through a surgical incision in the mother's lower abdominal wall and uterus, rather than through the vagina. This section will explain:

- Why you may need to have a cesarean section;
- How a cesarean section is performed;
- What to expect after the operation.

Remember that each individual is different, and the outcome of any operation depends upon the patient's individual condition.

This information is not intended to take the place of the professional expertise of a qualified obstetrician who is familiar with your situation. After reading this information, you should discuss any questions you may have openly and honestly with your obstetrician.

About Cesarean Section

A cesarean section is performed only after an obstetrician has carefully weighed the factors involved in a woman's pregnancy and has decided that performing a cesarean section is necessary. The indication for cesarean section may be evident at any time during the prenatal course. For the most part, the need for a cesarean section is evident only after the onset of labor, either in the early stage or after a woman has been in labor for a while.

Why Cesarean Section?

The presence of several conditions during pregnancy or labor may necessitate a cesarean section. Some of the most common conditions for which a cesarean section may be advised are:

- **Prolonged or ineffective labor:** When labor is prolonged for various reasons, including insufficient contractions of the uterus, a cesarean section may be necessary to speed the birth process.

- **Placenta previa:** This condition exists when the placenta (or afterbirth) becomes positioned abnormally low within the uterus and there is a possibility that it could completely block the cervix. This condition could prevent the baby from advancing through the birth canal and it also could cause hemorrhaging (severe bleeding).

- **Placenta abruptio:** Occasionally, the placenta can suddenly separate from the wall of the uterus prior to the delivery of the baby, possibly causing the mother to hemorrhage, and the baby to have an abnormal heart rate.

- **Disproportion:** This condition occurs when the baby's head is too large or the mother's birth canal is too small to allow for a safe vaginal delivery.

- **Abnormal presentation:** In some instances, the baby's position in the uterus may make vaginal delivery dangerous. This problem may occur when the baby is in a breech (buttocks or feet first) or traverse (side or shoulder first) position.

- **Prolapsed cord:** This condition exists when the umbilical cord precedes the baby through the vagina during labor. A prolapsed cord could strangle the baby as it is being born, or block the baby's progress through the vagina during a vaginal delivery.

- **Fetal distress:** If the baby has a slow or very rapid heart rate, deceleration of heart rate, or a heartbeat that does not fluctuate, it may be advisable to speed the delivery by performing a cesarean section.

- **Medical problems:** The mother may have medical problems, such as diabetes, genital herpes, hypertension, cardiac disease, toxemia, or ovarian or uterine cysts or tumors that could make labor hazardous to both the mother and the baby.

- **Multiple births:** Multiple births, such as twins and triplets, may sometimes be delivered more safely by cesarean section (particularly if one or more of the babies' position in the uterus will result in an abnormal presentation).

- **Previous cesarean delivery:** Previously, women who had one cesarean birth would deliver subsequent births by the same method. Now, however, it is estimated that as many as 60 percent of women who have had a cesarean section may be able to have a successful vaginal delivery. A subsequent vaginal delivery is an option that must be discussed with a qualified obstetrician.

- **Birth defects:** Some babies with birth defects diagnosed by ultrasound have a better outcome when delivered by cesarean section. The risks and benefits should be discussed with a qualified obstetrician.

Although any of these conditions may make a cesarean section advisable, they do not necessarily rule out the possibility of a normal vaginal delivery.

About the Operation

It is estimated that cesarean section is performed in approximately one out of every five deliveries in the United States; in most instances, it is not considered a dangerous or risky procedure.

While the type of anesthesia used for a cesarean section is determined by the condition of the mother and baby, in most cases either a spinal or epidural anesthetic is administered to numb the mother's legs and abdomen. Either anesthetic will allow the mother to remain awake without feeling pain. Sometimes, however, a general anesthetic that allows the mother to be asleep during the operation may be preferable.

Two types of abdominal skin incisions can be used for a cesarean section. The vertical or longitudinal incision extends from the navel to the pubic hair line. The transverse, or horizontal, incision (also known as the "bikini cut") runs across the pubic hair line. After making the first incision, the obstetrician usually makes a horizontal incision on the lower part of the uterus.

The obstetrician then gently removes the baby and the placenta from the uterus. The incision in the mother's uterus is then tightly sutured, and the abdomen is closed in the same manner that is used for any other operation.

Recovery

The average hospital stay after a cesarean section may be from three to five days. Most patients are encouraged to get out of bed the day after the operation or earlier and are able to return to normal activities in approximately four to six weeks.

Section 17.2

What to Expect in Labor and Delivery When Your Baby Has a Health Problem

Reprinted with permission from "When Your Baby Is Born With a Health Problem." This information was provided by KidsHealth, one of the largest resources online for medically reviewed health information written for parents, kids, and teens. For more articles like this one, visit www.KidsHealth.org, or www.TeensHealth.org. © 2005 The Nemours Center for Children's Health Media, a division of The Nemours Foundation.

If you are expecting a baby, it's likely that you are learning about everything you can do to make sure that your pregnancy, labor, and delivery go smoothly and leave you and your baby in good health. But it's also a good idea to understand that there are certain health problems and complications that can't be prevented, no matter how smoothly the pregnancy goes.

There is no way to completely prepare yourself for complications during delivery or for the discovery that your child has a birth defect. But you may be able to reduce some of your anxiety about the potential that something might go wrong if you understand some of the more common newborn health problems and how they are treated.

Gathering Information before Your Baby Is Born

With prenatal tests, doctors can detect certain birth defects, such as spina bifida, Down syndrome, congenital heart disease, exposed bowel, or cleft lip, before the baby is born. Other birth defects can't be discovered until after the baby is delivered. Delivery complications such as meconium aspiration (when a newborn inhales a mixture of meconium—the baby's first feces, ordinarily passed after birth—and amniotic fluid during labor and delivery) can occur.

If a birth defect is discovered prenatally, your doctor may discuss what will happen in the time right after you deliver the baby. You may want to ask about whether you can tour the intensive or special care unit at the hospital so that you can get familiar with the environment and meet the team of doctors who may be caring for your baby. This team may include a neonatologist, a pediatric anesthesiologist, or pediatric surgeon, as well as neonatal nurses and nurse practitioners.

Common Newborn Problems

It is very common for infants, particularly those who are born prematurely, to experience jaundice or breathing problems.

In the first days after delivery, premature infants or even full-term infants often develop jaundice, which may appear as a yellowish coloring of a baby's skin and whites of the eyes caused by excess bilirubin in the blood. Jaundice occurs in healthy babies when a baby's immature liver initially can't dispose of excess bilirubin (a yellow pigment produced by the normal breakdown of red blood cells) in the blood.

If your baby has jaundice, your doctor may order tests to determine what the bilirubin levels are in your baby's body and whether treatment is necessary. Usually, jaundice is treated by exposing the baby to special ultraviolet lights that help break down the extra bilirubin to help the baby's liver process it.

Another very common problem affecting preemies is immature lungs. Some preemies lack enough surfactant, a chemical that prevents the air sacs from collapsing when a baby exhales. Surfactant isn't usually fully in the fetal lungs until after thirty-four weeks' gestational age, so many premature babies require devices to assist their breathing, keep their air sacs open, and promote air exchange. One of these devices is a ventilator, a breathing machine that is hooked up to a small plastic tube that goes into the baby's windpipe to aid in breathing.

Synthetic surfactant is now routinely given (down a breathing tube) to very premature babies right after birth. This treatment allows infants to breathe on their own much sooner than in the past, and they sustain less lung damage because they do not require long-term ventilator use.

What Happens in the Delivery Room?

Most babies are born in a labor and delivery room. But if there are complications with the delivery, the mother may be transferred to a delivery room that contains additional medical equipment. The obstetrician, midwife, or family doctor, a nurse, or other specialists may also be there to provide any special medical attention that the baby might immediately need.

If a newborn has spina bifida (exposed spinal structures) or hydrocephalus (excess fluid inside of or surrounding the brain), the doctors will take special care to support the head or cover the opening in the spine. For a newborn who has an exposed bowel, the intestines are covered to protect them from infection and from heat and fluid losses.

In the case of meconium aspiration, usually the doctor tries to clear the baby's airways using a suction device to draw out any fluid that is interfering with the baby's ability to breathe. If the baby continues having trouble breathing or is very premature, he or she may require a breathing tube.

The medical staff, including a pediatrician or neonatologist, will monitor the baby's breathing and heart rate and make sure that the infant is kept warm. If necessary, they will perform a special kind of CPR for newborns. When your infant is stable enough to be moved, it's likely that he or she will be taken directly to the neonatal intensive care unit (NICU) for further treatment.

The obstetrics (OB) team will likely remain with the mother while the baby is being treated, providing any medical care that she may need. The OB team can make sure that the mother delivers the placenta, that she receives any needed stitches, and in the case of cesarean delivery, that the surgery is completed.

Communicating With the Doctor

The medical team that cares for your baby in the NICU should make every effort to communicate with you about the baby's condition. The doctor, obstetrician, midwife, or family practitioner is often the liaison between parents and the NICU team.

If the baby has a condition that was diagnosed prenatally, the doctor will explain any deviations from the original plan and continue to provide information about the baby's progress. For instance, the doctor might say, "Just like we talked about, the baby is having a problem breathing so we have put a tube into his windpipe to help him breathe—that's why you're not hearing him cry." When a problem is unanticipated, the doctor should explain what has occurred.

Beyond the Delivery Room

After the baby leaves the delivery room, the doctor may need to give the baby intravenous (IV) medications or fluids. And because a baby loses heat quickly, he or she will be put in a warmer to keep warm.

If the baby's breathing is too fast or labored, the medical team may order chest x-rays to determine what's causing it. If so, blood tests or a foot or hand oxygen monitor will tell the doctor how much help breathing the baby needs, and then put the baby on a ventilator to assist with that breathing.

When the baby's breathing and heartbeat are stabilized, treatment for any birth defects may begin. This evaluation and treatment period can last days or weeks, depending on the baby's condition.

Doctors may also want to take blood tests from your baby to rule out any other problems and check the baby's blood count and blood sugar levels. Sometimes blood tests can be taken from a baby's heel and other times the blood must come directly from a vein in the baby's arm.

Getting the Care You Need

Time away from a newborn is extremely difficult for the family—particularly the parents.

It is very common to feel disappointment and even guilt in these situations. It may help to talk about these feelings with a member of your baby's medical team or a hospital social worker. It may also help you to get as much information as possible about your child's medical problem, to ease any feelings of anxiety and powerlessness about your baby's condition.

Most hospitals encourage parents to spend as much time as they can with their babies. If the baby is transferred to a hospital with a special neonatal care unit, you might want to ask about whether the mother can get any necessary postpartum care at that hospital, too, so that if possible, the two can recover together.

As hard as it may be, parents should get plenty of rest and regular exercise and be sure to eat well during this time. If the mother is going to breastfeed, it's important to talk with a nurse or lactation consultant about getting a breast pump so she can freeze breast milk for when the baby comes home.

If your baby is born with a health problem, there are many sources for information and support. Start by asking your doctors for information on hospital- or community based resources.

Chapter 18

Medical Evaluations for the Newborn

Chapter Contents

Section 18.1—Apgar Score 254
Section 18.2—Newborn Screening Tests 256

Section 18.1

Apgar Score

Reprinted from "APGAR," © 2006 A.D.A.M., Inc.
Reprinted with permission.

Alternative Names: Newborn scoring

Definition: The Apgar score is a quick test performed at one and five minutes after birth to determine the physical condition of the newborn. The rating is based on a scale of 1 to 10. Ten suggests the healthiest infant, and scores below 5 indicate that the infant needs immediate assistance in adjusting to his or her new environment.

The test was designed in 1952 by Dr. Virginia Apgar at Columbia University's Babies Hospital.

How the Test Is Performed: Five categories are assessed:

- Heart rate;
- Respiratory effort;
- Muscle tone;
- Reflex irritability;
- Color.

Each of these categories is scored with 0, 1 or 2, depending on the observed condition of the newborn.

- Heart rate is evaluated by stethoscope. This is the most important assessment:

  - If there is no heartbeat, the infant scores 0 for heart rate.
  - If heart rate is less than one hundred beats per minute, the infant scores 1 for heart rate.
  - If heart rate is greater than one hundred beats per minute, the infant scores 2 for heart rate.

- Respiratory effort:
  - If there are no respirations, the infant scores 0 for respiratory effort.
  - If the respirations are slow or irregular, the infant scores 1 for respiratory effort.
  - If there is good crying, the infant scores 2 for respiratory effort.
- Muscle tone:
  - If the muscle tone is flaccid, the infant scores 0 for muscle tone.
  - If there is some flexion of the extremities, the infant scores 1 for muscle tone.
  - If there is active motion, the infant scores 2 for muscle tone.
- Reflex irritability is a term describing the level of newborn irritation in response to stimuli (such as a mild pinch):
  - If there is no reaction, the infant scores 0 for reflex irritability.
  - If there is grimacing, the infant scores 1 for reflex irritability.
  - If there is grimacing and a cough, sneeze, or a vigorous cry, the infant scores 2 for reflex irritability.
- Color:
  - If the color is pale blue, the infant scores 0 for color.
  - If the body is pink and the extremities are blue, the infant scores 1 for color.
  - If the entire body is pink, the infant scores 2 for color.

The one-minute APGAR score assesses how well the infant tolerated the birthing process. The five-minute APGAR score assesses how well the newborn is adapting to the environment.

Why the Test Is Performed: This test is a screening tool for health care providers to determine what assistance is immediately necessary to help your newborn stabilize.

Normal Values: A score of 8 or 9 is normal and indicates your newborn is in good condition. A score of 10 is very unusual—almost all newborns lose one point for blue hands and feet.

What Abnormal Results Mean: Any score lower than 8 indicates your child needs assistance stabilizing. A low score at one minute that normalizes by five minutes has not been associated with any long-term negative effects.

What the Risks Are: No risks are associated with the Apgar test.

Section 18.2

Newborn Screening Tests

What You Need to Know

All states screen newborns for certain metabolic birth defects. (Metabolic refers to chemical changes that take place within living cells.) These conditions cannot be seen in the newborn, but can cause physical problems, mental retardation, and, in some cases, death.

Fortunately, most babies receive a clean bill of health when tested. When test results show that the baby has a birth defect, early diagnosis and treatment can make the difference between lifelong disabilities and healthy development.

Many of the tests use a blood specimen taken before the baby leaves the hospital. The baby's heel is pricked to obtain a few drops of blood for laboratory analysis.

Tests for hearing loss use either a tiny, soft earphone or a microphone that is placed in the baby's ear.

The March of Dimes recommends that all newborns be screened for at least twenty-nine disorders, including hearing loss.

What You Can Do

Find out which tests are routinely done in your state by asking your health care provider or state health department.

Do not be overly alarmed if test results come back abnormal. The initial screening tests give only preliminary information that must be followed up by more precise testing.

Testing the Newborn for Metabolic Birth Defects

Metabolic birth defects can cause physical problems, mental retardation, and, in some cases, death. It is best for the baby and the family if these conditions are detected and treated early.

All states screen newborns for certain metabolic birth defects. (Metabolic refers to chemical changes that take place within living cells.) These conditions cannot be seen in the newborn, but can cause physical problems, mental retardation, and, in some cases, death.

What Do the Tests Look For?

Here is a description of some of the conditions and the available treatments:

- **Phenylketonuria (PKU):** Babies with this disorder cannot process a substance called phenylalanine that is found in almost all food. Without treatment, phenylalanine builds up in the bloodstream and causes brain damage and mental retardation. When PKU is detected early, mental retardation can be prevented by feeding the child a special diet. All states and U.S. territories screen for PKU.

- **Hypothyroidism:** Babies with this disorder have a hormone deficiency that slows growth and brain development. If it is detected in time, a baby can be treated with oral doses of the hormone to permit normal development. All states and U.S. territories screen for hypothyroidism.

- **Galactosemia:** Babies with this disorder cannot convert galactose, a sugar present in milk, into glucose, a sugar that the body uses as an energy source. Galactosemia can cause death in infancy, or blindness and mental retardation. The treatment for the condition is to eliminate milk and all other dairy products from the baby's diet.

- **Sickle Cell Anemia:** This inherited blood disease causes bouts of pain; damage to vital organs such as the lungs, kidneys, and brain; and sometimes serious infections and death in childhood. Early treatment can prevent some of the complications of sickle cell anemia.

- **Congenital adrenal hyperplasia (CAH):** Babies who have this group of disorders are deficient in certain hormones. CAH affects genital development and, in severe cases, can disturb kidney function and cause death. Lifelong treatment with the missing hormones suppresses the disease.

- **Hearing loss:** Early detection of hearing loss allows the baby to be fitted with hearing aids before six months of age. This early intervention helps prevent serious speech and language problems.

The March of Dimes recommends that all newborns be screened for twenty-nine disorders, including hearing loss.

How Are the Tests Done?

Most of the tests use a blood specimen taken before the baby leaves the hospital. The baby's heel is pricked to obtain a few drops of blood for laboratory analysis. The same blood sample can be used to screen for a number of disorders.

Usually, the baby's blood sample is sent to a state public health laboratory for testing. The health care provider responsible for the infant's care receives the results.

Hearing loss tests measure how a baby responds to sounds. The tests use either a tiny, soft earphone or a microphone that is placed in the baby's ear. If these tests show abnormal results, the baby may need more extensive testing to see if he or she has hearing loss.

What Should I Do if My Baby Is Diagnosed With One of the Conditions?

Your baby may need treatment at a specialized pediatric center. It is essential for your child's healthy development to follow the recommendations of his or her doctor.

Chapter 19

Perinatal Infections

Chapter Contents

Section 19.1—Group B Streptococcal Disease and
      Neonatal Risks 260
Section 19.2—Hepatitis B: Mother to Newborn Infection 266

Section 19.1

Group B Streptococcal Disease and Neonatal Risks

Reprinted from "Group B Strep Disease: Frequently Asked Questions,"
Centers for Disease Control and Prevention, November 8, 2002.

Group B streptococcus (group B strep) is a type of bacteria that causes illness in newborn babies, pregnant women, the elderly, and adults with other illnesses, such as diabetes or liver disease. Group B strep is the most common cause of life-threatening infections in newborns.

Newborns and Group B Strep

How common is group B strep disease in newborns?

Group B strep is the most common cause of sepsis (blood infection) and meningitis (infection of the fluid and lining around the brain) in newborns. Group B strep is a frequent cause of newborn pneumonia and is more common than other, more well known, newborn problems such as rubella, congenital syphilis, and spina bifida.

In the year 2001, there were about 1,700 babies in the United States less than one week old who got early-onset group B strep disease.

How does group B strep disease affect newborns?

About half of the cases of group B strep disease among newborns happen in the first week of life ("early-onset disease"), and most of these cases start a few hours after birth. Sepsis, pneumonia (infection in the lungs), and meningitis (infection of the fluid and lining around the brain) are the most common problems. Premature babies are more at risk of getting a group B strep infection, but most babies who become sick from group B strep are full-term.

Group B strep disease may also develop in infants one week to several months after birth ("late-onset disease"). Meningitis is more common with late-onset group B strep disease. Only about half of late-onset group B strep disease among newborns comes from a mother who is a group B strep carrier; the source of infection for others with late-onset group B strep disease can be hard to figure out. Late-onset disease is slightly less common than early-onset disease.

Can group B strep disease among newborns be prevented?

Yes! Most early-onset group B strep disease in newborns can be prevented by giving pregnant women antibiotics (medicine) by intravenous (IV) means during labor. Antibiotics help to kill some of the strep bacteria that are dangerous to the baby during birth. The antibiotics help during labor only—they can't be taken before labor, because the bacteria can grow back quickly. Any pregnant woman who had a baby with group B strep disease in the past, or who now has a bladder (urinary tract) infection caused by group B strep should receive antibiotics during labor.

Pregnant women who carry group B strep (test positive during this pregnancy) should be given antibiotics at the time of labor or when their water breaks.

What are the symptoms of group B strep in a newborn?

The symptoms for early-onset group B strep can seem like other problems in newborns. Some symptoms are fever, difficulty feeding, irritability, or lethargy (limpness or hard to wake up the baby). If you think your newborn is sick, get medical help right away.

How is group B strep disease diagnosed and treated in babies?

If a mother received antibiotics for group B strep during labor, the baby will be observed to see if he or she should get extra testing or treatment.

If the doctors suspect that a baby has group B strep infection, they will take a sample of the baby's sterile body fluids, such as blood or spinal fluid. Group B strep disease is diagnosed when the bacteria are grown from cultures of those fluids. Cultures take a few days to grow. Group B strep infections in both newborns and adults are usually treated with antibiotics (e.g., penicillin or ampicillin) given through a vein (by IV).

Pregnancy and Group B Strep Prevention

How will I know if I need antibiotics to prevent passing group B strep to my baby?

You should get a screening test late in pregnancy to see if you carry group B strep. If your test comes back positive, you should get antibiotics through the vein (by IV) during labor.

If you had a previous baby who got sick with group B strep disease, or if you had a urinary tract infection (bladder infection) during this pregnancy caused by group B strep, you also need to get antibiotics through the vein (by IV) when your labor starts.

How do you find out if you carry group B strep during pregnancy?

The Centers for Disease Control and Prevention (CDC)'s revised guidelines recommend that a pregnant woman be tested for group B strep in her vagina and rectum when she is thirty-five to thirty-seven weeks pregnant. The test is simple and does not hurt. A sterile swab ("Q-tip") is used to collect a sample from the vagina and the rectum. This is sent to a laboratory for testing.

What happens if my pregnancy screening test is positive for group B strep?

To prevent group B strep bacteria from being passed to the newborn, pregnant women who carry group B strep should be given antibiotics through the vein (by IV) at the time of labor or when their water breaks.

Are there any symptoms if you are a group B strep carrier?

Most pregnant women have no symptoms when they are carriers for group B strep bacteria.

Sometimes, group B strep can cause bladder infections during pregnancy, or infections in the womb during labor or after delivery.

Being a carrier (testing positive for group B strep, but having no symptoms) is quite common. Around 25 percent of women may carry the bacteria at any time. This doesn't mean that they have group B strep disease, but it does mean that they are at higher risk for giving their baby a group B strep infection during birth.

What if I don't know whether I am group B strep positive when my labor starts?

Talk to your doctor about your group B strep status. Pregnant women who do not know whether they are group B strep positive when labor starts should be given antibiotics if they have:

- labor starting at less than thirty-seven weeks (preterm labor);
- prolonged membrane rupture (water breaking more than eighteen hours before labor starts);
- fever during labor.

What are the risks of taking antibiotics to prevent group B strep disease in my newborn?

Penicillin is the most common antibiotic that is given. If you are allergic to penicillin, there are other antibiotics that can be given. Penicillin is very safe and effective at preventing group B strep disease in newborns. There can be side effects from penicillin for the woman, including a mild reaction to penicillin (about a 10 percent chance). There is a rare chance (about 1 in 10,000) of the mother having a severe allergic reaction that requires emergency treatment.

However, a pregnant woman who is a group B strep carrier (tested positive) at full-term delivery who gets antibiotics can feel confident knowing that she has only a 1 in 4,000 chance of delivering a baby with group B strep disease. If a pregnant woman who is a group B strep carrier does not get antibiotics at the time of delivery, her baby has a 1 in 200 chance of developing group B strep disease. This means that those infants whose mothers are group B strep carriers and do not get antibiotics have over twenty times the risk of developing disease than those who do receive treatment.

Can group B strep cause stillbirth, preterm delivery, or miscarriage?

There are many different factors that lead to stillbirth, preterm delivery, or miscarriage. Most of the time, the cause is not known. Group B strep can cause some stillbirths, and preterm babies are at greater risk of group B strep infections. However, the relationship between group B strep and premature babies is not always clear.

263

Will a C-section prevent group B strep in a newborn?

A C-section should not be used to prevent early-onset group B strep infection in infants. If you need to have a C-section for other reasons, and you are group B strep positive, you will not need antibiotics for group B strep only, unless you begin labor or your water breaks before the surgery begins.

What should I do if my water breaks early?

If your water breaks before term, get to the hospital right away. If your group B strep test has not been done, or if you don't know if you have been tested, you should talk with your doctor about group B strep disease prevention. If you have already tested positive for group B strep, remind the doctors and nurses during labor.

Can I breastfeed my baby if I am group B strep positive?

Yes. Women who are group B strep positive can breastfeed safely. There are many benefits for both the mother and child.

More about Group B Strep

Do people who are group B strep carriers feel sick?

Many people carry group B strep in their bodies, but they do not become sick or have any symptoms. Adults can have group B strep in the bowel, vagina, bladder, or throat. About 25 percent of pregnant women carry group B strep in the rectum or vagina. A person who is a "carrier" has the bacteria in her body but may not feel sick. However, her baby may come into contact with group B strep during birth. Group B strep bacteria may come and go in people's bodies without symptoms. A person does not have to be a carrier all of her life.

How does someone get group B strep?

The bacteria that cause group B strep disease normally live in the intestine, vagina, or rectal areas.

Group B strep colonization is not a sexually transmitted disease (STD). Approximately 25 percent (1 in 4) of pregnant women carry group B strep bacteria in their vagina or rectum. For most women there are no symptoms of carrying group B strep bacteria.

Will group B strep go away with antibiotics?

Antibiotics that are given when labor starts help to greatly reduce the number of group B strep bacteria present during labor. This reduces the chances of the newborn becoming exposed and infected.

However, for women who are group B strep carriers, antibiotics before labor starts are not a good way to get rid of group B strep bacteria. Since they naturally live in the gastrointestinal tract (guts), the bacteria can come back after antibiotics. A woman may test positive at certain times and not at others. That's why it's important for all pregnant women to be tested for group B strep carriage between thirty-five and thirty-seven weeks of every pregnancy. Talk to your doctor or nurse about the best way to prevent group B strep disease.

What if I'm allergic to some antibiotics?

Tell your doctor or nurse about your allergies during your checkup. Try to make a plan for delivery. When you get to the hospital, remind your doctor if you are allergic to any medicines. There are a variety of different antibiotics that can be used, even if you are allergic to some.

Is there a vaccine for group B strep?

There is not a vaccine right now to prevent group B strep. The federal government is supporting research on a vaccine for the prevention of group B strep disease.

Are yeast infections caused by group B strep?

Yeast infections are not caused by group B strep bacteria. Taking antibiotics can sometimes increase the chances of having a yeast infection. When bacteria that are normally found in the vagina are killed by antibiotics, yeast may have a chance to grow more quickly than usual.

Is group B strep the same as strep throat?

No. Strep throat is caused by group A streptococcus bacteria. Group A and group B streptococcus are different kinds of bacteria. They both belong to the same family, but they are different species.

Section 19.2

Hepatitis B: Mother to Newborn Infection

Reprinted from "HBV: Preventing Mother-to-Child Hepatitis B
Infection," with permission of the Hepatitis C Support Project, http://
www.hcvadvocate.org, © 2004. All rights reserved.

Pregnant women who have hepatitis B frequently infect their newborns. The concentration of hepatitis B virus (HBV) present in their blood and body fluids can be so high that up to 90 percent of their newborns may become infected due to contact with the virus in their mothers' blood and body fluids. Infants who are infected at birth face the highest risk of developing chronic or life-long hepatitis B infection because their young immune systems often fail to notice the viral invaders replicating in their livers. Years or even decades may pass before their immune systems finally notice the viral infection and try to eradicate the virus.

But whether or not newborns born to infected mothers contract hepatitis B depends primarily on their mothers' viral status, and whether they are immediately immunized against hepatitis B. The length of labor, whether or not membranes rupture, or the type of delivery (Cesarean vs. vaginal) apparently has little impact on mother-to-child transmission of hepatitis B.

According to a report issued by the Advisory Committee on Immunization Practices in the *Morbidity and Mortality Weekly Report*, infants born to mothers who tested positive for both the hepatitis B surface (HBsAg) and "e" (HBeAg) antigens faced a 70 to 90 percent risk of infection, with 85 to 90 percent of those infants becoming chronically infected. Infants born to mothers with the surface antigen and "e" antibody only faced a 31 percent risk of HBV infection.

Infections acquired during infancy, while estimated to represent only 1 to 3 percent of hepatitis B cases in the United States, account for 20 to 30 percent of chronic infections, according to the CDC.

But there is good news for HBV-infected women who are pregnant or planning to become pregnant. When a baby is born to an infected mother who has the surface and "e" antigens, if hepatitis B immune globulin (HBIG) and the first dose of the hepatitis B vaccine is administered to the newborn within twelve hours of birth, the baby's risk of HBV infection is reduced to only 5 to 15 percent.

HBIG contains antibodies to the hepatitis B virus and offers immediate but short-lived protection against HBV infection. When combined with the hepatitis B vaccine, HBIG reduces the risk of HBV infection by an additional 5 to 10 percent. In the United States, infants born to HB-infected mothers should receive HBIG and the first hepatitis B vaccination shot within twelve hours of birth.

But even if a baby does not receive HBIG, the vaccine is by itself highly effective in blocking HBV infection. In one study conducted in Thailand, ninety-seven babies born to HBV-infected women who had the "e" antigen received only the vaccination against hepatitis B at birth. Even without the added protection of HBIG, 82 to 86 percent of the immunized infants remained free of HBV infection.

It is recommended that obstetricians should screen all pregnant women for hepatitis B. If a doctor is not screening a pregnant woman for hepatitis B, she should ask for the test. According to the CDC, in 1999 about 19,000 women with chronic hepatitis B gave birth in the United States, and 1,455 of their newborns became infected because they were not immunized immediately after birth.

Infected mothers should make sure ahead of time that healthcare workers know they are infected so their newborns are immediately immunized and treated with HBIG.

To be fully protected, it is very important that babies must receive all three hepatitis B immunization shots. The second shot is administered two months after the first, and the third is administered about four months later.

Because of concerns about a mercury-based vaccine preservative called thimerosal, some parents unfortunately postponed immunizing their children against hepatitis B. However, today there is a thimerosal-free hepatitis B vaccine available and this immunization has repeatedly been found to be extremely safe.

The vaccine was recommended for all infants and unimmunized children and adolescents in 1991 by the CDC and the American Academy of Pediatrics. Since then, more than eighty-six million doses of hepatitis B vaccine have been given to children in the United States.

HBV-infected mothers can safely breastfeed their infants, according to the CDC. While the surface antigen—the outer coating of the virus—is found in breast milk, there are no intact viruses in breast milk that can infect infants. Studies have shown that breast-fed infants who were immunized immediately after birth were not at increased risk of HBV infection when compared to infants who were not breast-fed.

Immunization of newborns has been very successful in the United States in reducing hepatitis B. Hepatitis B infections have declined by two-thirds during the past decade due to routine childhood vaccination. CDC officials say the overall number of hepatitis B cases dropped 67 percent between 1990 and 2002, with the greatest decrease—89 percent—in the newborn-to-nineteen-year-old age group.

Chapter 20

What to Expect When Your Baby Has a Birth Defect

We see happy images of and tend to hear about only healthy babies. But many babies are born with problems called birth defects. These are abnormalities of structure, function, or body chemistry that will require medical or surgical care or could have some effect on a child's development.

About 150,000 babies are born in the United States each year with birth defects, according to the March of Dimes. There is a wide range of birth defects, from mild to severe, and they can be inherited or caused by something in the environment. In many cases, the cause is unknown. Often, doctors can detect a birth defect when they do prenatal tests.

If you've just found out that your child has a birth defect, you're probably experiencing many emotions. Parents in your situation often say that they feel overwhelmed and uncertain whether they will be able to care for their child properly. Fortunately, you aren't alone—with a little effort, you'll find that there are lots of people and resources to help you.

As the parent of a child with a birth defect, it's important for you to:

Reprinted from "When Your Baby Has a Birth Defect." This information was provided by KidsHealth, one of the largest resources online for medically reviewed health information written for parents, kids, and teens. For more articles like this one, visit www.Kidshealth.org, or www.TeensHealth.org. © 2006 The Nemours Center for Children's Health Media, a division of The Nemours Foundation.

Acknowledge your emotions. Parents of children with birth defects experience shock, denial, grief, and even anger. Acknowledge your feelings and give yourself permission to mourn the loss of the healthy child you thought you'd have. Talk about your feelings with your spouse or partner and with other family members. You might also consider seeing a counselor. Your doctor may be able to guide you to a social worker or psychologist in the area.

One of the best things you can do for yourself and your child is to seek support. Getting in touch with someone who's been through the same thing can be helpful; ask your doctor or a social worker at your hospital if they know any other parents in the area who have children with the same condition. Joining a support group may also help—consult your child's doctors or specialists for advice about finding a local or national support group.

Celebrate your child. Remember to let yourself enjoy your child the same way any parent would—by cuddling or playing, watching for developmental milestones (even if they're different from what they would be if your child didn't have a birth defect), and sharing your joy with family members and friends. Many parents of children with birth defects wonder if they should send out birth announcements. This is a personal decision—the fact that your child has a health problem doesn't mean you shouldn't be excited about the new addition to your family.

Seek information. The amount each person would like to learn varies from parent to parent, but try to educate yourself as much and as soon as you are able. Start by asking your child's doctors lots of questions. Record the answers as best as you can. If you're not satisfied with the answers—or if a doctor is unable to answer your questions thoroughly—don't be afraid to seek second opinions.

Additional places to get information include:

- books written for parents of children with birth defects;

- national organizations such as the March of Dimes, the National Information Center for Children and Youth With Disabilities, or those representing your child's specific birth defect;

- support groups or other parents.

Keep a binder with a running list of questions and the answers you find, as well as suggestions for further reading and any materials your child's doctor gives you. In addition, keep an updated list of all health care providers and their phone numbers, as well as emergency numbers, so you're able to reach them quickly and efficiently.

Part of this process of collecting information should involve exploring options for paying for treatment and ongoing care for your child. There may be extra medical and therapeutic costs associated with caring for a child with a birth defect. In addition to health insurance, there are many resources available to parents of children with birth defects, including nonprofit disability organizations, private foundations, Medicaid, and state and local programs. One of the hospital social workers should be able to help you learn more about these resources.

Seek early intervention. When your child has a birth defect, early intervention is usually the best strategy. Designed to bring a team of experts together to assess your child's needs and establish a program of treatment, early intervention services include feeding support, identification of assistive technology that may help your child, occupational therapy, physical therapy, speech therapy, nutrition services, and social work services. In addition to identifying, evaluating, and treating your child's needs, early intervention programs will:

- tell you where you can get information about your child's disability;

- help you to learn how to care for your child at home;

- help you determine your payment options and tell you where you can find services for free;

- help you make important decisions about your child's care;

- provide counseling to you and your family.

Your child's doctor or a social worker at the hospital where you gave birth should be able to connect you with the early intervention program in your area.

Use a team approach. Most children with birth defects require a team of professionals to treat them. Even if your child needs to see only one specialist, that person will need to coordinate care with your child's primary doctor. Although some hospitals already have teams in place to deal with problems such as heart defects, cleft lip and palate, or cerebral palsy, you may find yourself having to serve as both

271

the main point of contact between the different care providers and the coordinator of your child's appointments. As soon as you are able, get to know the different team members. Make sure they know who else will be caring for your child and that you intend to play a key role.

The Future of Birth Defects

Research into the environmental and genetic causes of birth defects is ongoing. Technology contributes to understanding and preventing defects in various ways—for example, prenatal testing is growing increasingly sophisticated. Safer and more accurate tests include:

- results of ultrasound tests and magnetic resonance imaging (MRI), which are sometimes combined with information from blood tests to determine the risk of having a child with certain birth defects;

- maternal blood screening to determine risk of chromosomal abnormalities;

- amniocentesis and chorionic villi sampling;

- preconception counseling to help you understand what risks you might have for having a child with a birth defect.

Although none of these tests can prevent birth defects, they give a clearer, safer, and more accurate diagnosis at an earlier stage of pregnancy—giving parents more time to seek advice and consider their options.

Genetics research is advancing quickly. The Human Genome Project is working on identifying all of the genes in the human body, including gene mutations that are associated with a high risk for birth defects.

Early surgery is becoming an option in the treatment of some birth defects—and can take place even while your child is still in the womb. Surgeons now operate on fetuses to repair structural defects, such as hernias of the diaphragm, spina bifida, and lung malformations. These treatments can be controversial, however, because they can cause premature labor. And it's still a bit unclear as to whether they ultimately improve the final outcome.

To get information on specific research about your child's disability, contact the national organization for that disability. The March of Dimes, the National Information Center for Children and Youth With Disabilities, and the National Organization for Rare Disorders, Inc. (NORD) also may have information about current research.

Part Three

Structural Abnormalities and Functional Impairments

Chapter 21

Cardiovascular Defects

Chapter Contents

Section 21.1—Diagnosing Congenital Heart Defects with
    Fetal Echocardiography 276
Section 21.2—Defects of the Heart and Blood Vessels 279
Section 21.3—Patent Foramen Ovale 290
Section 21.4—Arteriovenous Malformation 294
Section 21.5—Persistent Pulmonary Hypertension of the
    Newborn 305
Section 21.6—Vascular Rings 311

Section 21.1

Diagnosing Congenital Heart Defects with Fetal Echocardiography

From "Fetal Echocardiography," reproduced with permission from www.americanheart.org. © 2006 American Heart Association.

What is fetal echocardiography?

Fetal echocardiography is a test using sound waves (ultrasound) to study the structure of your baby's heart before birth. Your obstetrician may obtain a limited view of your baby's heart during a routine pregnancy ultrasound. However, a fetal echocardiogram is a very detailed evaluation of your baby's heart by a specialist in fetal echocardiography. There are no known risks to the mother or the fetus.

Who needs a detailed fetal echocardiogram?

Some pregnant women are at increased risk of giving birth to a baby with congenital heart disease (CHD). They should be considered for referral for a specialized fetal echocardiogram. Indications include the following:

- a family history of CHD—the risk if a previous child has CHD is about one in fifty, or about one in ten to one in twenty if the parent has CHD;

- an abnormal fetal heart rhythm;

- fetal heart abnormalities detected during a routine pregnancy ultrasound scan;

- abnormality of another major organ system;

- insulin-dependent (type 1) diabetes mellitus;

- exposure to some drugs in early pregnancy, for example, some anti-epileptic drugs can damage the developing heart;

- abnormal amniocentesis.

276

When can a fetal echocardiogram be performed?

The heart motion can be seen from about six weeks of gestation. However, details of heart structure cannot be seen until:

- fourteen weeks gestation using scanning through the vagina;
- eighteen weeks gestation using imaging through the abdomen.

Sometimes, repeat examinations are needed.

Who should do a fetal echocardiogram?

A limited cardiac evaluation is possible during regular obstetric scanning and is appropriate for women at low risk. However, some women should have a detailed fetal echocardiogram performed by a physician who is specially trained in fetal cardiac evaluation. They include women at increased risk of having a baby with a CHD or in whom a cardiac malformation is suspected by the initial ultrasound study.

What conditions can be identified?

- abnormalities of cardiac structure (CHD)
- cardiac rhythm disturbances (or arrhythmias)
- disorders of cardiac function

Are there limitations of fetal echocardiography?

Some heart abnormalities are not detectable prenatally even with a detailed expert examination. These tend to be minor defects, such as small holes in the heart, or mild valve abnormalities. In addition, some cardiac defects do not become evident until after birth.

The fetal echocardiogram focuses on the heart. The fetal echocardiographer may not see defects in other parts of the fetus.

What are the implications of fetal echocardiography?

- The detection of a heart defect increases the risk of finding other malformations in the child. A detailed ultrasound of the rest of the fetus is necessary. Also, amniocentesis to test the chromosomes may be recommended.

- A serious or even life-threatening heart abnormality may be identified. It may have a significant impact on the future of the child. You will want to discuss this with your doctor.

- Currently only cardiac rhythm disturbances are being treated before birth. In the future a number of structural cardiac defects may be treated before birth.

- In many cases of CHD diagnosed prenatally, it is safest to deliver the pregnancy at, or near, the center at which postnatal treatment will take place. This is especially true if surgery will be required soon after birth.

Who can counsel or advise me about cardiac findings?

- A perinatologist or obstetrician can advise you about the management of your pregnancy.

- A pediatric cardiologist is in the best position to give advice about the outlook for your child's heart problem.

- A geneticist can provide information about a fetus with an associated genetic syndrome, if present, and advise about future pregnancies.

- A cardiac surgeon can give details about surgical procedures that may be needed.

- A nurse who is familiar with heart disease in children can provide information about caring for a child with congenital heart disease.

Section 21.2

Defects of the Heart and Blood Vessels

What is a congenital cardiovascular defect?

Congenital means inborn or existing at birth. Among the terms you may hear are congenital heart defect, congenital heart disease, and congenital cardiovascular disease. The word "defect" is more accurate than "disease." A congenital cardiovascular defect occurs when the heart or blood vessels near the heart don't develop normally before birth.

What causes congenital cardiovascular defects?

Congenital cardiovascular defects are present in about 1 percent of live births. They're the most common congenital malformations in newborns. In most cases scientists don't know why they occur. Sometimes a viral infection causes serious problems. German measles (rubella) is an example. If a woman contracts German measles while pregnant, it can interfere with how her baby's heart develops or produce other malformations. Other viral diseases also may cause congenital defects.

Heredity sometimes plays a role in congenital cardiovascular defects. More than one child in a family may have a congenital cardiovascular defect, but this rarely occurs. Certain conditions affecting multiple organs, such as Down syndrome, can involve the heart, too. Some prescription drugs and over-the-counter medicines, as well as alcohol and "street" drugs, may increase the risk of having a baby with a heart defect. Researchers are studying other factors.

What are the types of congenital defects?

Most heart defects either obstruct blood flow in the heart or vessels near it, or cause blood to flow through the heart in an abnormal pattern. Rarely defects occur in which only one ventricle (single ventricle) is present, or both the pulmonary artery and aorta arise from the same ventricle (double outlet ventricle). A third rare defect occurs when the right or left side of the heart is incompletely formed—hypoplastic heart.

Patent ductus arteriosus (PDA). This defect (PA'tent DUK'tus ar-te"re-O'sis) allows blood to mix between the pulmonary artery and the aorta. Before birth an open passageway (the ductus arteriosus) exists between these two blood vessels. Normally this closes within a few hours of birth. When this doesn't happen, some blood that should flow through the aorta and on to nourish the body returns to the lungs. A ductus that doesn't close is quite common in premature infants but rather rare in full-term babies.

If the ductus arteriosus is large, a child may tire quickly, grow slowly, catch pneumonia easily, and breathe rapidly. In some children symptoms may not occur until after the first weeks or months of life. If the ductus arteriosus is small, the child seems well. If surgery is needed, the surgeon can close the ductus arteriosus by tying it, without opening the heart. If there's no other defect, this restores the circulation to normal.

Obstruction defects. An obstruction is a narrowing that partly or completely blocks the flow of blood. Obstructions called stenoses (sten-O'seez) can occur in heart valves, arteries or veins.

The three most common forms are pulmonary stenosis, aortic stenosis, and coarctation of the aorta. Related but less common forms include bicuspid aortic valve, subaortic stenosis, and Ebstein anomaly.

- Pulmonary stenosis (PUL'mo-nair-e sten-O'sis) (PS): The pulmonary or pulmonic valve is between the right ventricle and the pulmonary artery. It opens to allow blood to flow from the right ventricle to the lungs. A defective pulmonary valve that doesn't open properly is called stenotic (sten-OT'ik). This forces the right ventricle to pump harder than normal to overcome the obstruction. If the stenosis is severe, especially in babies, some cyanosis (si"ah-NO'sis) (blueness) may occur. Older children usually have no symptoms. Treatment is needed when the pressure in the right ventricle is higher than normal. In most children the obstruction can be relieved by a procedure called balloon valvuloplasty (VAL'vu-lo-plas-te). Others may need open-heart surgery. Surgery usually opens the valve satisfactorily. The outlook after balloon valvuloplasty or surgery is favorable, but follow-up is required to determine if heart function returns to normal. People with pulmonary stenosis, before and after treatment, are at risk for getting an infection of the valve (endocarditis). To help prevent this, they'll need to take antibiotics before certain dental and surgical procedures.

- Aortic stenosis (a-OR'tik sten-O'sis) (AS): The aortic valve, between the left ventricle and the aorta, is narrowed. The heart has difficulty pumping blood to the body. Aortic stenosis occurs when the aortic valve didn't form properly. A normal valve has three leaflets (cusps) but a stenotic (sten-OT'ik) valve may have only one cusp (unicuspid) or two cusps (bicuspid), which are thick and stiff. (See bicuspid aortic valve below.) Sometimes stenosis is severe and symptoms occur in infancy. Otherwise, most children with aortic stenosis have no symptoms. Some children may have chest pain, unusual tiring, dizziness, or fainting. The need for surgery depends on how bad the stenosis is. In children, a surgeon may be able to enlarge the valve opening. Surgery may improve the stenosis, but the valve remains deformed. Eventually the valve may need to be replaced with an artificial one. Balloon valvuloplasty (VAL'vu-lo-plaste) has been used in some children with aortic stenosis. The long-term results of this procedure are still being studied. Children with aortic stenosis need lifelong medical follow-up. Even mild stenosis may worsen over time, and surgical relief of a blockage is sometimes incomplete. Check with your pediatric cardiologist about limiting some kinds of exercise. People with aortic stenosis, before and after treatment, are at risk for getting an infection of the valve (endocarditis). To help prevent this, they'll need to take antibiotics before certain dental and surgical procedures.

- Coarctation (ko"ark-TA'shun) of the aorta ("Coarct"): The aorta is pinched or constricted. This obstructs blood flow to the lower body and increases blood pressure above the constriction. Usually there are no symptoms at birth, but they can develop as early as a baby's first week. A baby may develop congestive heart failure or high blood pressure that requires early surgery. Otherwise, surgery usually can be delayed. A child with a severe coarctation should have surgery in early childhood. This prevents problems such as developing high blood pressure as an adult. The outlook after surgery is favorable, but long-term follow-up is required. Rarely, coarctation of the aorta may recur. Some of these cases can be treated by balloon angioplasty. The long-term results are still being studied. Also, blood pressure may stay high even when the aorta's narrowing has been repaired. People with coarctation of the aorta, before and after treatment, are at risk for getting an infection within the aorta or the heart valves (endocarditis). To help prevent this, they'll need to take antibiotics before certain dental and surgical procedures.

- Bicuspid aortic (bi-KUS'pid a-OR'tik) valve: The normal aortic valve has three flaps (cusps) that open and close. A bicuspid valve has only two flaps. There may be no symptoms in childhood, but by adulthood (often middle age or older), the valve can become stenotic (sten-OT'ik) (narrowed), making it harder for blood to pass through it, or regurgitant (allowing blood to leak backward through it). Treatment depends on how well the valve works. People with bicuspid aortic valve, before and after treatment, are at risk for getting an infection within the aorta or the heart valves (endocarditis). To help prevent this, they'll need to take antibiotics before certain dental and surgical procedures.

- Subaortic stenosis (sub"a-OR'tik sten-O'sis): Stenosis means constriction or narrowing. Subaortic means below the aorta. Subaortic stenosis refers to a narrowing of the left ventricle just below the aortic valve, which blood passes through to go into the aorta. This stenosis limits the flow of blood out of the left ventricle. This condition may be congenital or may be due to a particular form of cardiomyopathy (kar"de-o-mi-OP'ah-the) known as "idiopathic hypertrophic (hi"per-TRO'fik) subaortic stenosis" (IHSS). Treatment depends on the cause and the severity of the narrowing. It can include drugs or surgery. People with subaortic stenosis, before and after treatment, are at risk for getting an infection within the aorta or the heart valves (endocarditis). To help prevent this, they'll need to take antibiotics before certain dental and surgical procedures.

- Ebstein anomaly (ah-NOM'ah-lee): This is a congenital downward displacement of the tricuspid valve (located between the heart's upper and lower chambers on the right side) into the heart's right bottom chamber (or right ventricle). It's usually associated with an atrial septal defect (see below). People with Ebstein anomaly, before and after treatment, are at risk for getting an infection within the heart valve (endocarditis). To help prevent this, they'll need to take antibiotics before certain dental and surgical procedures.

Septal defects. Some congenital cardiovascular defects let blood flow between the heart's right and left chambers. This happens when a baby is born with an opening between the wall (septum) that separates the right and left sides of the heart. This defect is sometimes called "a hole in the heart."

The two most common types of this defect are atrial septal defect and ventricular septal defect. Two variations are Eisenmenger complex and atrioventricular canal defect.

- Atrial septal (A'tre-al SEP'tal) defect (ASD): An opening exists between the heart's two upper chambers. This lets some blood from the left atrium (blood that's already been to the lungs) return via the hole to the right atrium instead of flowing through the left ventricle, out the aorta, and to the body. Many children with ASD have few, if any, symptoms. Closing the atrial defect by open-heart surgery in childhood can prevent serious problems later in life.

- Ventricular septal (ven-TRIK'u-ler SEP'tal) defect (VSD): An opening exists between the heart's two lower chambers. Some blood that's returned from the lungs and been pumped into the left ventricle flows to the right ventricle through the hole instead of being pumped into the aorta. Because the heart has to pump extra blood and is overworked, it may enlarge. If the opening is small, it doesn't strain the heart. In that case, the only abnormal finding is a loud murmur. But if the opening is large, open-heart surgery is recommended to close the hole and prevent serious problems. Some babies with a large ventricular septal defect don't grow normally and may become undernourished. Babies with VSD may develop severe symptoms or high blood pressure in their lungs. Repairing a ventricular septal defect with surgery usually restores normal blood circulation. The long-term outlook is good, but long-term follow-up is required. People with a ventricular septal defect are at risk for getting an infection of the heart's walls or valves (endocarditis). To help prevent this, they'll need to take antibiotics before certain dental and surgical procedures. After a VSD has been successfully fixed with surgery, antibiotics should no longer be needed.

- Eisenmenger complex: This is a ventricular septal defect coupled with pulmonary high blood pressure, the passage of blood from the right side of the heart to the left (right to left shunt), an enlarged right ventricle, and a latent or clearly visible bluish discoloration of the skin called cyanosis (si"ah-NO'sis). It may also include a malpositioned aorta that receives ejected blood from both the right and left ventricles (an overriding aorta). People with Eisenmenger complex, before and after treatment, are at risk for getting an infection within the aorta or the heart valves (endocarditis). To help prevent this, they'll need to take antibiotics before certain dental and surgical procedures.

- Atrioventricular (A'tre-o-ven-TRIK'u-ler) (A-V) canal defect (also called endocardial cushion defect or atrioventricular septal defect): A large hole in the center of the heart exists where the wall between the upper chambers joins the wall between the lower chambers. Also, the tricuspid and mitral valves that normally separate the heart's upper and lower chambers aren't formed as individual valves. Instead, a single large valve forms that crosses the defect. The large opening in the center of the heart lets oxygen-rich (red) blood from the heart's left side— blood that's just gone through the lungs—pass into the heart's right side. There, the oxygen-rich blood, along with venous (bluish) blood from the body, is sent back to the lungs. The heart must pump an extra amount of blood and may enlarge. Most babies with an atrioventricular canal don't grow normally and may become undernourished. Because of the large amount of blood flowing to the lungs, high blood pressure may occur there and damage the blood vessels. In some babies the common valve between the upper and lower chambers doesn't close properly. This lets blood leak backward from the heart's lower chambers to the upper ones. This leak, called regurgitation or insufficiency, can occur on the right side, left side, or both sides of the heart. With a valve leak, the heart pumps an extra amount of blood, becomes overworked, and enlarges. In babies with severe symptoms or high blood pressure in the lungs, surgery usually must be done in infancy. The surgeon closes the large hole with one or two patches and divides the single valve between the heart's upper and lower chambers to make two separate valves. Surgical repair of an atrioventricular canal usually restores the blood circulation to normal. However, the reconstructed valve may not work normally. Rarely, the defect may be too complex to repair in infancy. In this case, the surgeon may do a procedure called pulmonary artery banding to reduce the blood flow and high pressure in the lungs. When a child is older, the band is removed and corrective surgery is done. More medical or surgical treatment is sometimes needed. People with atrioventricular canal defect, before and after treatment, are at risk for getting an infection within the heart's walls or valves (endocarditis). To help prevent this, they'll need to take antibiotics before certain dental and surgical procedures.

Cyanotic defects. Another type of heart defect is congenital cyanotic (si"ah-NOT'ik) heart defects. In these defects, blood pumped to the body contains less oxygen than normal. This causes a condition called cyanosis (si"ah-NO'sis), a blue discoloration of the skin. Infants with cyanosis are often called "blue babies."

Examples of cyanotic defects are tetralogy of Fallot, transposition of the great arteries, tricuspid atresia, pulmonary atresia, truncus arteriosus, and total anomalous pulmonary venous connection.

- Tetralogy of Fallot (TE'TRAL'o-je of fal-O'): This defect has four components. The two major ones are a large hole, or ventricular septal defect, that lets blood pass from the right to the left ventricle without going through the lungs; and a narrowing (stenosis) at or just beneath the pulmonary valve. This narrowing partially blocks the blood flow from the heart's right side to the lungs. The other two components are: the right ventricle is more muscular than normal; and the aorta lies directly over the ventricular septal defect. This results in cyanosis (blueness), which may appear soon after birth, in infancy, or later in childhood. These "blue babies" may have sudden episodes of severe cyanosis with rapid breathing. They may even become unconscious. During exercise, older children may become short of breath and faint. These symptoms occur because not enough blood flows to the lungs to supply the child's body with oxygen. Some infants with severe tetralogy of Fallot may need an operation to give temporary relief by increasing blood flow to the lungs with a shunt. This is done by making a connection between the aorta and the pulmonary artery. Then some blood from the aorta flows into the lungs to get more oxygen. This reduces the cyanosis and allows the child to grow and develop until the problem can be fixed when the child is older. Most children with tetralogy of Fallot have open-heart surgery before school age. The operation involves closing the ventricular septal defect and removing the obstructing muscle. After surgery the long-term outlook varies, depending largely on how severe the defects were before surgery. Lifelong medical follow-up is needed. People with tetralogy of Fallot, before and after treatment, are at risk for getting an infection within the aorta or the heart valves (endocarditis). To help prevent this, they'll need to take antibiotics before certain dental and surgical procedures.

- Transposition of the great arteries: The positions of the pulmonary artery and the aorta are reversed. The aorta is connected to the right ventricle, so most of the blood returning to the heart from the body is pumped back out without first going to the lungs. The pulmonary artery is connected to the left ventricle, so most of the blood returning from the lungs goes back to the lungs again. Infants born with transposition survive only if they have one or more connections that let oxygen-rich blood reach the body. One such connection may be a hole between the two atria, called atrial septal defect, or between the two ventricles, called ventricular (ven-TRIK'u-ler) septal defect. Another may be a vessel connecting the pulmonary artery with the aorta, called patent ductus arteriosus (PA'tent DUK'tus ar-te"re-O'sis). Most babies with transposition of the great arteries are extremely blue (cyanotic) (si"ah-NOT'ik) soon after birth because these connections are inadequate. To improve the body's oxygen supply, a special procedure called balloon atrial septostomy (sep-TOS'to-me) is used. Two general types of surgery may be used to help fix the transposition. One is a venous switch or intra-atrial baffle procedure that creates a tunnel inside the atria. Another is an arterial switch. After surgery, the long-term outlook varies quite a bit. It depends largely on how severe the defects were before surgery. Lifelong follow-up is needed. People with transposition of the great arteries, before and after treatment, are at risk for getting an infection on the heart's walls or valves (endocarditis). To help prevent this, they'll need to take antibiotics before certain dental and surgical procedures.

- Tricuspid atresia (tri-KUS'pid ah-TRE'zhuh): In this condition, there's no tricuspid valve. That means no blood can flow from the right atrium to the right ventricle. As a result, the right ventricle is small and not fully developed. The child's survival depends on there being an opening in the wall between the atria called an atrial septal defect and usually an opening in the wall between the two ventricles called a ventricular (ven-TRIK'u-ler) septal defect. Because the circulation is abnormal, the blood can't get enough oxygen, and the child looks blue (cyanotic) (si"ah-NOT'ik). Often a surgical shunting procedure is needed to increase blood flow to the lungs. This reduces the cyanosis. Some children with tricuspid atresia have too much blood flowing to the lungs. They may need a procedure (pulmonary artery banding) to reduce blood flow to the lungs. Other children with tricuspid atresia may have a more functional repair (Fontan procedure). Children with tricuspid atresia require lifelong follow-up by a cardiologist. People with tricuspid atresia, before and after treatment, are at risk for getting an infection of the valves (endocarditis). To help prevent this, they'll need to take antibiotics before certain dental and surgical procedures.

- Pulmonary atresia (PUL'mo-nair-e ah-TRE'zhuh): No pulmonary valve exists, so blood can't flow from the right ventricle into the pulmonary artery and on to the lungs. The right ventricle acts as a blind pouch that may stay small and not well developed. The tricuspid valve is often poorly developed, too. An opening in the atrial septum lets blood exit the right atrium, so venous (bluish) blood mixes with the oxygen-rich (red) blood in the left atrium. The left ventricle pumps this mixture of oxygen-poor blood into the aorta and out to the body. The baby appears blue (cyanotic) (si"ah-NOT'ik) because there's less oxygen in the blood circulating through the arteries. The only source of lung blood flow is the patent ductus arteriosus (PA'tent DUK'tus ar-te"re-O'sis) (PDA), an open passageway between the pulmonary artery and the aorta. If the PDA narrows or closes, the lung blood flow is reduced to critically low levels. This can cause very severe cyanosis. Early treatment often includes using a drug to keep the PDA from closing. A surgeon can create a shunt between the aorta and the pulmonary artery to help increase blood flow to the lungs. A more complete repair depends on the size of the pulmonary artery and right ventricle. If they're very small, it may not be possible to correct the defect with surgery. In cases where the pulmonary artery and right ventricle are a more normal size, open-heart surgery may produce a good improvement in how the heart works. If the right ventricle stays too small to be a good pumping chamber, the surgeon can compensate by connecting the right atrium directly to the pulmonary artery. The atrial defect also can be closed to relieve the cyanosis. This is called a Fontan procedure. Children with tricuspid atresia require lifelong follow-up by a cardiologist. People with pulmonary atresia, before and after treatment, are at risk for getting an infection on the heart's walls or valves (endocarditis). To help prevent this, they'll need to take antibiotics before certain dental and surgical procedures.

- Truncus arteriosus (TRUN'kus ar-te"re-O'sis): This is a complex malformation where only one artery arises from the heart and forms the aorta and pulmonary artery. Surgery for this condition usually is required early in life. It includes closing a large ventricular (ven-TRIK'u-ler) septal defect within the heart, detaching the pulmonary arteries from the large common artery, and connecting the pulmonary arteries to the right ventricle with a tube graft. Children with truncus arteriosus need lifelong follow-up to see how well the heart is working. People with truncus arteriosus, before and after treatment, are at risk for getting an infection on the heart's walls or valves (endocarditis). To help prevent this, they'll need to take antibiotics before certain dental and surgical procedures.

- Total anomalous pulmonary venous (ah-NOM'ah-lus PUL'monair-e VE'nus) (P-V) connection: The pulmonary veins that bring oxygen-rich (red) blood from the lungs back to the heart aren't connected to the left atrium. Instead, the pulmonary veins drain through abnormal connections to the right atrium. In the right atrium, oxygen-rich (red) blood from the pulmonary veins mixes with venous (bluish) blood from the body. Part of this mixture passes through the atrial septum (atrial septal defect) into the left atrium. From there it goes into the left ventricle, to the aorta and out to the body. The rest of the poorly oxygenated mixture flows through the right ventricle, into the pulmonary artery and on to the lungs. The blood passing through the aorta to the body doesn't have enough oxygen, which causes the child to look blue (cyanotic) (si"ah-NOT'ik). This defect must be surgically repaired in early infancy. The pulmonary veins are reconnected to the left atrium and the atrial septal defect is closed. When surgical repair is done in early infancy, the long-term outlook is very good. Still, lifelong follow-up is needed to make sure that any remaining problems, such as an obstruction in the pulmonary veins or irregularities in heart rhythm, are treated properly. It's important to make certain that a blockage doesn't develop in the pulmonary veins or where they're attached to the left atrium. Heart rhythm irregularities (arrhythmias) also may occur at any time after surgery.

Hypoplastic left heart syndrome. In hypoplastic (hi"po-PLAS'tik) left heart syndrome, the left side of the heart is underdeveloped—including the aorta, aortic valve, left ventricle, and mitral valve. Blood returning from the lungs must flow through an opening in the wall between the atria, called an atrial septal defect. The right ventricle pumps the blood into the pulmonary artery, and blood reaches the aorta through a patent ductus arteriosus (PA'tent DUK'tus ar-te"re-O'sis).

The baby often seems normal at birth, but will come to medical attention within a few days as the ductus closes. Babies with this syndrome become ashen, have rapid and difficult breathing, and have difficulty feeding. This heart defect is usually fatal within the first days or months of life without treatment.

This defect isn't correctable, but some babies can be treated with a series of operations or with a heart transplant. Until an operation is performed, the ductus is kept open by intravenous (IV) medication. Because these operations are complex and different for each patient, you need to discuss all the medical and surgical options with your child's doctor. Your doctor will help you decide which is best for your baby.

If you and your child's doctor choose surgery, it will be done in several stages. The first stage, called the Norwood procedure, allows the right ventricle to pump blood to both the lungs and the body. It must be performed soon after birth. The final stage(s) has many names including bi-directional Glenn, Fontan operation, and lateral tunnel. These operations create a connection between the veins returning blue blood to the heart and the pulmonary artery. The overall goal is to allow the right ventricle to pump only oxygenated blood to the body and to prevent or reduce mixing of the red and blue blood. Some infants require several intermediate operations to achieve the final goal.

Some doctors will recommend a heart transplant to treat this problem. Although it provides the infant with a heart that has normal structure, the infant will require lifelong medications to prevent rejection.

Many other problems related to transplants can develop. You should discuss these with your doctor.

Children with hypoplastic left heart syndrome require lifelong follow-up by a cardiologist for repeated checks of how their heart is working. Virtually all the children will require heart medicines.

People with hypoplastic left heart syndrome, before and after treatment, are at risk for getting an infection on the heart's inner lining or valves (endocarditis). To help prevent this, they'll need to take antibiotics before certain dental and surgical procedures.

Good dental hygiene also lowers the risk of endocarditis. For more information about dental hygiene and preventing endocarditis, ask your pediatric cardiologist.

Section 21.3

Patent Foramen Ovale

Reprinted from "Patent Foramen Ovale (PFO)," © 2004 The Cleveland Clinic Foundation, 9500 Euclid Avenue, Cleveland, OH 44195, www .clevelandclinic.org. Additional information is available from the Cleveland Clinic Health Information Center, 216-444-3771, toll-free 800-223-2273 extension 43771, or at http://www.clevelandclinic.org/health.

What is a patent foramen ovale (PFO)?

A patent foramen ovale (PFO) is a defect in the septum (wall) between the two upper (atrial) chambers of the heart. Specifically, the defect is an incomplete closure of the atrial septum that results in the creation of a flap or a valve-like opening in the atrial septal wall (see Figure 21.1). A PFO is frequent in everyone before birth but seals shut in about 80 percent of people.

When a person with this defect creates pressure inside his or her chest—such as when coughing, sneezing, or straining during a bowel movement—the flap can open, and blood can flow in either direction directly between the right and left atrium. When blood moves directly from the right atrium to the left atrium, this blood bypasses the filtering system of the lungs. If debris is present in the blood, such as small blood clots, it can pass through the left atrium and lodge in the brain, causing a stroke, or in another organ, such as the heart, eyes, or kidneys.

What are the symptoms of a PFO?

PFOs are not uncommon and usually cause no symptoms at all. One in five people have a PFO but less than 1 percent have a stroke or other cause to have the PFO closed.

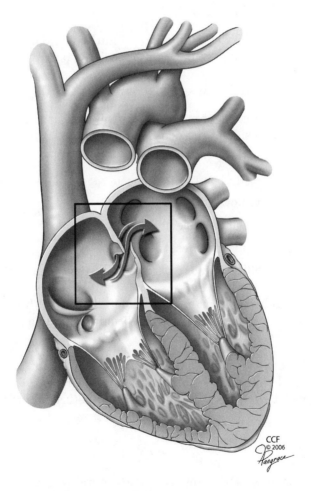

Figure 21.1. Patent foramen ovale.

What causes a PFO?

A PFO is congenital, meaning it is a defect that is inborn or exists at birth. Stated another way, the defect is an abnormality, not a disease. The septum between the two atria of the heart developed normally before birth but the flap did not seal completely after birth.

Sometimes a viral infection can cause heart defects to develop, and other causes include genetic factors, certain other medical conditions (Down syndrome, for example), and some prescription and nonprescription drugs, but 95 percent of the time a cause cannot be identified.

How is a PFO diagnosed?

Frequently a PFO is not diagnosed until a child or adult with this defect has a transient ischemic attack (TIA) (symptoms of a stroke that last for less than twenty-four hours) or a stroke. Symptoms of a TIA or stroke include any of the following:

- Sudden numbness or weakness in the face, arm, or leg (especially on one side of the body)
- Difficulty speaking or understanding words or simple sentences
- Sudden blurred vision or decreased vision in one or both eyes
- Difficulty swallowing
- Dizziness, loss of balance or coordination
- Brief loss of consciousness
- Sudden inability to move part of the body (paralysis)

A PFO can be detected only by a specialized test. It does not cause a heart murmur. If a PFO is suspected, your doctor will order tests that can include:

- **electrocardiogram (ECG or EKG):** a test that records the electrical changes that occur during a heartbeat; reveals abnormal heart rhythms (arrhythmias) and detects heart muscle stress;

- **chest x-ray:** a test to show the size and shape of the heart and lungs;

- **echocardiogram:** a test that uses sound waves to create a moving picture of the heart's internal structures;

- **Doppler ultrasound:** a test that uses sound waves to measure blood flow; often combined with echocardiogram to evaluate both the internal structure of the heart and blood flow across the heart's valves;

- **transesophageal echocardiography:** an ultrasound test used to visualize the heart and defect, where an imaging probe with a camera is placed into the esophagus;

- **cardiac magnetic resonance imaging (MRI):** a test that uses three-dimensional imaging to reveal how blood flows through the heart and how the heart is working;

- **cardiac catheterization:** a procedure that involves inserting a thin tube (a catheter) into a vein or artery and passing it into the heart to sample the level of oxygen, measure pressure changes, and make x-ray movies of the heart and its internal structures;

- **angiography:** a dye-enhanced x-ray of the heart's internal structures.

Additional tests may be ordered as necessary.

How are PFOs treated?

If you or your child is diagnosed with a PFO, your primary care doctor will recommend that you meet with a congenital heart specialist (a doctor who has the training and equipment to determine the heart problem) who will order the necessary special tests, medical care, and follow-up checkups. A careful assessment of the patient's stroke (if he or she has already experienced one) by a neurologist will first need to be done to determine the best course of action for the PFO.

The usual care for a patient who has had a stroke is the use of blood-thinning medications, such as aspirin or the prescription drugs warfarin (Coumadin) or clopidogrel (Plavix). These drugs keep the blood cells from sticking together, reducing the risk of blood clot development that could lead to new TIAs or stroke.

However, there are risks and inconveniences associated with the long-term use of blood-thinning medications, including:

- development of ulcers;
- internal bleeding;
- bleeding in the brain;

- blood in the urine;

- bleeding in the rectal tissue;

- the need to avoid activities that could result in injury, which could trigger internal or external bleeding.

An alternative for patients unable to take blood-thinning drugs or those who have a second stroke while on blood-thinning drugs is non-surgical (catheter based) closure of the hole.

Section 21.4

Arteriovenous Malformation

Reprinted from "Arteriovenous Malformations and Other Vascular Lesions of the Central Nervous System Fact Sheet," National Institute of Neurological Disorders and Stroke, National Institutes of Health, January 23, 2006.

What are arteriovenous malformations?

Arteriovenous malformations (AVMs) are defects of the circulatory system that are generally believed to arise during embryonic or fetal development or soon after birth. They are comprised of snarled tangles of arteries and veins. Arteries carry oxygen-rich blood away from the heart to the body's cells; veins return oxygen-depleted blood to the lungs and heart. The presence of an AVM disrupts this vital cyclical process. Although AVMs can develop in many different sites, those located in the brain or spinal cord—the two parts of the central nervous system—can have especially widespread effects on the body.

AVMs of the brain or spinal cord (neurological AVMs) are believed to affect approximately 300,000 Americans. They occur in males and females of all racial or ethnic backgrounds at roughly equal rates.

What are the symptoms?

Most people with neurological AVMs experience few, if any, significant symptoms, and the malformations tend to be discovered only incidentally, usually either at autopsy or during treatment for an unrelated disorder. But for about 12 percent of the affected population (about 36,000 of the estimated 300,000 Americans with AVMs), these abnormalities cause symptoms that vary greatly in severity. For a small fraction of the individuals within this group, such symptoms are severe enough to become debilitating or even life threatening. Each year about 1 percent of those with AVMs will die as a direct result of the AVM.

Seizures and headaches are the most generalized symptoms of AVMs, but no particular type of seizure or headache pattern has been identified. Seizures can be partial or total, involving a loss of control over movement, convulsions, or a change in a person's level of consciousness. Headaches can vary greatly in frequency, duration, and intensity, sometimes becoming as severe as migraines. Sometimes a headache consistently affecting one side of the head may be closely linked to the site of an AVM. More frequently, however, the location of the pain is not specific to the lesion and may encompass most of the head.

AVMs also can cause a wide range of more specific neurological symptoms that vary from person to person, depending primarily upon the location of the AVM. Such symptoms may include muscle weakness or paralysis in one part of the body; a loss of coordination (ataxia) that can lead to such problems as gait disturbances; apraxia, or difficulties carrying out tasks that require planning; dizziness; visual disturbances such as a loss of part of the visual field; an inability to control eye movement; papilledema (swelling of a part of the optic nerve known as the optic disk); various problems using or understanding language (aphasia); abnormal sensations such as numbness, tingling, or spontaneous pain (paresthesia or dysesthesia); memory deficits; and mental confusion, hallucinations, or dementia. Researchers have recently uncovered evidence that AVMs may also cause subtle learning or behavioral disorders in some people during their childhood or adolescence, long before more obvious symptoms become evident.

One of the more distinctive signs indicating the presence of an AVM is an auditory phenomenon called a bruit, coined from the French word meaning noise. (A sign is a physical effect observable by a physician, but not by a patient.) Doctors use this term to describe the rhythmic, whooshing sound caused by excessively rapid blood flow through the arteries and veins of an AVM. The sound is similar to that made by a torrent of water rushing through a narrow pipe. A bruit can sometimes become a symptom—that is, an effect experienced by a patient—when it is especially severe. When audible to patients, the bruit may compromise hearing, disturb sleep, or cause significant psychological distress.

Symptoms caused by AVMs can appear at any age, but because these abnormalities tend to result from a slow buildup of neurological damage over time they are most often noticed when people are in their twenties, thirties, or forties. If AVMs do not become symptomatic by the time people reach their late forties or early fifties, they tend to remain stable and rarely produce symptoms. In women, pregnancy sometimes causes a sudden onset or worsening of symptoms, due to accompanying cardiovascular changes, especially increases in blood volume and blood pressure.

In contrast to the vast majority of neurological AVMs, one especially severe type causes symptoms to appear at, or very soon after, birth. Called a vein of Galen defect after the major blood vessel involved, this lesion is located deep inside the brain. It is frequently associated with hydrocephalus (an accumulation of fluid within certain spaces in the brain, often with visible enlargement of the head), swollen veins visible on the scalp, seizures, failure to thrive, and congestive heart failure. Children born with this condition who survive past infancy often remain developmentally impaired.

How do AVMs damage the brain and spinal cord?

AVMs become symptomatic only when the damage they cause to the brain or spinal cord reaches a critical level. This is one of the reasons why a relatively small fraction of people with these lesions experiences significant health problems related to the condition. AVMs damage the brain or spinal cord through three basic mechanisms: by reducing the amount of oxygen reaching neurological tissues; by causing bleeding (hemorrhage) into surrounding tissues; and by compressing or displacing parts of the brain or spinal cord.

AVMs compromise oxygen delivery to the brain or spinal cord by altering normal patterns of blood flow. Arteries and veins are normally interconnected by a series of progressively smaller blood vessels that control and slow the rate of blood flow. Oxygen delivery to surrounding tissues takes place through the thin, porous walls of the smallest of these interconnecting vessels, known as capillaries, where the blood flows most slowly. The arteries and veins that make up AVMs, however, lack this intervening capillary network. Instead, arteries dump blood directly into veins through a passageway called a fistula. The flow rate is uncontrolled and extremely rapid—too rapid to allow oxygen to be dispersed to surrounding tissues. When starved of normal amounts of oxygen, the cells that make up these tissues begin to deteriorate, sometimes dying off completely.

This abnormally rapid rate of blood flow frequently causes blood pressure inside the vessels located in the central portion of an AVM directly adjacent to the fistula—an area doctors refer to as the nidus, from the Latin word for nest—to rise to dangerously high levels. The arteries feeding blood into the AVM often become swollen and distorted; the veins that drain blood away from it often become abnormally constricted (a condition called stenosis). Moreover, the walls of the involved arteries and veins are often abnormally thin and weak. Aneurysms—balloon-like bulges in blood vessel walls that are susceptible to rupture—may develop in association with approximately half of all neurological AVMs due to this structural weakness.

Bleeding can result from this combination of high internal pressure and vessel wall weakness. Such hemorrhages are often microscopic in size, causing limited damage and few significant symptoms. Even many nonsymptomatic AVMs show evidence of past bleeding. But massive hemorrhages can occur if the physical stresses caused by extremely high blood pressure, rapid blood flow rates, and vessel wall weakness are great enough. If a large enough volume of blood escapes from a ruptured AVM into the surrounding brain, the result can be a catastrophic stroke. AVMs account for approximately 2 percent of all hemorrhagic strokes that occur each year.

Even in the absence of bleeding or significant oxygen depletion, large AVMs can damage the brain or spinal cord simply by their presence. They can range in size from a fraction of an inch to more than 2.5 inches in diameter, depending on the number and size of the blood vessels making up the lesion. The larger the lesion, the greater the amount of pressure it exerts on surrounding brain or spinal cord structures. The largest lesions may compress several inches of the spinal cord or distort the shape of an entire hemisphere of the brain. Such massive AVMs can constrict the flow of cerebrospinal fluid—a clear liquid that normally nourishes and protects the brain and spinal cord—by distorting or closing the passageways and open chambers (ventricles) inside the brain that allow this fluid to circulate freely. As cerebrospinal fluid accumulates, hydrocephalus results. This fluid buildup further increases the amount of pressure on fragile neurological structures, adding to the damage caused by the AVM itself.

Where do neurological AVMs tend to form?

AVMs can form virtually anywhere in the brain or spinal cord—wherever arteries and veins exist. Some are formed from blood vessels located in the dura mater or in the pia mater, the outermost and innermost, respectively, of the three membranes surrounding the brain and spinal cord. (The third membrane, called the arachnoid, lacks blood vessels.) AVMs affecting the spinal cord are of two types, AVMs of the dura mater, which affect the function of the spinal cord by transmitting excess pressure to the venous system of the spinal cord, and AVMs of the spinal cord itself, which affect the function of the spinal cord by hemorrhage, by reducing blood flow to the spinal cord, or by causing excess venous pressure. Spinal AVMs frequently cause attacks of sudden, severe back pain, often concentrated at the roots of nerve fibers where they exit the vertebrae; the pain is similar to that caused by a slipped disk. These lesions also can cause sensory disturbances, muscle weakness, or paralysis in the parts of the body served by the spinal cord or the damaged nerve fibers. Spinal cord injury by the AVM by either of the mechanisms described above can lead to degeneration of the nerve fibers within the spinal cord below the level of the lesion, causing widespread paralysis in parts of the body controlled by those nerve fibers.

Dural and pial AVMs can appear anywhere on the surface of the brain. Those located on the surface of the cerebral hemispheres—the uppermost portions of the brain—exert pressure on the cerebral cortex, the brain's "gray matter." Depending on their location, these AVMs may damage portions of the cerebral cortex involved with thinking, speaking, understanding language, hearing, taste, touch, or initiating and controlling voluntary movements. AVMs located on the frontal lobe close to the optic nerve or on the occipital lobe, the rear portion of the cerebrum where images are processed, may cause a variety of visual disturbances.

AVMs also can form from blood vessels located deep inside the interior of the cerebrum. These AVMs may compromise the functions of three vital structures: the thalamus, which transmits nerve signals between the spinal cord and upper regions of the brain; the basal ganglia surrounding the thalamus, which coordinate complex movements; and the hippocampus, which plays a major role in memory.

AVMs can affect other parts of the brain besides the cerebrum. The hindbrain is formed from two major structures: the cerebellum, which is nestled under the rear portion of the cerebrum, and the brainstem, which serves as the bridge linking the upper portions of the brain with the spinal cord. These structures control finely coordinated movements, maintain balance, and regulate some functions of internal organs, including those of the heart and lungs. AVM damage to these parts of the hindbrain can result in dizziness, giddiness, vomiting, a loss of the ability to coordinate complex movements such as walking, or uncontrollable muscle tremors.

What are the health consequences of AVMs?

The greatest potential danger posed by AVMs is hemorrhage. Researchers believe that each year between 2 and 4 percent of all AVMs hemorrhage. Most episodes of bleeding remain undetected at the time they occur because they are not severe enough to cause significant neurological damage. But massive, even fatal, bleeding episodes do occur. The present state of knowledge does not permit doctors to predict whether or not any particular person with an AVM will suffer an extensive hemorrhage. The lesions can remain stable or can suddenly begin to grow. In a few cases, they have been observed to regress spontaneously. Whenever an AVM is detected, the individual should be carefully and consistently monitored for any signs of instability that may indicate an increased risk of hemorrhage.

A few physical characteristics appear to indicate a greater-than-usual likelihood of clinically significant hemorrhage. Smaller AVMs have a greater likelihood of bleeding than do larger ones. Impaired drainage by unusually narrow or deeply situated veins also increases the chances of hemorrhage. Pregnancy also appears to increase the likelihood of clinically significant hemorrhage, mainly because of increases in blood pressure and blood volume. Finally, AVMs that have hemorrhaged once are about nine times more likely to bleed again during the first year after the initial hemorrhage than are lesions that have never bled.

The damaging effects of a hemorrhage are related to lesion location. Bleeding from AVMs located deep inside the interior tissues, or parenchyma, of the brain typically causes more severe neurological damage than does hemorrhage by lesions that have formed in the dural or pial membranes or on the surface of the brain or spinal cord. (Deeply located bleeding is usually referred to as an intracerebral or parenchymal hemorrhage; bleeding within the membranes or on the surface of the brain is known as subdural or subarachnoid hemorrhage.) Thus, location is an important factor to consider when weighing the relative risks of surgical versus nonsurgical treatment of AVMs.

What other types of vascular lesions affect the central nervous system?

Besides AVMs, three other main types of vascular lesion can arise in the brain or spinal cord: cavernous malformations, capillary telangiectases, and venous malformations. These lesions may form virtually anywhere within the central nervous system, but unlike AVMs, they are not caused by high-velocity blood flow from arteries into veins. In contrast, cavernous malformations, telangiectases, and venous malformations are all low-flow lesions. Instead of a combination of arteries and veins, each one involves only one type of blood vessel. These lesions are less unstable than AVMs and do not pose the same relatively high risk of significant hemorrhage. In general, low-flow lesions tend to cause fewer troubling neurological symptoms and require less aggressive treatment than do AVMs.

- **Cavernous malformations.** These lesions are formed from groups of tightly packed, abnormally thin-walled, small blood vessels that displace normal neurological tissue in the brain or spinal cord. The vessels are filled with slow-moving or stagnant blood that is usually clotted or in a state of decomposition. Like AVMs, cavernous malformations can range in size from a few fractions of an inch to several inches in diameter, depending on the number of blood vessels involved. Some people develop multiple lesions. Although cavernous malformations usually do not hemorrhage as severely as AVMs do, they sometimes leak blood into surrounding neurological tissues because the walls of the involved blood vessels are extremely fragile. Although they are often not as symptomatic as AVMs, cavernous malformations can cause seizures in some people. After AVMs, cavernous malformations are the type of vascular lesion most likely to require treatment.

- **Capillary telangiectases.** These lesions consist of groups of abnormally swollen capillaries and usually measure less than an inch in diameter. Capillaries are the smallest of all blood vessels, with diameters smaller than that of a human hair; they have the capacity to transport only small quantities of blood, and blood flows through these vessels very slowly. Because of these factors, telangiectases rarely cause extensive damage to surrounding brain or spinal cord tissues. Any isolated hemorrhages that occur are microscopic in size. Thus, the lesions are usually benign. However, in some inherited disorders in which people develop large numbers of these lesions (see following), telangiectases can contribute to the development of nonspecific neurological symptoms such as headaches or seizures.

- **Venous malformations.** These lesions consist of abnormally enlarged veins. The structural defect usually does not interfere with the function of the blood vessels, which is to drain oxygen-depleted blood away from the body's tissues and return it to the lungs and heart. Venous malformations rarely hemorrhage. As with telangiectases, most venous malformations do not produce symptoms, remain undetected, and follow a benign course.

What causes vascular lesions?

Although the cause of these vascular anomalies of the central nervous system is not yet well understood, scientists believe that they most often result from mistakes that occur during embryonic or fetal development. These mistakes may be linked to genetic mutations in some cases. A few types of vascular malformations are known to be hereditary and thus are known to have a genetic basis. Some evidence also suggests that at least some of these lesions are acquired later in life as a result of injury to the central nervous system.

During fetal development, new blood vessels continuously form and then disappear as the human body changes and grows. These changes in the body's vascular map continue after birth and are controlled by angiogenic factors, chemicals produced by the body that stimulate new blood vessel formation and growth. Researchers have recently identified changes in the chemical structures of various angiogenic factors in some people who have AVMs or other vascular abnormalities of the central nervous system. However, it is not yet clear how these chemical changes actually cause changes in blood vessel structure.

By studying patterns of familial occurrence, researchers have established that one type of cavernous malformation involving multiple lesion formation is caused by a genetic mutation in chromosome 7. This genetic mutation appears in many ethnic groups, but it is especially frequent in a large population of Hispanic Americans living in the Southwest; these individuals share a common ancestor in whom the genetic change occurred. Some other types of vascular defects of the central nervous system are part of larger medical syndromes known to be hereditary. They include hereditary hemorrhagic telangiectasia (also known as Osler-Weber-Rendu disease), Sturge-Weber syndrome, Klippel-Trenaunay syndrome, Parkes Weber syndrome, and Wyburn-Mason syndrome.

How are AVMs and other vascular lesions detected?

Physicians now use an array of traditional and new imaging technologies to uncover the presence of AVMs. Angiography provides the most accurate pictures of blood vessel structure in AVMs. The technique requires injecting a special water-soluble dye, called a contrast agent, into an artery. The dye highlights the structure of blood vessels so that it can be recorded on conventional x-rays. Although angiography can record fine details of vascular lesions, the procedure is somewhat invasive and carries a slight risk of causing a stroke. Its safety, however, has recently been improved through the development of more precise techniques for delivering dye to the site of an AVM. Superselective angiography involves inserting a thin, flexible tube called a catheter into an artery; a physician guides the tip of the catheter to the site of the lesion and then releases a small amount of contrast agent directly into the lesion.

Two of the most frequently employed noninvasive imaging technologies used to detect AVMs are computed axial tomography (CT) and magnetic resonance imaging (MRI) scans. CT scans use x-rays to create a series of cross-sectional images of the head, brain, or spinal cord and are especially useful in revealing the presence of hemorrhage. MRI imaging, however, offers superior diagnostic information by using magnetic fields to detect subtle changes in neurological tissues. A recently developed application of MRI technology—magnetic resonance angiography (MRA)—can record the pattern and velocity of blood flow through vascular lesions as well as the flow of cerebrospinal fluid throughout the brain and spinal cord. CT, MRI, and MRA can provide three-dimensional representations of AVMs by taking images from multiple angles.

How can AVMs and other vascular lesions be treated?

Medication can often alleviate general symptoms such as headache, back pain, and seizures caused by AVMs and other vascular lesions. However, the definitive treatment for AVMs is either surgery or focused irradiation therapy. Venous malformations and capillary telangiectases rarely require surgery; moreover, their structures are diffuse and usually not suitable for surgical correction and they usually do not require treatment anyway. Cavernous malformations are usually well defined enough for surgical removal, but surgery on these lesions is less common than for AVMs because they do not pose the same risk of hemorrhage.

The decision to perform surgery on any individual with an AVM requires a careful consideration of possible benefits versus risks. The natural history of an individual AVM is difficult to predict; however, left untreated, they have the potential of causing significant hemorrhage, which may result in serious neurological deficits or death. On the other hand, surgery on any part of the central nervous system carries its own risks as well; AVM surgery is associated with an estimated 8 percent risk of serious complications or death. There is no easy formula that can allow physicians and their patients to reach a decision on the best course of therapy—all therapeutic decisions must be made on a case-by-case basis.

Today, three surgical options exist for the treatment of AVMs: conventional surgery, endovascular embolization, and radiosurgery. The choice of treatment depends largely on the size and location of an AVM.

Conventional surgery involves entering the brain or spinal cord and removing the central portion of the AVM, including the fistula, while causing as little damage as possible to surrounding neurological structures. This surgery is most appropriate when an AVM is located in a superficial portion of the brain or spinal cord and is relatively small in size. AVMs located deep inside the brain generally cannot be approached through conventional surgical techniques because there is too great a possibility that functionally important brain tissue will be damaged or destroyed.

Endovascular embolization and radiosurgery are less invasive than conventional surgery and offer safer treatment options for some AVMs located deep inside the brain. In endovascular embolization the surgeon guides a catheter though the arterial network until the tip reaches the site of the AVM. The surgeon then introduces a substance that will plug the fistula, correcting the abnormal pattern of blood flow. This process is known as embolization because it causes an embolus (a blood clot) to travel through blood vessels, eventually becoming lodged in a vessel and obstructing blood flow. The materials used to create an artificial blood clot in the center of an AVM include fast-drying biologically inert glues, fibered titanium coils, and tiny balloons. Since embolization usually does not permanently obliterate the AVM, it is usually used as an adjunct to surgery or to radiosurgery to reduce the blood flow through the AVM and make the surgery safer.

Radiosurgery is an even less invasive therapeutic approach. It involves aiming a beam of highly focused radiation directly on the AVM. The high dose of radiation damages the walls of the blood vessels making up the lesion. Over the course of the next several months, the irradiated vessels gradually degenerate and eventually close, leading to the resolution of the AVM.

Embolization frequently proves incomplete or temporary, although in recent years new embolization materials have led to improved results. Radiosurgery often has incomplete results as well, particularly when an AVM is large, and it poses the additional risk of radiation damage to surrounding normal tissues. Moreover, even when successful, complete closure of an AVM takes place over the course of many months following radiosurgery. During that period, the risk of hemorrhage is still present. However, both techniques now offer the possibility of treating deeply situated AVMs that had previously been inaccessible. And in many patients, staged embolization followed by conventional surgical removal or by radiosurgery is now performed, resulting in further reductions in mortality and complication rates.

Because so many variables are involved in treating AVMs, doctors must assess the danger posed to individual patients largely on a case-by-case basis. The consequences of hemorrhage are potentially disastrous, leading many clinicians to recommend surgical intervention whenever the physical characteristics of an AVM appear to indicate a greater-than-usual likelihood of significant bleeding and resultant neurological damage.

What research is being done?

Within the federal government, the National Institute of Neurological Disorders and Stroke (NINDS), a division of the National Institutes of Health (NIH), has primary responsibility for sponsoring research on neurological disorders. As part of its mission, the NINDS conducts research on AVMs and other vascular lesions of the central nervous system and supports studies through grants to major medical institutions across the country.

In partnership with the medical school of Columbia University, the NINDS has established a long-term Arteriovenous Study Group to learn more about the natural course of AVMs in patients and to improve the surgical treatment of these lesions.

Another group of NINDS -sponsored researchers is currently studying large populations of patients with AVMs to formulate criteria that will allow doctors to predict more accurately the risk of hemorrhage in individual patients. Of particular importance is the role that high blood pressure within the lesion plays in the onset of hemorrhage. Other scientists are examining the genetic basis of familial cavernous malformations and other hereditary syndromes that cause neurological vascular lesions, including ataxia telangiectasia.

Other scientists are seeking to refine the techniques now available to treat AVMs. Radiosurgery is a special area of interest because this technology is still in its infancy. An ongoing study is closely examining the precise effects that radiation exposure has on vascular tissue in order to improve the predictability and consistency of treatment results.

Finally, several ongoing studies are devoted to developing new noninvasive neuroimaging technologies to increase the effectiveness and safety of AVM surgery. Some scientists are pioneering the use of MRI to measure amounts of oxygen present in the brain tissue of patients with vascular lesions in order to predict the brain's response to surgical therapies. Others are developing a new micro-imager that may be inserted into catheters to increase the accuracy of angiography. In addition, new types of noninvasive imaging devices are being developed that detect functional brain activity through changes in tissue light emission or reflectance. This technology may prove more sensitive than MRI and other imaging devices currently available, giving surgeons a new tool for improving the efficacy and safety of AVM surgery.

Section 21.5

Persistent Pulmonary Hypertension of the Newborn

This information was provided by KidsHealth, one of the largest resources online for medically reviewed health information written for parents, kids, and teens. For more articles like this one, visit www.KidsHealth.org, or www.TeensHealth.org. © 2001 The Nemours Center for Children's Health Media, a division of The Nemours Foundation.

After you endure labor and delivery, the first few cries of your newborn are a sweet reward that indicates your baby is healthy and strong. After all, a hearty yell means your infant was born with a healthy set of lungs, right?

But some newborns may experience breathing and lung function problems immediately after birth. Most of the time, these babies recover quickly and uneventfully, especially if they are full term. But others continue to have breathing complications that are more serious and require a longer course of treatment and intensive care.

Although persistent pulmonary hypertension of the newborn (PPHN) isn't common, it can seriously compromise a newborn's health and have long-term complications. Fortunately, better understanding of newborn lung function and technology has improved the outcome for infants affected by this serious condition. Keep reading to learn more about causes and treatment of PPHN.

What Is Persistent Pulmonary Hypertension of the Newborn?

In the womb, the pathway of your baby's blood circulation is different than it is after birth.

In the uterus, a baby's circulation bypasses the lungs. The lungs are not needed to exchange oxygen because the placenta (the organ that nourishes and protects your developing baby) supplies the baby with oxygen through the umbilical cord. The pulmonary artery—which, after birth, will carry blood from the heart to the lungs—instead sends blood directly back to the heart through a fetal blood vessel called the ductus arteriosus.

Normally, when a baby is born and begins to breathe air, his circulatory system quickly adapts to the outside world. The pressure in the lungs changes as air enters and inflates the lungs. As a result, the ductus arteriosus, which previously supplied the fetal heart with blood, permanently closes. Blood returning to the heart from the body can now be pumped into the lungs, where oxygen and carbon dioxide are exchanged. The blood is then returned to the heart and pumped back out to the body in an oxygen-rich state.

In a baby with PPHN, however, the fetal circulatory system doesn't "switch over." The ductus arteriosus remains open, and the baby's blood flow continues to bypass the lungs. Even though the baby is breathing, oxygen in the breathed air will not reach the bloodstream. Because the blood returning from the body is unable to enter the lungs properly—and instead flows through the still-open ductus arteriosus—it returns to the heart in an oxygen-poor state. This condition is known as persistent fetal circulation, or PFC.

"The baby's circulation has not made the normal transition from fetal circulation to normal newborn circulation, because pressure in the lungs is increased and this causes distress," says Neal Cohn, M.D., a pediatrician. Depending on the degree of PPHN causing the persistent fetal circulation, the oxygen in the air your baby breathes into his lungs is not adequately picked up and carried by the blood to other areas of the body that need it (such as the brain, kidneys, liver, and other organs). These organs soon become stressed from lack of oxygen.

PPHN sometimes develops as the result of another event during delivery or from a disease or congenital condition affecting the newborn (usually one that directly affects either the lungs or oxygen supply to the baby before or during birth). Often, however, PPHN occurs as an isolated condition, and its cause is not known. It is usually seen soon after birth, often within twelve hours after birth. PPHN occurs in approximately one in seven hundred births.

What Causes PPHN?

In an otherwise healthy newborn, the cause of PPHN is usually unknown. Some researchers believe that stress while the baby is in the uterus (associated with certain pregnancy complications, such as maternal diabetes, high blood pressure or anemia, or delivery after forty weeks) may increase the risk of developing PPHN.

PPHN may occur with certain diseases or congenital conditions of the infant that affect the lungs in some way. Meconium aspiration syndrome, anemia, severe pneumonia, infection, hypoglycemia (low blood sugar), and birth asphyxia (when the baby is deprived of oxygen during a complicated delivery) have all been associated with PPHN.

These conditions may cause the pressure in the blood vessels leading to the lungs to increase to the point where the baby's blood continues to bypass the lungs after birth, resulting in PFC. These conditions are often temporary and reversible, with intensive care and time for the lungs and body to heal. Certain congenital conditions that result in immature or incomplete lung development (such as diaphragmatic hernia) may also be associated with PPHN.

Signs and Symptoms

The following signs and symptoms may indicate a baby has PPHN:

- rapid breathing (also called tachypnea)

- rapid heart rate

- respiratory distress, including signs such as flaring nostrils and grunting

- cyanosis (when the skin has a bluish tinge), even while the baby is receiving extra oxygen to breathe

Sometimes when examining a baby with PPHN, the doctor will hear a heart murmur (an extra or abnormal heart sound). With PPHN, a baby may also continue to have low oxygen levels in the blood while receiving 100 percent oxygen.

How Is It Diagnosed and Treated?

For any newborn having difficulty breathing and showing signs of poor oxygen delivery to the body's tissues, several tests will be performed to determine possible causes. Various imaging and laboratory tests can help determine if a baby has PPHN.

Imaging tests will be done to get a better look at the lungs, heart, and circulation, and to check for other possible causes of the baby's problems:

- Chest x-rays can show whether the baby has lung disease and whether the heart is enlarged.

- An ultrasound of the heart (an echocardiogram) can show whether the baby has heart or lung disease and can determine the direction of blood flow in those organs. This test is often very helpful in diagnosing PPHN because it will show the doctor the baby's circulating blood flow, including whether the ductus arteriosus is open or closed, and can determine if PFC exists.

- An ultrasound of the head may be used to look for bleeding in the brain.

Laboratory tests can also assist doctors in making a diagnosis of PPHN:

- An arterial blood gas (ABG) determines how much oxygen, carbon dioxide, and acid buildup are in the arterial blood. Arteries normally contain high levels of oxygen, and this test is the most accurate way to determine how well oxygen is being delivered to the body.

- A complete blood count (CBC) measures the number of oxygen-carrying red blood cells, white blood cells (which help fight infection), and platelets (which are involved in blood clotting). A CBC usually shows if anemia or possible infection is causing the baby to be ill.

- Serum electrolyte tests evaluate the balance of minerals in the blood.

- A lumbar puncture (spinal tap) and other blood tests can help determine whether an infection is present.

- Pulse oximetry, which measures oxygen levels in the blood, can help doctors monitor whether the baby's tissues are receiving an adequate amount of oxygen.

A doctor who specializes in newborn problems, called a neonatologist, will direct the treatment for a child with PPHN. Babies with PPHN usually need to be cared for in a neonatal intensive care unit (NICU). NICUs are usually found in larger hospitals or children's hospitals.

The first step in PPHN treatment is to maximize the amount of oxygen delivered to the baby's lungs (and, in turn, to the blood), so 100 percent oxygen will be given through a tube inserted directly into the baby's trachea (windpipe). The oxygen is administered by a mechanical ventilator, which does the work of breathing for the baby. This treatment is given in conjunction with other treatments for the illnesses that may have contributed to the initial development of PPHN (such as low blood sugar, pneumonia, or other infections).

If your child has PPHN caused by a lung problem, his breathing rate may be set at a higher than usual rate and pressure through the mechanical ventilator. This is known as high-frequency oscillatory ventilation (HFOV). This ventilation technique improves oxygen delivery to the lungs, reduces acid buildup in the blood, and often helps open up the blood vessels leading the lungs—thus allowing more blood to flow to the lungs. Because PPHN is worsened by narrowed lung blood vessels and raised acid levels in the body (a condition called acidosis), sodium bicarbonate may also be given with this form of ventilation to lower acid levels and help dilate blood vessels.

Recent research shows that supplying inhaled nitric oxide to babies with PPHN may also be successful. Nitric oxide has been shown to have a relaxing effect on contracted lung blood vessels, thus improving blood flow to the lungs in some babies with PPHN.

If other methods can't reverse the PPHN and raise the baby's oxygen levels to the necessary range, a type of intensive procedure called extracorporeal membrane oxygenation (ECMO) may be needed. ECMO requires major surgery, is complicated to monitor, and has potentially serious side effects associated with it. It is reserved for the sickest babies who are not responding to other forms of treatment.

The ECMO machine acts as an artificial heart and lung for the baby for several days while the baby's lungs heal and recover. Although

ECMO is very successful in treating PPHN, fewer than one hundred hospitals (mostly children's hospitals) in the United States have facilities that can provide this treatment.

Complications and Prognosis

PPHN is a serious condition and intensive monitoring and treatment are critical. Even with prompt recognition and treatment, an infant with PPHN may continue to supply an inadequate amount of oxygen to the body's tissues, resulting in shock, heart failure, brain hemorrhage, seizures, kidney failure, multiple organ damage, and possibly even death.

Some causes of PPHN are treatable and reversible; others are associated with a poor survival rate, even if nitric oxide and ECMO are used. In some newborns with PPHN, the lungs are too diseased or malformed to heal adequately, even if the baby stays on ECMO for a longer period of time.

Periods of inadequate oxygenation can have long-term effects on infants who survive PPHN, such as bronchopulmonary dysplasia (a chronic lung disease associated with scarred, stiffened lungs) and breathing difficulties. Seizure disorders, developmental delay, and neurological deficits may also be seen.

For several weeks following treatment, infants who've had PPHN may not be able to take feedings by mouth. A temporary feeding tube may have to be inserted into the baby's nose, or for longer-term feeding problems, directly into the stomach through the skin on the abdomen. Feeding tubes will be needed if the baby cannot eat enough to meet his nutritional requirements for growth.

Hearing problems are another common condition associated with PPHN. If your child had PPHN, he will probably need to be evaluated by a hearing specialist during early childhood to check for hearing loss, and the development of his speech will also need to be followed closely.

Medical treatments such as high frequency ventilation, nitric oxide, and ECMO have significantly decreased the percentage of children who die from PPHN. Fifteen years ago, almost half of infants diagnosed with PPHN died; today, less than 20 percent of infants with PPHN die, and only about one-fifth of surviving infants experience long-term physical or developmental complications.

Section 21.6

Vascular Rings

What Is a Vascular Ring?

A vascular ring is a type of vascular compression syndrome, which represents a mixed bag of anomalies that share the common feature of compromise of the esophagus or airway by adjacent arterial structures.

These arteries may be those carrying blood to the body, to the lungs, or both. They are most easily segregated into three main groups: Vascular rings, the innominate compression syndrome, and pulmonary arterial slings.

Vascular rings include a number of anatomic variations of abnormal development of the aortic arch complex resulting in vascular structures completely encircling both the trachea and esophagus.

The aorta originally develops as a series of arches with bilateral symmetry.

By the end of the second month of fetal development, parts of the arch complex have regressed, leaving the "typical" anatomy of a left aortic arch with three arch branches (innominate, left common carotid, and left subclavian) and a left-sided ductus arteriosus from the proximal left pulmonary artery to the aorta in the general vicinity of the left subclavian artery origin.

Vascular rings can virtually all be explained by abnormal regression or persistence of different components of the bilateral aortic arch complex.

The two most common anatomic variants of true vascular rings, occurring in nearly equal frequency, are persistent double aortic arch and right aortic arch with anomalous origin of the left subclavian artery.

In the latter, the left-sided ligamentum arteriosum completes the vascular ring as it passes from the left pulmonary artery to the left

311

subclavian artery as it travels its abnormal course behind the esophagus.

Problems Caused by Vascular Rings

The symptoms seen with vascular rings can be quite varied. They may occasionally be noted in the newborn, but more often are recognized later.

Many cases have been described with no or minimal symptoms attributed to the anomaly. When symptoms occur early in life they are most commonly related to the airway, typically stridor (noisy breathing). Worsening of breathing difficulties with feeding or during upper respiratory infections may be seen.

Children with double aortic arch anomalies tend to present earlier than those with right aortic arch variants. Swallowing problems are uncommon in the first months of life while children are on a liquid diet.

Choking or swallowing difficulties are more common in older children as the predominant symptoms. Occasionally, a vascular ring is discovered during evaluation of a seemingly unrelated problem.

Diagnosing Vascular Rings

Physical examination may help characterize the "noisy breathing" and help differentiate it from other more common problems such as asthma.

With a vascular ring, the noisy breathing may be heard both during inspiration and expiration, while in asthma, the noise is mainly at the end of expiration.

Occasionally, physical examination will detect an abnormally weak pulse in an arm or the legs due to narrowing in a part of the anomalous blood vessels. Listening to the chest for murmurs is often included to assess the need for more thorough evaluation for associated cardiac anomalies (which are uncommon).

A chest x-ray is often performed as a part of the initial evaluation, and if the aortic arch appears to be right-sided, a vascular ring should be suspected. The identification of the side of the aortic arch on the plain chest x-ray, though, may be difficult in some children, particularly infants.

Patients with swallowing difficulties should undergo a barium swallow as part of the initial evaluation. This will typically demonstrate abnormal compression of the middle part of the esophagus characteristic for a vascular ring.

A barium study demonstrating classic features of a vascular ring, coupled with a chest x-ray showing a right-sided aortic arch is generally all that is necessary to proceed with operation.

Computed axial tomography (CT) and magnetic resonance imaging (MRI) of the chest will generally demonstrate the details of the arch anatomy extremely well and will often be ordered if the side of the aortic arch is unclear from plain x-rays.

When breathing symptoms predominate, bronchoscopy may be performed which will often demonstrate extrinsic, sometime pulsatile compression of the trachea.

Treating Vascular Rings

Operation to divide the vascular ring is indicated in all symptomatic cases. It may be argued that when the vascular ring anomaly is found "incidentally" that continued observation is appropriate.

While the symptoms prompting evaluation leading to the diagnosis may not be "classic" stridor or dysphagia (swallowing difficulty), many feel that unusual presentations such as a "barky" cough or frequent upper respiratory infections may be associated with the vascular anomaly and constitute indications for surgery.

Given the low risk associated with surgical division of a vascular ring, it is difficult to recommend continued observation, particularly in younger patients.

The goal of surgical intervention for vascular rings is to convert a restrictive, closed ring into one that is open, realizing that there may still be an abnormal course of some of the blood vessels. With the ring open in at least one direction, symptoms related to esophageal and tracheal compression will be relieved.

In most cases the operation is performed using an incision on the left side of the chest, entering between the ribs. In the case of double aortic arch, the left side of the ring (which is usually the smaller side) is divided where it is compressing the esophagus.

With a right aortic arch and anomalous left subclavian artery, the ligamentum arteriosum (a ligament that was a blood vessel during fetal life) is divided between the descending aorta and the pulmonary artery. Hospitalization after surgery is rarely more than a day or two.

Vascular Ring Treatment Results

Complete relief of symptoms may be noted immediately following operation, although persistence of some findings is not uncommon.

In infants, there may be some degree of tracheomalacia (floppiness of the trachea) associated with the vascular anomaly and persistence of some stridor, particularly during times of great activity or during upper respiratory infections, may be seen.

Depending on the specific anatomy, division of the ring may still leave either the subclavian artery or a segment of the aorta itself in an abnormal position behind the esophagus. Improvement of swallowing symptoms in such cases may be seen only gradually.

Chapter 22

Congenital Brain Defects

Chapter Contents

Section 22.1—Hydrocephalus 316
Section 22.2—Other Cephalic Disorders 322
Section 22.3—Agenesis of the Corpus Callosum 333
Section 22.4—Chiari Malformation 334
Section 22.5—Craniosynostosis 336
Section 22.6—Dandy-Walker Syndrome 337

Section 22.1

Hydrocephalus

Reprinted from "Hydrocephalus Fact Sheet,"
National Institute of Neurological Disorders and Stroke,
National Institutes of Health, NIH Publication No. 05-385,
January 25, 2006.

What is hydrocephalus?

The term hydrocephalus is derived from the Greek words "hydro," meaning water, and "cephalus," meaning head. As its name implies, it is a condition in which the primary characteristic is excessive accumulation of fluid in the brain. Although hydrocephalus was once known as "water on the brain," the "water" is actually cerebrospinal fluid (CSF)—a clear fluid surrounding the brain and spinal cord. The excessive accumulation of CSF results in an abnormal dilation of the spaces in the brain called ventricles. This dilation causes potentially harmful pressure on the tissues of the brain.

The ventricular system is made up of four ventricles connected by narrow pathways. Normally, CSF flows through the ventricles, exits into cisterns (closed spaces that serve as reservoirs) at the base of the brain, bathes the surfaces of the brain and spinal cord, and then is absorbed into the bloodstream.

CSF has three important life-sustaining functions: 1) to keep the brain tissue buoyant, acting as a cushion or "shock absorber"; 2) to act as the vehicle for delivering nutrients to the brain and removing waste; and 3) to flow between the cranium and spine to compensate for changes in intracranial blood volume (the amount of blood within the brain).

The balance between production and absorption of CSF is critically important. Ideally, the fluid is almost completely absorbed into the bloodstream as it circulates; however, there are circumstances that, when present, will prevent or disturb the production or absorption of CSF, or that will inhibit its normal flow. When this balance is disturbed, hydrocephalus is the result.

What are the different types of hydrocephalus?

Hydrocephalus may be congenital or acquired. Congenital hydrocephalus is present at birth and may be caused by either environmental influences during fetal development or genetic predisposition. Acquired hydrocephalus develops at the time of birth or at some point afterward. This type of hydrocephalus can affect individuals of all ages and may be caused by injury or disease.

Hydrocephalus may also be communicating or noncommunicating. Communicating hydrocephalus occurs when the flow of CSF is blocked after it exits from the ventricles. This form is called communicating because the CSF can still flow between the ventricles, which remain open. Noncommunicating hydrocephalus—also called "obstructive" hydrocephalus—occurs when the flow of CSF is blocked along one or more of the narrow pathways connecting the ventricles. One of the most common causes of hydrocephalus is "aqueductal stenosis." In this case, hydrocephalus results from a narrowing of the aqueduct of Sylvius, a small passageway between the third and fourth ventricles in the middle of the brain.

There are two other forms of hydrocephalus which do not fit distinctly into the categories mentioned above and primarily affect adults: hydrocephalus ex vacuo and normal pressure hydrocephalus.

Hydrocephalus ex vacuo occurs when there is damage to the brain caused by stroke or traumatic injury. In these cases, there may be actual shrinkage (atrophy or wasting) of brain tissue. Normal pressure hydrocephalus can occur in people of any age, but it is most common in the elderly population. It may result from a subarachnoid hemorrhage, head trauma, infection, tumor, or complications of surgery. However, many people develop normal pressure hydrocephalus even when none of these factors are present. In these cases the cause of the disorder is unknown.

Who gets this disorder?

Incidence and prevalence data are difficult to establish as there is no existing national registry or database of people with hydrocephalus and closely associated disorders; however, hydrocephalus is believed to affect approximately one in every five hundred children. At present, most of these cases are diagnosed prenatally, at the time of delivery, or in early childhood. Advances in diagnostic imaging technology allow more accurate diagnoses in individuals with atypical presentations, including adults with conditions such as normal pressure hydrocephalus.

What causes hydrocephalus?

The causes of hydrocephalus are not all well understood. Hydrocephalus may result from genetic inheritance (aqueductal stenosis) or developmental disorders such as those associated with neural tube defects including spina bifida and encephalocele. Other possible causes include complications of premature birth such as intraventricular hemorrhage, diseases such as meningitis, tumors, traumatic head injury, or subarachnoid hemorrhage blocking the exit from the ventricles to the cisterns and eliminating the cisterns themselves.

What are the symptoms?

Symptoms of hydrocephalus vary with age, disease progression, and individual differences in tolerance to CSF. For example, an infant's ability to tolerate CSF pressure differs from an adult's. The infant skull can expand to accommodate the buildup of CSF because the sutures (the fibrous joints that connect the bones of the skull) have not yet closed.

In infancy, the most obvious indication of hydrocephalus is often the rapid increase in head circumference or an unusually large head size. Other symptoms may include vomiting, sleepiness, irritability, downward deviation of the eyes (also called "sunsetting"), and seizures.

Older children and adults may experience different symptoms because their skulls cannot expand to accommodate the buildup of CSF. In older children or adults, symptoms may include headache followed by vomiting, nausea, papilledema (swelling of the optic disk, which is part of the optic nerve), blurred vision, diplopia (double vision), sunsetting of the eyes, problems with balance, poor coordination, gait disturbance, urinary incontinence, slowing or loss of development, lethargy, drowsiness, irritability, or other changes in personality or cognition including memory loss.

Symptoms of normal pressure hydrocephalus include progressive mental impairment and dementia, problems with walking, and impaired bladder control leading to urinary frequency and/or incontinence. The person also may have a general slowing of movements or may complain that his or her feet feel "stuck." Because these symptoms are similar to those of other disorders such as Alzheimer disease, Parkinson disease, and Creutzfeldt-Jakob disease, the disorder is often misdiagnosed. Many cases go unrecognized and are never properly treated. Doctors may use a variety of tests, including brain scans (computed tomography [CT] and/or magnetic resonance imaging

[MRI]), a spinal tap or lumbar catheter, intracranial pressure moni-toring, and neuropsychological tests, to help them diagnose normal pressure hydrocephalus and rule out other conditions.

The symptoms described in this section account for the most typi-cal ways in which progressive hydrocephalus manifests itself; it is, however, important to remember that symptoms vary significantly from individual to individual.

How is hydrocephalus diagnosed?

Hydrocephalus is diagnosed through clinical neurological evalua-tion and by using cranial imaging techniques such as ultrasonogra-phy, computed tomography (CT), magnetic resonance imaging (MRI), or pressure-monitoring techniques. A physician selects the appropri-ate diagnostic tool based on the patient's age, clinical presentation, and the presence of known or suspected abnormalities of the brain or spinal cord. In September 2005 an international team of scientists developed clinical guidelines to help physicians diagnose normal pres-sure hydrocephalus. The guidelines were published as a supplement to the journal *Neurosurgery* ("Diagnosing Idiopathic Normal-pressure Hydrocephalus," vol. 57(3), supplement: S2-4–S2-16, 2005).

What is the current treatment?

Hydrocephalus is most often treated with the surgical placement of a shunt system. This system diverts the flow of CSF from a site within the central nervous system (CNS) to another area of the body where it can be absorbed as part of the circulatory process.

A shunt is a flexible but sturdy silastic tube. A shunt system con-sists of the shunt, a catheter, and a valve. One end of the catheter is placed in the CNS—most usually within a ventricle inside the brain, but also potentially within a cyst or in a site close to the spinal cord. The other end of the catheter is commonly placed within the perito-neal (abdominal) cavity, but may also be placed at other sites within the body such as a chamber of the heart or a cavity in the lung where the CSF can drain and be absorbed. A valve located along the cath-eter maintains one-way flow and regulates the rate of CSF flow.

A limited number of patients can be treated with an alternative procedure called third ventriculostomy. In this procedure, a neuro-endoscope—a small camera designed to visualize small and difficult to reach surgical areas—allows a doctor to view the ventricular sur-face using fiber optic technology. The scope is guided into position so that a small hole can be made in the floor of the third ventricle, allowing the CSF to bypass the obstruction and flow toward the site of resorption around the surface of the brain.

What are the possible complications of a shunt system?

Shunt systems are not perfect devices. Complications may include mechanical failure, infections, obstructions, and the need to lengthen or replace the catheter. Generally, shunt systems require monitoring and regular medical follow-up. When complications do occur, usually the shunt system will require some type of revision.

Some complications can lead to other problems such as overdraining or underdraining. Overdraining occurs when the shunt allows CSF to drain from the ventricles more quickly than it is produced. This overdraining can cause the ventricles to collapse, tearing blood vessels and causing headache, hemorrhage (subdural hematoma), or slit-like ventricles (slit ventricle syndrome). Underdraining occurs when CSF is not removed quickly enough and the symptoms of hydrocephalus recur. In addition to the common symptoms of hydrocephalus, infections from a shunt may also produce symptoms such as a low-grade fever, soreness of the neck or shoulder muscles, and redness or tenderness along the shunt tract. When there is reason to suspect that a shunt system is not functioning properly (for example, if the symptoms of hydrocephalus return), medical attention should be sought immediately.

What is the prognosis?

The prognosis for patients diagnosed with hydrocephalus is difficult to predict, although there is some correlation between the specific cause of the hydrocephalus and the patient's outcome. Prognosis is further complicated by the presence of associated disorders, the timeliness of diagnosis, and the success of treatment. The degree to which decompression (relief of CSF pressure or buildup) following shunt surgery can minimize or reverse damage to the brain is not well understood.

Affected individuals and their families should be aware that hydrocephalus poses risks to both cognitive and physical development. However, many children diagnosed with the disorder benefit from rehabilitation therapies and educational interventions and go on to lead normal lives with few limitations. Treatment by an interdisciplinary team of medical professionals, rehabilitation specialists, and educational experts is critical to a positive outcome. Left untreated, progressive hydrocephalus is, with rare exceptions, fatal.

The symptoms of normal pressure hydrocephalus usually get worse over time if the condition is not treated, although some people may experience temporary improvements. While the success of treatment with shunts varies from person to person, some people recover almost completely after treatment and have a good quality of life. Early diagnosis and treatment improves the chance of a good recovery.

What research is being done?

Within the federal government, the leading supporter of research on hydrocephalus is the National Institute of Neurological Disorders and Stroke (NINDS). The NINDS, a part of the National Institutes of Health (NIH), is responsible for supporting and conducting research on the brain and the central nervous system. NINDS conducts research in its laboratories at NIH and also supports studies through grants to major medical institutions across the country.

One NINDS-supported study examined cognitive development, academic achievement, and behavioral adjustment in children with hydrocephalus. With further research, investigators hope to shed new light on the influence of hydrocephalus on development as well as the more general issue of the effect of early brain injury.

The NINDS also conducts and supports a wide range of fundamental studies that explore the complex mechanisms of normal brain development. The knowledge gained from these studies provides the foundation for understanding how this process can go awry and, thus, offers hope for new means to treat and prevent developmental brain disorders such as hydrocephalus.

Section 22.2

Other Cephalic Disorders

Reprinted from "Cephalic Disorders Fact Sheet," National Institute of Neurological Disorders and Stroke, National Institutes of Health, NIH Publication No. 98-4339, January 25, 2006.

What are cephalic disorders?

Cephalic disorders are congenital conditions that stem from damage to, or abnormal development of, the budding nervous system. Cephalic is a term that means "head" or "head end of the body." Congenital means the disorder is present at, and usually before, birth. Although there are many congenital developmental disorders, this section briefly describes only cephalic conditions.

Cephalic disorders are not necessarily caused by a single factor but may be influenced by hereditary or genetic conditions or by environmental exposures during pregnancy such as medication taken by the mother, maternal infection, or exposure to radiation. Some cephalic disorders occur when the cranial sutures (the fibrous joints that connect the bones of the skull) join prematurely. Most cephalic disorders are caused by a disturbance that occurs very early in the development of the fetal nervous system.

The human nervous system develops from a small, specialized plate of cells on the surface of the embryo. Early in development, this plate of cells forms the neural tube, a narrow sheath that closes between the third and fourth weeks of pregnancy to form the brain and spinal cord of the embryo. Four main processes are responsible for the development of the nervous system: cell proliferation, the process in which nerve cells divide to form new generations of cells; cell migration, the process in which nerve cells move from their place of origin to the place where they will remain for life; cell differentiation, the process during which cells acquire individual characteristics; and cell death, a natural process in which cells die. Understanding the normal development of the human nervous system, one of the research priorities of the National Institute of Neurological Disorders and Stroke, may lead to a better understanding of cephalic disorders.

Damage to the developing nervous system is a major cause of chronic, disabling disorders and, sometimes, death in infants, children, and even adults. The degree to which damage to the developing nervous system harms the mind and body varies enormously. Many disabilities are mild enough to allow those afflicted to eventually function independently in society. Others are not. Some infants, children, and adults die, others remain totally disabled, and an even larger population is partially disabled, functioning well below normal capacity throughout life.

What are the different kinds of cephalic disorders?

Anencephaly is a neural tube defect that occurs when the cephalic (head) end of the neural tube fails to close, usually between the twenty-third and twenty-sixth days of pregnancy, resulting in the absence of a major portion of the brain, skull, and scalp. Infants with this disorder are born without a forebrain—the largest part of the brain, consisting mainly of the cerebrum, which is responsible for thinking and coordination. The remaining brain tissue is often exposed—not covered by bone or skin.

Infants born with anencephaly are usually blind, deaf, unconscious, and unable to feel pain. Although some individuals with anencephaly may be born with a rudimentary brainstem, the lack of a functioning cerebrum permanently rules out the possibility of ever gaining consciousness. Reflex actions such as breathing and responses to sound or touch may occur. The disorder is one of the most common disorders of the fetal central nervous system. Approximately one thousand to two thousand American babies are born with anencephaly each year. The disorder affects females more often than males.

The cause of anencephaly is unknown. Although it is believed that the mother's diet and vitamin intake may play a role, scientists agree that many other factors are also involved.

There is no cure or standard treatment for anencephaly and the prognosis for affected individuals is poor. Most infants do not survive infancy. If the infant is not stillborn, then he or she will usually die within a few hours or days after birth. Anencephaly can often be diagnosed before birth through an ultrasound examination.

Recent studies have shown that the addition of folic acid to the diet of women of childbearing age may significantly reduce the incidence of neural tube defects. Therefore it is recommended that all women of childbearing age consume 0.4 mg of folic acid daily.

Colpocephaly is a disorder in which there is an abnormal enlargement of the occipital horns—the posterior or rear portion of the lateral ventricles (cavities or chambers) of the brain. This enlargement occurs when there is an underdevelopment or lack of thickening of the white matter in the posterior cerebrum. Colpocephaly is characterized by microcephaly (abnormally small head) and mental retardation. Other features may include motor abnormalities, muscle spasms, and seizures.

Although the cause is unknown, researchers believe that the disorder results from an intrauterine disturbance that occurs between the second and sixth months of pregnancy. Colpocephaly may be diagnosed late in pregnancy, although it is often misdiagnosed as hydrocephalus (excessive accumulation of cerebrospinal fluid in the brain). It may be more accurately diagnosed after birth when signs of mental retardation, microcephaly, and seizures are present.

There is no definitive treatment for colpocephaly. Anticonvulsant medications can be given to prevent seizures, and doctors try to prevent contractures (shrinkage or shortening of muscles). The prognosis for individuals with colpocephaly depends on the severity of the associated conditions and the degree of abnormal brain development. Some children benefit from special education.

Holoprosencephaly is a disorder characterized by the failure of the prosencephalon (the forebrain of the embryo) to develop. During normal development the forebrain is formed and the face begins to develop in the fifth and sixth weeks of pregnancy. Holoprosencephaly is caused by a failure of the embryo's forebrain to divide to form bilateral cerebral hemispheres (the left and right halves of the brain), causing defects in the development of the face and in brain structure and function.

There are three classifications of holoprosencephaly. Alobar holoprosencephaly, the most serious form, in which the brain fails to separate, is usually associated with severe facial anomalies. Semilobar holoprosencephaly, in which the brain's hemispheres have a slight tendency to separate, is an intermediate form of the disease. Lobar holoprosencephaly, in which there is considerable evidence of separate brain hemispheres, is the least severe form. In some cases of lobar holoprosencephaly, the patient's brain may be nearly normal.

Holoprosencephaly, once called arrhinencephaly, consists of a spectrum of defects or malformations of the brain and face. At the most severe end of this spectrum are cases involving serious malformations of the brain, malformations so severe that they are incompatible with life and often cause spontaneous intrauterine death. At the other end of the spectrum are individuals with facial defects—which may affect the eyes, nose, and upper lip—and normal or near-normal brain development. Seizures and mental retardation may occur.

The most severe of the facial defects (or anomalies) is cyclopia, an abnormality characterized by the development of a single eye, located in the area normally occupied by the root of the nose, and a missing nose or a nose in the form of a proboscis (a tubular appendage) located above the eye.

Ethmocephaly is the least common facial anomaly. It consists of a proboscis separating narrow-set eyes with an absent nose and microphthalmia (abnormal smallness of one or both eyes). Cebocephaly, another facial anomaly, is characterized by a small, flattened nose with a single nostril situated below incomplete or underdeveloped closely set eyes.

The least severe in the spectrum of facial anomalies is the median cleft lip, also called premaxillary agenesis.

Although the causes of most cases of holoprosencephaly remain unknown, researchers know that approximately one-half of all cases have a chromosomal cause. Such chromosomal anomalies as Patau syndrome (trisomy 13) and Edwards syndrome (trisomy 18) have been found in association with holoprosencephaly. There is an increased risk for the disorder in infants of diabetic mothers.

There is no treatment for holoprosencephaly and the prognosis for individuals with the disorder is poor. Most of those who survive show no significant developmental gains. For children who survive, treatment is symptomatic. Although it is possible that improved management of diabetic pregnancies may help prevent holoprosencephaly, there is no means of primary prevention.

Hydranencephaly is a rare condition in which the cerebral hemispheres are absent and replaced by sacs filled with cerebrospinal fluid. Usually the cerebellum and brainstem are formed normally. An infant with hydranencephaly may appear normal at birth. The infant's head size and spontaneous reflexes such as sucking, swallowing, crying, and moving the arms and legs may all seem normal. However, after a few weeks the infant usually becomes irritable and has increased muscle tone (hypertonia). After several months of life, seizures and hydrocephalus may develop. Other symptoms may include visual impairment, lack of growth, deafness, blindness, spastic quadriparesis (paralysis), and intellectual deficits.

Hydranencephaly is an extreme form of porencephaly (a rare disorder, discussed later in this section, characterized by a cyst or cavity in the cerebral hemispheres) and may be caused by vascular insult (such as stroke) or injuries, infections, or traumatic disorders after the twelfth week of pregnancy.

Diagnosis may be delayed for several months because the infant's early behavior appears to be relatively normal. Transillumination, an examination in which light is passed through body tissues, usually confirms the diagnosis. Some infants may have additional abnormalities at birth, including seizures, myoclonus (involuntary sudden, rapid jerks), and respiratory problems.

There is no standard treatment for hydranencephaly. Treatment is symptomatic and supportive. Hydrocephalus may be treated with a shunt.

The outlook for children with hydranencephaly is generally poor, and many children with this disorder die before age one. However, in rare cases, children with hydranencephaly may survive for several years or more.

Iniencephaly is a rare neural tube defect that combines extreme retroflexion (backward bending) of the head with severe defects of the spine. The affected infant tends to be short, with a disproportionately large head. Diagnosis can be made immediately after birth because the head is so severely retroflexed that the face looks upward. The skin of the face is connected directly to the skin of the chest and the scalp is directly connected to the skin of the back. Generally, the neck is absent.

Most individuals with iniencephaly have other associated anomalies such as anencephaly, cephalocele (a disorder in which part of the cranial contents protrudes from the skull), hydrocephalus, cyclopia, absence of the mandible (lower jaw bone), cleft lip and palate, cardiovascular disorders, diaphragmatic hernia, and gastrointestinal malformation. The disorder is more common among females.

The prognosis for those with iniencephaly is extremely poor. Newborns with iniencephaly seldom live more than a few hours. The distortion of the fetal body may also pose a danger to the mother's life.

Lissencephaly, which literally means "smooth brain," is a rare brain malformation characterized by microcephaly and the lack of normal convolutions (folds) in the brain. It is caused by defective neuronal migration, the process in which nerve cells move from their place of origin to their permanent location.

The surface of a normal brain is formed by a complex series of folds and grooves. The folds are called gyri or convolutions, and the grooves are called sulci. In children with lissencephaly, the normal convolutions are absent or only partly formed, making the surface of the brain smooth.

Symptoms of the disorder may include unusual facial appearance, difficulty swallowing, failure to thrive, and severe psychomotor retardation. Anomalies of the hands, fingers, or toes, muscle spasms, and seizures may also occur.

Lissencephaly may be diagnosed at or soon after birth. Diagnosis may be confirmed by ultrasound, computed tomography (CT), or magnetic resonance imaging (MRI).

Lissencephaly may be caused by intrauterine viral infections or viral infections in the fetus during the first trimester, insufficient blood supply to the baby's brain early in pregnancy, or a genetic disorder. There are two distinct genetic causes of lissencephaly—X-linked and chromosome 17–linked.

The spectrum of lissencephaly is only now becoming more defined as neuroimaging and genetics have provided more insights into migration disorders. Other causes that have not yet been identified are likely as well.

Lissencephaly may be associated with other diseases including isolated lissencephaly sequence, Miller-Dieker syndrome, and Walker-Warburg syndrome.

Treatment for those with lissencephaly is symptomatic and depends on the severity and locations of the brain malformations. Supportive care may be needed to help with comfort and nursing needs. Seizures may be controlled with medication and hydrocephalus may require shunting. If feeding becomes difficult, a gastrostomy tube may be considered.

The prognosis for children with lissencephaly varies depending on the degree of brain malformation. Many individuals show no significant development beyond a three- to five-month-old level. Some may have near-normal development and intelligence. Many will die before the age of two. Respiratory problems are the most common causes of death.

Megalencephaly, also called macrencephaly, is a condition in which there is an abnormally large, heavy, and usually malfunctioning brain. By definition, the brain weight is greater than average for the age and gender of the infant or child. Head enlargement may be evident at birth or the head may become abnormally large in the early years of life.

Megalencephaly is thought to be related to a disturbance in the regulation of cell reproduction or proliferation. In normal development, neuron proliferation—the process in which nerve cells divide to form new generations of cells—is regulated so that the correct number of cells is formed in the proper place at the appropriate time.

Symptoms of megalencephaly may include delayed development, convulsive disorders, corticospinal (brain cortex and spinal cord) dysfunction, and seizures. Megalencephaly affects males more often than females.

The prognosis for individuals with megalencephaly largely depends on the underlying cause and the associated neurological disorders. Treatment is symptomatic. Megalencephaly may lead to a condition called macrocephaly (defined later in this section). Unilateral megalencephaly or hemimegalencephaly is a rare condition characterized by the enlargement of one-half of the brain. Children with this disorder may have a large, sometimes asymmetrical head. Often they suffer from intractable seizures and mental retardation. The prognosis for those with hemimegalencephaly is poor.

Microcephaly is a neurological disorder in which the circumference of the head is smaller than average for the age and gender of the infant or child. Microcephaly may be congenital or it may develop in the first few years of life. The disorder may stem from a wide variety of conditions that cause abnormal growth of the brain, or from syndromes associated with chromosomal abnormalities.

Infants with microcephaly are born with either a normal or a reduced head size. Subsequently the head fails to grow while the face continues to develop at a normal rate, producing a child with a small head, a large face, a receding forehead, and a loose, often wrinkled scalp. As the child grows older, the smallness of the skull becomes more obvious, although the entire body also is often underweight and dwarfed. Development of motor functions and speech may be delayed. Hyperactivity and mental retardation are common occurrences, although the degree of each varies. Convulsions may also occur. Motor ability varies, ranging from clumsiness in some to spastic quadriplegia in others.

Generally there is no specific treatment for microcephaly. Treatment is symptomatic and supportive.

In general, life expectancy for individuals with microcephaly is reduced and the prognosis for normal brain function is poor. The prognosis varies depending on the presence of associated abnormalities.

Porencephaly is an extremely rare disorder of the central nervous system involving a cyst or cavity in a cerebral hemisphere. The cysts or cavities are usually the remnants of destructive lesions, but are sometimes the result of abnormal development. The disorder can occur before or after birth.

Porencephaly most likely has a number of different, often unknown causes, including absence of brain development and destruction of brain tissue. The presence of porencephalic cysts can sometimes be detected by transillumination of the skull in infancy. The diagnosis may be confirmed by CT, MRI, or ultrasonography.

More severely affected infants show symptoms of the disorder shortly after birth, and the diagnosis is usually made before age one. Signs may include delayed growth and development, spastic paresis (slight or incomplete paralysis), hypotonia (decreased muscle tone), seizures (often infantile spasms), and macrocephaly or microcephaly.

Individuals with porencephaly may have poor or absent speech development, epilepsy, hydrocephalus, spastic contractures (shrinkage or shortening of muscles), and mental retardation. Treatment may include physical therapy, medication for seizure disorders, and a shunt for hydrocephalus. The prognosis for individuals with porencephaly varies according to the location and extent of the lesion. Some patients with this disorder may develop only minor neurological problems and have normal intelligence, while others may be severely disabled. Others may die before the second decade of life.

Schizencephaly is a rare developmental disorder characterized by abnormal slits, or clefts, in the cerebral hemispheres. Schizencephaly is a form of porencephaly. Individuals with clefts in both hemispheres, or bilateral clefts, are often developmentally delayed and have delayed speech and language skills and corticospinal dysfunction. Individuals with smaller, unilateral clefts (clefts in one hemisphere) may be weak on one side of the body and may have average or near-average intelligence. Patients with schizencephaly may also have varying degrees of microcephaly, mental retardation, hemiparesis (weakness or paralysis affecting one side of the body), or quadriparesis (weakness or paralysis affecting all four extremities), and may have reduced muscle tone (hypotonia). Most patients have seizures and some may have hydrocephalus.

In schizencephaly, the neurons border the edge of the cleft, implying a very early disruption in development. There is now a genetic origin for one type of schizencephaly. Causes of this type may include environmental exposures during pregnancy such as medication taken by the mother, exposure to toxins, or a vascular insult. Often there are associated heterotopias (isolated islands of neurons), which indicate a failure of migration of the neurons to their final position in the brain.

Treatment for individuals with schizencephaly generally consists of physical therapy, treatment for seizures, and, in cases that are complicated by hydrocephalus, a shunt.

The prognosis for individuals with schizencephaly varies depending on the size of the clefts and the degree of neurological deficit.

What are other less common cephalies?

Acephaly literally means absence of the head. It is a much rarer condition than anencephaly. The acephalic fetus is a parasitic twin attached to an otherwise intact fetus. The acephalic fetus has a body but lacks a head and a heart; the fetus's neck is attached to the normal twin. The blood circulation of the acephalic fetus is provided by the heart of the twin. The acephalic fetus cannot exist independently of the fetus to which it is attached.

Exencephaly is a condition in which the brain is located outside of the skull. This condition is usually found in embryos as an early stage of anencephaly. As an exencephalic pregnancy progresses, the neural tissue gradually degenerates. It is unusual to find an infant carried to term with this condition because the defect is incompatible with survival.

Macrocephaly is a condition in which the head circumference is larger than average for the age and gender of the infant or child. It is a descriptive rather than a diagnostic term and is a characteristic of a variety of disorders. Macrocephaly also may be inherited. Although one form of macrocephaly may be associated with mental retardation, in approximately one-half of cases mental development is normal. Macrocephaly may be caused by an enlarged brain or hydrocephalus. It may be associated with other disorders such as dwarfism, neurofibromatosis, and tuberous sclerosis.

Micrencephaly is a disorder characterized by a small brain and may be caused by a disturbance in the proliferation of nerve cells. Micrencephaly may also be associated with maternal problems such as alcoholism, diabetes, or rubella (German measles). A genetic factor may play a role in causing some cases of micrencephaly. Affected newborns generally have striking neurological defects and seizures. Severely impaired intellectual development is common, but disturbances in motor functions may not appear until later in life.

Otocephaly is a lethal condition in which the primary feature is agnathia—a developmental anomaly characterized by total or virtual absence of the lower jaw. The condition is considered lethal because of a poorly functioning airway. In otocephaly, agnathia may occur alone or together with holoprosencephaly.

Another group of less common cephalic disorders are the craniostenoses. Craniostenoses are deformities of the skull caused by the premature fusion or joining together of the cranial sutures. Cranial sutures are fibrous joints that join the bones of the skull together. The nature of these deformities depends on which sutures are affected.

Brachycephaly occurs when the coronal suture fuses prematurely, causing a shortened front-to-back diameter of the skull. The coronal suture is the fibrous joint that unites the frontal bone with the two parietal bones of the skull. The parietal bones form the top and sides of the skull.

Oxycephaly is a term sometimes used to describe the premature closure of the coronal suture plus any other suture, or it may be used to describe the premature fusing of all sutures. Oxycephaly is the most severe of the craniostenoses.

Plagiocephaly results from the premature unilateral fusion (joining of one side) of the coronal or lambdoid sutures. The lambdoid suture unites the occipital bone with the parietal bones of the skull. Plagiocephaly is a condition characterized by an asymmetrical distortion (flattening of one side) of the skull. It is a common finding at birth and may be the result of brain malformation, a restrictive intrauterine environment, or torticollis (a spasm or tightening of neck muscles).

Scaphocephaly applies to premature fusion of the sagittal suture. The sagittal suture joins together the two parietal bones of the skull. Scaphocephaly is the most common of the craniostenoses and is characterized by a long, narrow head.

Trigonocephaly is the premature fusion of the metopic suture (part of the frontal suture which joins the two halves of the frontal bone of the skull) in which a V-shaped abnormality occurs at the front of the skull. It is characterized by the triangular prominence of the forehead and closely set eyes.

What research is being done?

Within the federal government, the National Institute of Neurological Disorders and Stroke (NINDS), one of the National Institutes of Health (NIH), has primary responsibility for conducting and supporting research on normal and abnormal brain and nervous system development, including congenital anomalies. The National Institute of Child Health and Human Development, the National Institute of Mental Health, the National Institute of Environmental Health Sciences, the National Institute of Alcohol Abuse and Alcoholism, and the National Institute on Drug Abuse also support research related to disorders of the developing nervous system. Gaining basic knowledge about how the nervous system develops and understanding the role of genetics in fetal development are major goals of scientists studying congenital neurological disorders.

Scientists are rapidly learning how harmful insults at various stages of pregnancy can lead to developmental disorders. For example, a critical nutritional deficiency or exposure to an environmental insult during the first month of pregnancy (when the neural tube is formed) can produce neural tube defects such as anencephaly.

Scientists are also concentrating their efforts on understanding the complex processes responsible for normal early development of the brain and nervous system and how the disruption of any of these processes results in congenital anomalies such as cephalic disorders. Understanding how genes control brain cell migration, proliferation, differentiation, and death, and how radiation, drugs, toxins, infections, and other factors disrupt these processes will aid in preventing many congenital neurological disorders.

Currently, researchers are examining the mechanisms involved in neurulation—the process of forming the neural tube. These studies will improve our understanding of this process and give insight into how the process can go awry and cause devastating congenital disorders. Investigators are also analyzing genes and gene products necessary for human brain development to achieve a better understanding of normal brain development in humans.

Section 22.3

Agenesis of the Corpus Callosum

Reprinted from "Agenesis of the Corpus Callosum Information Page,"
National Institute of Neurological Disorders and Stroke, National
Institutes of Health, January 23, 2006.

What is agenesis of the corpus callosum?

Agenesis of the corpus callosum (ACC) is a birth defect in which
the structure that connects the two hemispheres of the brain (the corpus callosum) is partially or completely absent. ACC can occur as an
isolated condition or in combination with other cerebral abnormalities, including Arnold-Chiari malformation, Dandy-Walker syndrome,
Andermann syndrome, schizencephaly (clefts or deep divisions in
brain tissue), and holoprosencephaly (failure of the forebrain to divide into lobes). Girls may have a gender-specific condition called
Aicardi syndrome, which causes severe mental retardation, seizures,
abnormalities in the vertebra of the spine, and lesions on the retina
of the eye. ACC can also be associated with malformations in other
parts of the body, such as midline facial defects. The effects of the disorder range from subtle or mild to severe, depending on associated
brain abnormalities. Intelligence may be normal with mild compromise of skills requiring matching of visual patterns. But children with
the most severe brain malformations may have intellectual retardation, seizures, hydrocephalus, and spasticity.

Is there any treatment?

There is no standard course of treatment for ACC. Treatment usually involves management of symptoms and seizures if they occur.

What is the prognosis?

Prognosis depends on the extent and severity of malformations.
ACC does not cause death in the majority of children. Mental retardation does not worsen. Although many children with the disorder

have average intelligence and lead normal lives, neuropsychological testing reveals subtle differences in higher cortical function compared to individuals of the same age and education without ACC.

What research is being done?

The National Institute of Neurological Disorders and Stroke (NINDS) conducts and supports a wide range of studies that explore the complex mechanisms of normal brain development. The knowledge gained from these fundamental studies helps researchers understand how the process can go awry and provides opportunities for more effectively treating, and perhaps even preventing, developmental brain disorders such as ACC.

Section 22.4

Chiari Malformation

Reprinted from "Chiari Malformation Information Page," National Institute of Neurological Disorders and Stroke, National Institutes of Health, January 23, 2006.

What is Chiari Malformation?

Arnold-Chiari malformation is a condition in which the cerebellum portion of the brain protrudes into the spinal canal. It may or may not be apparent at birth. Arnold-Chiari I type malformation usually causes symptoms in young adults and is often associated with syringomyelia, in which a tubular cavity develops within the spinal cord. Arnold-Chiari II type malformation is associated with myelomeningocele (a defect of the spine) and hydrocephalus (increased cerebrospinal fluid and pressure within the brain), which usually are apparent at birth. Myelomeningocele usually causes paralysis of the legs and, less commonly, the arms. If left untreated, hydrocephalus can cause mental impairment. Either type of Arnold-Chiari malformation can cause symptoms of headache, vomiting, difficulty swallowing, and hoarseness.

Adults and adolescents who are unaware they have Arnold-Chiari I type malformation may develop headache that is predominantly located in the back of the head and is increased by coughing or straining. Symptoms of progressive brain impairment may include dizziness, an impaired ability to coordinate movement, double vision, and involuntary, rapid, downward eye movements.

Is there any treatment?

Infants and children with myelomeningocele may require surgery to repair protrusion of the meningeal sac into the spinal cord. Hydrocephalus may be treated with surgical implantation of a shunt to relieve increased pressure on the brain. Some adults with Arnold-Chiari malformation may benefit from surgery in which the existing opening in the back of the skull is enlarged.

What is the prognosis?

Infants with very severe malformations may have life-threatening complications. Most patients who have surgery experience a reduction in their symptoms. Some patients may experience prolonged periods of relative stability.

What research is being done?

Research supported by the National Institute of Neurological Disorders and Stroke (NINDS) includes studies to understand how the brain and nervous system normally develop and function and how they are affected by disease and trauma. These studies contribute to a greater understanding of congenital birth defects, such as Arnold-Chiari malformation, and open promising new doors to potential treatments.

Section 22.5

Craniosynostosis

Reprinted from "Craniosynostosis Information Page,"
National Institute of Neurological Disorders and Stroke,
National Institutes of Health, January 23, 2006.

What is craniosynostosis?

Craniosynostosis is a birth defect of the brain characterized by the premature closure of one or more of the fibrous joints between the bones of the skull (called the cranial sutures) before brain growth is complete. Closure of a single suture is most common. The abnormally shaped skull that results is due to the brain not being able to grow in its natural shape because of the closure. Instead it compensates with growth in areas of the skull where the cranial sutures have not yet closed. The condition can be gene-linked, or caused by metabolic diseases, such as rickets or an overactive thyroid. Some cases are associated with other disorders such as microcephaly (abnormally small head) and hydrocephalus (excessive accumulation of cerebrospinal fluid in the brain). The first sign of craniosynostosis is an abnormally shaped skull. Other features can include signs of increased intracranial pressure, developmental delays, or mental retardation, which are caused by constriction of the growing brain. Seizures and blindness may also occur.

Is there any treatment?

Treatment for craniosynostosis generally consists of surgery to relieve pressure on the brain and the cranial nerves. For some children with less severe problems, cranial molds can reshape the skull to accommodate brain growth and improve the appearance of the head.

What is the prognosis?

The prognosis for craniosynostosis varies depending on whether single or multiple cranial sutures are involved or other abnormalities are present. The prognosis is better for those with single suture involvement and no associated abnormalities.

What research is being done?

The National Institute of Neurological Disorders and Stroke (NINDS) conducts and supports a wide range of studies that explore the complex mechanisms of early neurological development. The knowledge gained from these fundamental studies provides the foundation for understanding how this process can go awry and offers hope for new ways to treat and prevent brain birth defects, including craniosynostosis.

Section 22.6

Dandy-Walker Syndrome

Reprinted from "Dandy-Walker Syndrome Information Page,"
National Institute of Neurological Disorders and Stroke, National
Institutes of Health, January 24, 2006.

What is Dandy-Walker syndrome?

Dandy-Walker syndrome is a congenital brain malformation involving the cerebellum (an area at the back of the brain that controls movement) and the fluid filled spaces around it. The key features of this syndrome are an enlargement of the fourth ventricle (a small channel that allows fluid to flow freely between the upper and lower areas of the brain and spinal cord), a partial or complete absence of the cerebellar vermis (the area between the two cerebellar hemispheres), and cyst formation near the internal base of the skull. An increase in the size of the fluid spaces surrounding the brain as well as an increase in pressure may also be present. The syndrome can appear dramatically or develop unnoticed. Symptoms, which often occur in early infancy, include slow motor development and progressive enlargement of the skull. In older children, symptoms of increased intracranial pressure such as irritability, vomiting, and convulsions, and signs of cerebellar dysfunction such as unsteadiness, lack of muscle coordination, or jerky movements of the eyes may occur. Other symptoms include increased head circumference; bulging at the back of the skull; problems with the nerves that control the eyes, face, and neck; and abnormal breathing patterns. Dandy-Walker syndrome is frequently associated with disorders of other areas of the central nervous system including absence of the corpus callosum (the connecting area between the two cerebral hemispheres) and malformations of the heart, face, limbs, fingers, and toes.

Is there any treatment?

Treatment for individuals with Dandy-Walker syndrome generally consists of treating the associated problems, if needed. A special tube to reduce intracranial pressure may be placed inside the skull to control swelling. Parents of children with Dandy Walker syndrome may benefit from genetic counseling if they intend to have more children.

What is the prognosis?

Children with Dandy-Walker syndrome may never have normal intellectual development, even when the hydrocephalus is treated early and correctly. Longevity depends on the severity of the syndrome and associated malformations. The presence of multiple congenital defects may shorten life span.

What research is being done?

The National Institute of Neurological Disorders and Stroke (NINDS) conducts and supports a wide range of studies that explore the complex mechanisms of normal brain development. The knowledge gained from these fundamental studies provides the foundation for understanding abnormal brain development and offers hope for new ways to treat and prevent developmental brain disorders such as Dandy-Walker syndrome.

Chapter 23

Craniofacial Defects

Chapter Contents

Section 23.1—Cleft Lip and Palate 340
Section 23.2—Facial Palsy 347
Section 23.3—Goldenhar Syndrome 351
Section 23.4—Hemifacial Microsomia 353
Section 23.5—Microtia 355
Section 23.6—Pierre Robin Sequence 357

Section 23.1

Cleft Lip and Palate

"Cleft Lip and Palate" is reprinted with permission from The Nemours
Foundation. This information was provided by KidsHealth, one of the larg-
est resources online for medically reviewed health information written
for parents, kids, and teens. For more articles like this one, visit www.Kids
Health.org, or www.TeensHealth.org. © 2005 The Nemours Center for
Children's Health Media, a division of The Nemours Foundation. "Parent's
Age and Risk of Conceiving a Child with Oral Clefts" is reprinted from
"Does a Parent's Age Increase Risk of Conceiving Child with Oral Clefts?"
National Institute of Dental and Craniofacial Research, National Insti-
tutes of Health, May 2005.

Cleft Lip and Palate

Oral-facial clefts are birth defects in which the tissues of the mouth
or lip don't form properly during fetal development. In the United
States, clefts occur in one in seven hundred to one thousand births,
making it the one of the most common major birth defects. Clefts occur more often in children of Asian, Latino, or Native American descent.

The good news is that both cleft lip and cleft palate are treatable
birth defects. Most kids who are born with these conditions can have
reconstructive surgery within the first twelve to eighteen months of
life to correct the defect and significantly improve facial appearance.

What Is Oral Clefting?

Oral clefting occurs when the tissues of the lip and/or palate of a
fetus don't grow together early in pregnancy. Children with clefts often don't have enough tissue in their mouths, and the tissue they do
have isn't fused together properly to form the roof of their mouths.

A cleft lip appears as a narrow opening or gap in the skin of the
upper lip that extends all the way to the base of the nose. A cleft palate is an opening between the roof of the mouth and the nasal cavity.
Some children have clefts that extend through both the front and rear
part of the palates, while others have only partial clefting.

340

There are generally three different kinds of clefts:

- cleft lip without a cleft palate
- cleft palate without a cleft lip
- cleft lip and cleft palate together

In addition, clefts can occur on one side of the mouth (unilateral clefting) or on both sides of the mouth (bilateral clefting).

More boys than girls have a cleft lip, while more girls have cleft palate without a cleft lip.

Because clefting causes specific visible symptoms, it's easy to diagnose. It can be detected through a prenatal ultrasound. If the clefting has not been detected prior to the baby's birth, it's identified immediately afterward.

What Causes Oral Clefting?

Doctors don't know exactly why a baby develops cleft lip or cleft palate, but believe it may be a combination of genetic (inherited) and environmental factors (such as certain drugs, illnesses, and the use of alcohol or tobacco while a woman is pregnant). The risk may be higher for kids whose sibling or parents have a cleft or who have a history of clefting in their families. Both mothers and fathers can pass on a gene or genes that cause cleft palate or cleft lip.

Complications Related to Oral Clefting

A child with a cleft lip or palate tends to be more susceptible to colds, hearing loss, and speech defects. Dental problems—such as missing, extra, malformed, or displaced teeth, and cavities—also are common in children born with cleft palate.

Many children with clefts are especially vulnerable to ear infections because their eustachian tubes don't drain fluid properly from the middle ear into the throat. Fluid accumulates, pressure builds in the ears, and infection may set in. For this reason, a child with cleft lip or palate may have special tubes surgically inserted into his or her ears at the time of the first reconstructive surgery.

Feeding can be another complication for an infant with a cleft lip or palate. A cleft lip can make it more difficult for a child to suck on a nipple, while a cleft palate may cause formula or breast milk to be accidentally taken up into the nasal cavity. Special nipples and other devices can help make feeding easier; you will probably be given information on how to use them and where to buy them before you take your baby home from the hospital. And in some cases, a child with a cleft lip or palate may need to wear a prosthetic palate called an obturator to help him or her eat properly.

If you're experiencing problems with feeding, your doctor may be able to offer other suggestions or feeding aids to help you and your baby.

Treating Clefts

The good news is that there have been many medical advancements in the treatment of oral clefting. Reconstructive surgery can repair cleft lips and palates, and in severe cases, plastic surgery can address specific appearance-related concerns.

A child with oral clefting will need to see a variety of specialists who will work together as a team to treat the condition. Treatment usually begins in the first few months of an infant's life, depending on the health of the infant and the extent of the cleft.

Members of a child's cleft lip and palate treatment team usually include:

- a geneticist;
- a plastic surgeon;
- an ear, nose, and throat physician (otolaryngologist);
- an oral surgeon;
- an orthodontist;
- a dentist;
- a speech pathologist (often called a speech therapist);
- an audiologist;
- a nurse coordinator;
- a social worker and/or psychologist.

The team specialists will evaluate your child's progress regularly, examining your child's hearing, speech, nutrition, teeth, and emotional state. They will share their recommendations with you, and can forward their evaluation to your child's school and any speech therapists that your child may be working with.

In addition to treating your child's cleft, the specialists will work with your child on any issues related to feeding, social problems, speech, and how you approach the condition with your child. They'll provide feedback and recommendations to help you through the phases of your child's growth and treatment.

Surgery for Oral Clefting

Surgery is usually performed during the first twelve to eighteen months to repair cleft lip and/or cleft palate. Both types of surgery are performed in the hospital under general anesthesia.

Cleft lip often requires only one reconstructive surgery, especially if the cleft is unilateral. The surgeon will make an incision on each side of the cleft from the lip to the nostril. The two sides of the lip will then be sutured together. Bilateral cleft lips may be repaired in two surgeries, about a month apart, and usually require a short hospital stay.

Cleft palate surgery involves drawing tissue from either side of the mouth to rebuild the palate. It requires two or three nights in the hospital, with the first night spent in the intensive care unit. The initial surgery is intended to create a functional palate, reduce the chances that fluid will develop in the middle ears, and help the child's teeth and facial bones develop properly. In addition, this functional palate will help your child's speech development and feeding abilities.

The necessity for more operations depends on the skill of the surgeon as well as the severity of the cleft, its shape, and the thickness of available tissue that can be used to create the palate. Some children with a cleft palate require more surgeries to help improve their speech. Additional surgeries may also improve the appearance of the lip and nose, close openings between the mouth and nose, help breathing, and stabilize and realign the jaw. Subsequent surgeries are usually scheduled at least six months apart to allow a child time to heal and to reduce the chances of serious scarring.

It's a good idea to meet regularly with your child's plastic surgeon to determine what's most appropriate in your child's case. Final repairs of the scars left by the initial surgery may not be performed until adolescence, when facial structure is more fully developed. Surgery is designed to aid in normalizing function and cosmetic appearance so that the child will have as few difficulties as possible.

Dental Care and Orthodontia

Children with oral clefting often undergo dental and orthodontic treatment to help align the teeth and take care of any gaps that exist because of the cleft.

Routine dental care may get lost in the midst of these major procedures, but healthy teeth are critical for a child with clefting because they're needed for proper speech.

A child with oral clefting generally needs the same dental care as other children—regular brushing supplemented with flossing once the child's six-year molars come in. Depending on the shape of your child's mouth and teeth, your child's dentist may recommend a toothette, a soft sponge that contains mouthwash, rather than a toothbrush. As your child grows, you may be able to switch to a soft children's toothbrush. The key is to make sure that your child brushes regularly and well.

Children with cleft palate often have an alveolar ridge defect. The alveolus is the bony upper gum that contains teeth, and defects can:

- displace, tip, or rotate permanent teeth;

- prevent permanent teeth from appearing;

- prevent the alveolar ridge from forming.

These problems can be fixed by grafting bone matter onto the alveolus, which allows the placement of your child's teeth to be corrected orthodontically.

Orthodontic treatment usually involves a number of phases, with the first phase beginning as the permanent teeth start to come in. In the first phase, which is called an orthopalatal expansion, the upper dental arch is rounded out and the width of the upper jaw is increased. A device called an expander is placed inside the child's mouth. The widening of the jaw may be followed by a bone graft in the alveolus.

Your child's orthodontist may wait until the remainder of your child's permanent teeth come in before beginning the second phase of orthodontic treatment. The second phase may involve removing extra teeth, adding dental implants if teeth are missing, or applying braces to straighten teeth.

In about 25 percent of children with a unilateral cleft lip and palate, the upper jaw growth does not keep up with the lower jaw growth. If this occurs, your child may need orthognathic surgery to align the teeth and help the upper jaw to develop.

For these children, phase-two orthodontics may include an operation called an osteotomy on the upper jaw that moves the upper jaw both forward and down. This usually requires another bone graft for stability.

Speech Therapy

A child with oral clefting may have trouble speaking—the clefting can make the voice nasal and difficult to understand. Some will find that surgery fixes the problem completely.

Catching speech problems early can be a key part of solving them. It's a good idea to take your child to a speech therapist between the ages of eighteen months and two years. Many speech therapists like to talk with parents at least once during the child's first six months to provide an overview of the treatment and suggest specific language- and speech-stimulation games to play with the baby.

Shortly after the initial surgery is completed, the speech pathologist will see your child for a complete assessment. The therapist will evaluate your child's developing communication skills by assessing the number of sounds he or she makes and the actual words your child tries to use, and by observing interaction and play behavior.

This analysis helps determine what, if any, speech exercises your child needs and if further surgery is required. The speech pathologist will often continue to work with your child through additional surgeries. Many children who have clefts work with a speech therapist throughout their grade-school years.

Dealing with Emotional and Social Issues

Our society often focuses on people's appearances, and this can make childhood—and, especially, the teen years—very difficult for someone with a physical difference. Because a child with oral clefting has a prominent facial difference, your child may experience painful teasing, which can damage self-esteem. Part of the cleft palate and lip treatment team includes psychiatric and emotional support personnel.

Here are some ways that you can support your child:

- Try not to focus on your child's cleft and do not allow it to define your child as an individual.

- Create a warm and supportive home environment, where each person's individual worth is openly celebrated.

- Let your child know that you feel good about who he or she is by showing acceptance and by not trying to make your child into your idea of who he or she should be.

- Encourage your child to develop friendships with people from diverse backgrounds. The best way to do this is to lead by example and to be open to all people yourself.

- Point out positive attributes in others that do not involve physical appearance.

- Encourage autonomy by giving your child the freedom to make decisions and take appropriate risks, letting your child's own accomplishments lead to a sense of personal value. By providing opportunities for your child to make decisions early on—like picking out what clothes to wear—he or she can gain more confidence and the ability to make bigger decisions down the road.

You might also consider encouraging your child to present information about clefting to his or her class with a special presentation that you arrange with the teacher. Or perhaps your child would like you to talk to the class. This can be especially effective with young children.

If your child does experience teasing, encourage discussions about it and be a patient listener. Give your child the tools to confront the teasers by asking what he or she would like to say and then practicing those statements.

If your child seems to have ongoing self-esteem problems, you may want to consult with a child psychologist or social worker for support and information. Together with the members of your child's treatment team, you can help your child through tough times.

Also, it's important to keep the lines of communication open as your child approaches adolescence so that you can address any concerns he or she may have about appearance.

Parent's Age and Risk of Conceiving a Child with Oral Clefts

Doctors have long recognized that the older a woman is during pregnancy, the greater are the chances her baby will be born with a birth defect. What remains unclear is whether parental age—including the age of the father—is a risk factor for cleft lip and/or palate or the genetically distinct cleft palate. To answer this question, National Institute of Dental and Craniofacial Research (NIDCR) grantees and colleagues identified 2,876 Danish babies born with isolated oral clefts from 1973 to 1996. According to the data, 1,920 babies had cleft lip and/or palate, while 956 infants were born with cleft palate alone. The researchers then turned to Denmark's highly reliable Civil Registration System to determine the ages of the parents of these children. Based on their analyses, the scientists determined that the age of both parents is a risk factor for both conditions. However, the group offered two interesting qualifiers from the data. One, in a joint analysis comparing the mother's and father's ages, they found that the contribution of each parent to the baby's risk was dependent on the age of their partner. Secondly, they found that the age of the father was a risk factor for cleft palate only, while it was not for the mother.

Section 23.2

Facial Palsy

What is facial palsy?

Facial palsy is a congenital deformity, which dates from birth, or an acquired deformity, which causes complete or partial paralysis of the facial motion. The act of facial motion starts in the brain and travels through the facial nerves to the muscles in the face. These muscles then contract in response to a stimulus. Inside the skull, the facial nerve is a single nerve. Once the nerve is traced outside the skull, it branches into many smaller limbs that go to many different facial muscles. These muscles control facial expression. The coordinated activity of this nerve and these muscles causes motions such as smiling, blinking, frowning, and a full range of normal facial motions. Diseases or injuries affecting the brain, the facial nerve, or the muscles of the face can cause facial palsy.

Are there other names for this condition?

Facial palsy is also called paresis. Paresis suggests a weakness in facial motion. Palsy is usually a complete lack of motion. Moebius syndrome is a subtype of facial palsy. This syndrome involves a weakness of the muscles responsible for facial expression and side-to-side eye movement. Moebius syndrome may also involve abnormalities of the limbs.

What causes facial palsy?

A variety of things can cause facial palsy. Congenital facial palsy is a condition present at birth. Moebius syndrome is a congenital condition. In most cases the exact cause of congenital palsy is uncertain. A lack of proper nerve and/or muscle development causes some cases of congenital palsy. The reason for this is unknown. Other palsies may result from stretching of the muscles or nerves during the birthing process. Most congenital palsies involve one side of the face with the exception of Moebius, which is typically bilateral. This means that it affects both sides of the face. A large number of cases of facial palsy develop when a weakness or complete palsy occurs later in life despite a normal facial movement at birth. This group is called the acquired group. Causes of acquired palsy include trauma to the facial nerve and muscle, certain inflammatory or infectious diseases such as Lyme disease, and tumors in and around the regions of the head and neck.

What are the chances of producing a child with this condition?

The incidence of facial palsy is rare. The chance of producing a child with Moebius syndrome is very rare. The incidence of other forms of congenital facial palsy is approximately two in every one thousand births. Most congenital facial palsies have no apparent cause but can occasionally be associated with syndromes of the head and neck.

Does facial palsy ever improve?

In most cases, other than Moebius syndrome, the condition does improve. However, the return of function is usually only a partial one. In most cases of congenital palsy, the weakness is incomplete, and some motion is present. Moebius syndrome is usually an incomplete palsy, and some patients have movement of the lower face and the lip region. It does not improve with time. However, 90 percent of the other congenital palsy patients can expect an improvement. With acquired facial palsy, patients may experience improvement if the cause of the palsy is trauma to the nerve or muscle, or if the pressure from a tumor on the nerve can be treated.

What are problems caused by facial palsy?

With children there are no immediate effects. This is due to the normal elastic skin tone. Therefore, the structures of the face do not sag.

With adults, however, the sudden onset of facial palsy generally results in a significant loss of tone in the tissues and considerable facial sagging. One of the most important functions of the facial nerves and muscles is helping the eyelid to close. If the eyelid does not close, the eye is more prone to injury such as scratches. Injury can then result in scarring and visual loss. It is critical for young children with this condition to be evaluated by an ophthalmologist so that appropriate eye protection and lubrication can be started.

Facial palsy can cause problems with normal sucking and chewing. Drooling may also be a problem. Appearance is a major concern. Asymmetry of the face can cause the face to be significantly distorted. Occasionally a child discovers that smiling frequently causes facial imbalance. For that reason, he may avoid smiling altogether.

What can be done surgically to correct this condition?

for infants with newly diagnosed facial palsy, eye protection is the primary concern. Lubricants are usually sufficient to prevent injury to the eye. When lubrication is not adequate, then the eyelids are partially sewn shut. This procedure, called tarsorrhaphy, does not block the child's vision.

A watchful, conservative approach is usually best for a child with congenital facial palsy. Since many children improve, treatment should not start before the age of five or six except in the case of the eye as mentioned above. Once the child has reached the age of five or six, there are several treatment options available.

Two methods of treatment are static slings and dynamic muscle transfers. Static slings involve procedures in which a patient's own tissue is used to elevate the sagging portions of the face. These slings may be applied to the portion of the face that produces a smile, as well as the eyelid region. These static slings improve facial balance and eyelid closure. Dynamic procedures include muscle transfers and man-made devices to improve lid closure. Muscle transfers involve moving locally available muscles, such as those for chewing, to substitute for nonfunctioning or absent facial muscles. Once the transfer is made, the patient relies on the act of biting to contract and bring on a smile or to cause the eyelid to close.

Very sophisticated methods of muscle transfers have been developed. The "gold standard" at the present is a two-staged procedure. Nerves are first transferred from "the good side of the face" to the paralyzed side of the face. After this, a muscle transfer is done to reproduce a smile effect. Using a microscope, this muscle is transferred and hooked up to the nerve grafts. If this is successful, nerve activity from the "good side of the face" travels instantly through the nerve grafts to the new muscle on the opposite side. This can then cause a motion. However, this motion is, at best, unrefined because a few nerves and one muscle are being asked to take the place of many muscles that work together during normal facial expression.

When there is not a side of the face with normal motion, as in the case of Moebius syndrome or bilateral facial palsy, muscles can be transferred using a microscopic technique. They are then connected to nerves that activate biting muscles if done in a sequence on both sides. Facial motion can be restored, but the patient must bite in order to activate the muscles. Procedures have also been developed to improve eyelid closure. One method involves placing gold weights in the upper eyelid to help it close when the lid is relaxed. The use of surgical springs can accomplish the same thing.

How successful are the surgeries?

The success of the operations varies from patient to patient. The success is dictated by the severity of the facial weakness. Normal facial motion depends on multiple facial muscles and nerves working together to produce a full spectrum of motion. Presently, procedures result in a replacement of a portion of this facial activity. Complete normalization of the facial motion is rarely possible. Due to the many microscopic techniques, there is a chance that nerve growth may not be complete or that circulation to the transferred muscle may fail. This can result in no marked improvement. This occurs in 5 to 10 percent of patients.

If my child needs surgery, when is the best time?

Generally, early surgery is not necessary unless eye exposure is a problem. In this case, surgery can be done at any age. The most complicated muscle transfers and static slings require a high degree of patient cooperation. This is true during the surgery and the rehabilitation process. For that reason, these procedures are best accomplished after the age of five or six.

Where should my child go for treatment?

Surgeons who are familiar with facial nerve paralysis are frequently a part of a craniofacial team. There are a number of microsurgeons in the United States who have a great deal of experience with facial paralysis. A craniofacial team can guide you to the appropriate physician.

Facial reanimation procedures are extremely complex. It is important to seek care from a team of surgeons specialized and experienced in the area of facial palsy.

Section 23.3

Goldenhar Syndrome

"Goldenhar Syndrome," written by Lynn Mayfield. Reproduced with permission from FACES: The National Craniofacial Association, www.faces-cranio.org. All rights reserved.

What is Goldenhar Syndrome?

Goldenhar Syndrome is a congenital birth defect which involves deformities of the face. It usually affects one side of the face only. Characteristics include:

- a partially formed or totally absent ear (microtia);
- the chin may be closer to the affected ear;
- one corner of the mouth may be higher than the other;
- benign growths of the eye;
- a missing eye.

Goldenhar is also known as oculoauricular dysplasia or OAV.

Why did this happen?

Doctors are uncertain why Goldenhar occurs. However, they do not believe it is the result of anything the mother did while she was pregnant. Environmental factors may play a part and there does seem to be an increased incidence of Goldenhar among the children of Gulf War Veterans. Currently, a scientific study is being conducted by the University of Texas Southwestern Medical Center at Dallas and the Association of Birth Defect Children, Inc. They are trying to locate all children with Goldenhar syndrome who were born since July 1, 1991, and who had a parent who served in the U.S. military in any capacity in 1990 or 1991. If you are interested in this study, please contact the Association of Birth Defect Children by e-mail at abdc@birthdefects .org or call (407) 895-0802.

Will this happen to children I have in the future?

The chances of having another child with Goldenhar is less than 1 percent. Your child has about a 3 percent chance of passing it on to his or her children.

What kinds of problems could my child have?

In addition to the physical characteristics common to Goldenhar, your child may have the following problems:

- hearing problems;
- weakness in moving the side of the face that is smaller;
- dental problems—the soft palate may move to the unaffected side of the face;
- the tongue may be smaller on the affected side of the face;
- fusion of the bones of the neck.

Will my child need surgery?

Depending on the severity of Goldenhar Syndrome, your child may have some or all of the following surgeries:

- lowering of the jaw on the affected side;
- lengthening of the lower jaw;
- three to four operations to rebuild the outer ear;
- addition of bone to build up the cheeks;
- addition of soft tissue may to the face.

New advances in procedures to correct the symptoms of Goldenhar Syndrome are constantly being developed. Be an advocate for your child!

How do I get help for my child?

Your child should be treated by a qualified craniofacial medical team at a craniofacial center.

Section 23.4

Hemifacial Microsomia

What is hemifacial microsomia?

Hemifacial microsomia is a condition in which the lower half of one side of the face is underdeveloped and does not grow normally. It is sometimes also referred to as first and second brachial arch syndrome, oral-mandibular-auricular syndrome, lateral facial dysplasia, or oto-mandibular dysostosis. The syndrome varies in severity, but always includes the maldevelopment of the ear and the mandible. This is the second most common facial birth defect after clefts.

Why did this happen?

Researchers are still not sure why this happens, however, most agree that something occurred in the early stages of development such as a disturbance of the blood supply to the first and second brachial arches in the first six to eight weeks of pregnancy. Studies do *not* link this condition with the mother's activities or actions during her pregnancy.

Will this happen to children I have in the future?

For parents with one child with hemifacial microsomia, the chances are between 0 and 1 percent. Adults with this condition have a 3 percent chance of passing it to their children.

Will my child need surgery?

The surgeries recommended for children with hemifacial microsomia have a goal to improve facial symmetry, by reconstructing the bony and soft tissue and establishing normal occlusion and joint junction. The timing for such surgeries varies depending upon the surgeons and the severity of the problems. Common surgeries include the following:

* lowering the upper jaw to match the opposite side and lengthening the lower jaw. Sometimes a bone graft is used to lengthen the jaw and sometimes a distraction device is used.

* ear reconstruction at about five to six years of age, involving three to four surgeries.

* addition of bone to build up the cheekbone.

* addition of soft tissues to further balance the face.

What kinds of problems could my child have?

Your child may have skin tags in front of the ear or on different parts of the face. Hearing problems depend on the structures that are involved. Some children have some weakness in movement on the affected side of the face.

New advances in procedures to correct the symptoms of hemifacial microsomia are constantly being developed. Be an advocate for your child!

How do I get help for my child?

Your child should be treated by a qualified craniofacial medical team at a craniofacial center.

Section 23.5

Microtia

What is microtia?

Microtia is an incompletely formed ear. It ranges in severity from a bump of tissue to a partially formed ear. In most cases, only one ear is affected. In that case, it is called unilateral microtia. If both ears are affected, it is called bilateral microtia. Unilateral microtia occurs in one out of eight thousand births and bilateral microtia occurs in one out of twenty-five thousand births.

Why did this happen?

At this time, no one knows why microtia occurs; however, there is nothing to suggest that the mother's actions during pregnancy caused the microtia. Further research is necessary to determine the exact cause.

Will this happen to other children I have in the future?

The possibility of passing microtia on to another child is believed to be less than 6 percent.

What kinds of problems could my child have?

In addition to the physical characteristics, your child may have some or all of these problems:

- about a 40 percent reduction of hearing in the affected ear;
- problems locating the direction from which a sound comes;
- ear infections.

Will my child need surgery?

Your child will either require reconstructive surgery to rebuild the outer ear or he or she may wish to wear a prosthesis. The prosthesis is glued to the head. If you choose reconstructive surgery, it is a three- to four-step process, usually done two to three months apart. Surgical procedures usually begin around six years of age, because the ear is 90 percent of its adult size, so it is easier to determine the size of the ear that must be made.

Portions of ribs 5, 6, 7, and 8 are carved into the shape of the external ear. The ear is then grafted into place and the overlying skin is draped onto the graft. Other operations may be needed to rotate the lobule and possibly to reposition the cartilage framework into its final position.

New advances in procedures to treat microtia are constantly being made. Be an advocate for your child!

How do I get help for my child?

Your child should be treated by a qualified craniofacial medical team at a craniofacial center.

Section 23.6

Pierre Robin Sequence

What is Pierre Robin?

Pierre Robin is not a syndrome or a disease. It is usually referred to as Pierre Robin sequence, although it is also known as "Pierre Robin malformation sequence," "Robin anomalad," and "cleft palate, micrognathia, and glossoptosis." It is the name given to the following birth defects if they appear together:

- small lower jaw (micrognathia);
- a tongue which tends to ball up at the back of the mouth and fall back toward the throat (glossoptosis);
- breathing problems;
- horseshoe-shaped cleft palate may or may not be present.

Why did this happen?

Doctors do not know exactly why Pierre Robin occurs. They do not believe it is the result of anything the mother did or did not do during pregnancy. If the child has only Pierre Robin, many experts believe that it is the result of the positioning of the fetus in the early weeks of pregnancy.

Will this happen to children I have in the future?

Pierre Robin does not tend to run in families. The chances of you having another child with Pierre Robin are very small, unless the Pierre Robin sequence is a part of a syndrome.

What kinds of problems could my child have?

In addition to the physical characteristics common to Pierre Robin, your child may have the following problems:

- feeding problems in infancy;
- ear infections;
- reduced hearing.

About 40 percent of infants with Pierre Robin have Stickler syndrome and about 15 percent have velocardiofacial syndrome. FACES recommends genetic testing be done to determine if your infant has either of these associated syndromes. The Pierre Robin Network has excellent information concerning genetic testing for babies born with Pierre Robin sequence.

Will my child need surgery?

Depending on the severity of Pierre Robin, your child may have some or all of the following surgeries:

- surgery to repair the cleft palate;
- special devices to protect the airway and aid in feeding;
- surgery to improve breathing.

The small jaw associated with Pierre Robin usually grows out on its own during the first two years, and usually no surgery is necessary on the jaw.

New advances in procedures to correct the problems associated with Pierre Robin are constantly being made. Be an advocate for your child!

How do I get help for my child?

Your child should be treated by a qualified craniofacial medical team at a craniofacial center.

Chapter 24

Cerebral Palsy

Chapter Contents

Section 24.1—What You Should Know about Cerebral
Palsy 360
Section 24.2—Botox in the Management of Children with
Cerebral Palsy 384
Section 24.3—Hyperbaric Oxygen Therapy for Cerebral
Palsy 386
Section 24.4—Hypothermia in the Prevention of Cerebral
Palsy among Newborn Infants 391

Section 24.1

What You Should
Know about Cerebral Palsy

Excerpted from "Cerebral Palsy: Hope Through Research,"
National Institute of Neurological Disorders and Stroke, National
Institutes of Health, NIH Publication No. 93-159, January 23, 2006.

In the 1860s, an English surgeon named William Little wrote the
first medical descriptions of a puzzling disorder that struck children
in the first years of life, causing stiff, spastic muscles in their legs and,
to a lesser degree, their arms. These children had difficulty grasping
objects, crawling, and walking. They did not get better as they grew
up nor did they become worse. Their condition, which was called Little
disease for many years, is now known as spastic diplegia. It is just
one of several disorders that affect control of movement and are
grouped together under the term cerebral palsy.

Because it seemed that many of these children were born following premature or complicated deliveries, Little suggested their condition resulted from a lack of oxygen during birth. This oxygen
shortage damaged sensitive brain tissues controlling movement, he
proposed. But in 1897, the famous psychiatrist Sigmund Freud dis-
agreed. Noting that children with cerebral palsy often had other problems such as mental retardation, visual disturbances, and seizures,
Freud suggested that the disorder might sometimes have roots earlier in life, during the brain's development in the womb. "Difficult
birth, in certain cases," he wrote, "is merely a symptom of deeper effects that influence the development of the fetus."

Despite Freud's observation, the belief that birth complications
cause most cases of cerebral palsy was widespread among physicians,
families, and even medical researchers until very recently. In the
1980s, however, scientists analyzed extensive data from a government study of more than thirty-five thousand births and were surprised to discover that such complications account for only a fraction
of cases—probably less than 10 percent. In most cases of cerebral
palsy, no cause of the factors explored could be found. These findings

from the National Institute of Neurological Disorders and Stroke (NINDS) perinatal study have profoundly altered medical theories about cerebral palsy and have spurred today's researchers to explore alternative causes.

At the same time, biomedical research has also led to significant changes in understanding, diagnosing, and treating persons with cerebral palsy. Risk factors not previously recognized have been identified, notably intrauterine exposure to infection and disorders of coagulation, and others are under investigation. Identification of infants with cerebral palsy very early in life gives youngsters the best opportunity to receive treatment for sensory disabilities and for prevention of contractures. Biomedical research has led to improved diagnostic techniques such as advanced brain imaging and modern gait analysis. Certain conditions known to cause cerebral palsy, such as rubella (German measles) and jaundice, can now be prevented or treated. Physical, psychological, and behavioral therapies that assist with such skills as movement and speech and foster social and emotional development can help children who have cerebral palsy to achieve and succeed. Medications, surgery, and braces can often improve nerve and muscle coordination, help treat associated medical problems, and either prevent or correct deformities.

What is cerebral palsy?

Cerebral palsy is an umbrella-like term used to describe a group of chronic disorders impairing control of movement that appear in the first few years of life and generally do not worsen over time. The term cerebral refers to the brain's two halves, or hemispheres, and palsy describes any disorder that impairs control of body movement. Thus, these disorders are not caused by problems in the muscles or nerves. Instead, faulty development or damage to motor areas in the brain disrupts the brain's ability to adequately control movement and posture.

Symptoms of cerebral palsy lie along a spectrum of varying severity. An individual with cerebral palsy may have difficulty with fine motor tasks, such as writing or cutting with scissors; experience trouble with maintaining balance and walking; or be affected by involuntary movements, such as uncontrollable writhing motion of the hands or drooling. The symptoms differ from one person to the next, and may even change over time in the individual. Some people with cerebral palsy are also affected by other medical disorders, including seizures or mental impairment. Contrary to common belief, however, cerebral palsy does not always cause profound handicap. While a child with severe cerebral palsy might be unable to walk and need extensive, lifelong care, a child with mild cerebral palsy might be only slightly awkward and require no special assistance. Cerebral palsy is not contagious nor is it usually inherited from one generation to the next. At this time, it cannot be cured, although scientific research continues to yield improved treatments and methods of prevention.

How many people have this disorder?

The United Cerebral Palsy Associations estimate that more than five hundred thousand Americans have cerebral palsy. Despite advances in preventing and treating certain causes of cerebral palsy, the number of children and adults it affects has remained essentially unchanged or perhaps risen slightly over the past thirty years. This is partly because more critically premature and frail infants are surviving through improved intensive care. Unfortunately, many of these infants have developmental problems of the nervous system or suffer neurological damage. Research is under way to improve care for these infants, as in ongoing studies of technology to alleviate troubled breathing and trials of drugs to prevent bleeding in the brain before or soon after birth.

What are the different forms?

Spastic diplegia, the disorder first described by Dr. Little in the 1860s, is only one of several disorders called cerebral palsy. Today doctors classify cerebral palsy into four broad categories—spastic, athetoid, ataxic, and mixed forms—according to the type of movement disturbance.

Spastic cerebral palsy. In this form of cerebral palsy, which affects 70 to 80 percent of patients, the muscles are stiffly and permanently contracted. Doctors will often describe which type of spastic cerebral palsy a patient has based on which limbs are affected. The names given to these types combine a Latin description of affected limbs with the term plegia or paresis, meaning paralyzed or weak.

When both legs are affected by spasticity, they may turn in and cross at the knees. As these individuals walk, their legs move awkwardly and stiffly and nearly touch at the knees. This causes a characteristic walking rhythm, known as the scissors gait.

Individuals with spastic hemiparesis may also experience hemiparetic tremors, in which uncontrollable shaking affects the limbs on one side of the body. If these tremors are severe, they can seriously impair movement.

Athetoid, or dyskinetic, cerebral palsy. This form of cerebral palsy is characterized by uncontrolled, slow, writhing movements. These abnormal movements usually affect the hands, feet, arms, or legs and, in some cases, the muscles of the face and tongue, causing grimacing or drooling. The movements often increase during periods of emotional stress and disappear during sleep. Patients may also have problems coordinating the muscle movements needed for speech, a condition known as dysarthria. Athetoid cerebral palsy affects about 10 to 20 percent of patients.

Ataxic cerebral palsy. This rare form affects the sense of balance and depth perception. Affected persons often have poor coordination; walk unsteadily with a wide-based gait, placing their feet unusually far apart; and experience difficulty when attempting quick or precise movements, such as writing or buttoning a shirt. They may also have intention tremor. In this form of tremor, beginning a voluntary movement, such as reaching for a book, causes a trembling that affects the body part being used and that worsens as the individual gets nearer to the desired object. The ataxic form affects an estimated 5 to 10 percent of cerebral palsy patients.

Mixed forms. It is common for patients to have symptoms of more than one of the previous three forms. The most common mixed form includes spasticity and athetoid movements but other combinations are also possible.

What other medical disorders are associated with cerebral palsy?

Many individuals who have cerebral palsy have no associated medical disorders. However, disorders that involve the brain and impair its motor function can also cause seizures and impair an individual's intellectual development, attentiveness to the outside world, activity and behavior, and vision and hearing. Medical disorders associated with cerebral palsy include:

- **Mental impairment.** About one-third of children who have cerebral palsy are mildly intellectually impaired, one-third are moderately or severely impaired, and the remaining third are intellectually normal. Mental impairment is even more common among children with spastic quadriplegia.

- **Seizures or epilepsy.** As many as half of all children with cerebral palsy have seizures. During a seizure, the normal, orderly pattern of electrical activity in the brain is disrupted by uncontrolled bursts of electricity. When seizures recur without a direct trigger, such as fever, the condition is called epilepsy. In the person who has cerebral palsy and epilepsy, this disruption may be spread throughout the brain and cause varied symptoms all over the body—as in tonic-clonic seizures—or may be confined to just one part of the brain and cause more specific symptoms—as in partial seizures. Tonic-clonic seizures generally cause patients to cry out and are followed by loss of consciousness, twitching of both legs and arms, convulsive body movements, and loss of bladder control. Partial seizures are classified as simple or complex. In simple partial seizures, the individual has localized symptoms, such as muscle twitches, chewing movements, and numbness or tingling. In complex partial seizures, the individual may hallucinate, stagger, perform automatic and purposeless movements, or experience impaired consciousness or confusion.

- **Growth problems.** A syndrome called failure to thrive is common in children with moderate-to-severe cerebral palsy, especially those with spastic quadriparesis. Failure to thrive is a general term physicians use to describe children who seem to lag behind in growth and development despite having enough food. In babies, this lag usually takes the form of too little weight gain; in young children, it can appear as abnormal shortness; in teenagers, it may appear as a combination of shortness and lack of sexual development. Failure to thrive probably has several causes, including, in particular, poor nutrition and damage to the brain centers controlling growth and development. In addition, the muscles and limbs affected by cerebral palsy tend to be smaller than normal. This is especially noticeable in some patients with spastic hemiplegia, because limbs on the affected side of the body may not grow as quickly or as large as those on the more normal side. This condition usually affects the hand and foot most severely. Since the involved foot in hemiplegia is often smaller than the unaffected foot even among patients who walk, this size difference is probably not due to lack of use.

Scientists believe the problem is more likely to result from disruption of the complex process responsible for normal body growth.

- **Impaired vision or hearing.** A large number of children with cerebral palsy have strabismus, a condition in which the eyes are not aligned because of differences in the left and right eye muscles. In an adult, this condition causes double vision. In children, however, the brain often adapts to the condition by ignoring signals from one of the misaligned eyes. Untreated, this can lead to very poor vision in one eye and can interfere with certain visual skills, such as judging distance. In some cases, physicians may recommend surgery to correct strabismus. Children with hemiparesis may have hemianopia, which is defective vision or blindness that impairs the normal field of vision of one eye. For example, when hemianopia affects the right eye, a child looking straight ahead might have perfect vision except on the far right. In homonymous hemianopia, the impairment affects the same part of the visual field of both eyes. Impaired hearing is also more frequent among those with cerebral palsy than in the general population.

- **Abnormal sensation and perception.** Some children with cerebral palsy have impaired ability to feel simple sensations like touch and pain. They may also have stereognosia, or difficulty perceiving and identifying objects using the sense of touch. A child with stereognosia, for example, would have trouble identifying a hard ball, sponge, or other object placed in his hand without looking at the object.

What causes cerebral palsy?

Cerebral palsy is not one disease with a single cause, like chicken pox or measles. It is a group of disorders with similar problems in control of movement, but probably with different causes. When physicians try to uncover the cause of cerebral palsy in an individual child, they look at the form of cerebral palsy, the mother's and child's medical history, and onset of the disorder.

In the United States, about 10 to 20 percent of children who have cerebral palsy acquire the disorder after birth. (The figures are higher in underdeveloped countries.) Acquired cerebral palsy results from brain damage in the first few months or years of life and can follow brain infections, such as bacterial meningitis or viral encephalitis, or result from head injury—most often from a motor vehicle accident, a fall, or child abuse.

Congenital cerebral palsy, on the other hand, is present at birth, although it may not be detected for months. In most cases, the cause of congenital cerebral palsy is unknown. Thanks to research, however, scientists have pinpointed some specific events during pregnancy or around the time of birth that can damage motor centers in the developing brain. Some of these causes of congenital cerebral palsy include:

- **Infections during pregnancy.** German measles, or rubella, is caused by a virus that can infect pregnant women and, therefore, the fetus in the uterus, to cause damage to the developing nervous system. Other infections that can cause brain injury in the developing fetus include cytomegalovirus and toxoplasmosis. There is relatively recent evidence that placental and perhaps other maternal infection can be associated with cerebral palsy.

- **Jaundice in the infant.** Bile pigments, compounds that are normally found in small amounts in the bloodstream, are produced when blood cells are destroyed. When many blood cells are destroyed in a short time, as in the condition called Rh incompatibility, the yellow-colored pigments can build up and cause jaundice. Severe, untreated jaundice can damage brain cells.

- **Rh incompatibility.** In this blood condition, the mother's body produces immune cells called antibodies that destroy the fetus's blood cells, leading to a form of jaundice in the newborn.

- **Severe oxygen shortage in the brain or trauma to the head during labor and delivery.** The newborn infant's blood is specially equipped to compensate for low levels of oxygen, and asphyxia (lack of oxygen caused by interruption in breathing or poor oxygen supply) is common in babies during the stresses of labor and delivery. But if asphyxia severely lowers the supply of oxygen to the infant's brain for lengthy periods, the child may develop brain damage called hypoxic-ischemic encephalopathy. A significant proportion of babies with this type of brain damage die, and others may develop cerebral palsy, which is then often accompanied by mental impairment and seizures. In the past, physicians and scientists attributed most cases of cerebral palsy to asphyxia or other complications during birth if they could not identify another cause. However, extensive research by NINDS scientists and others has shown that very few babies who experience asphyxia during birth develop encephalopathy soon after birth. Research also shows that a large proportion of babies who experience asphyxia do not grow up to have cerebral palsy or other neurological disorders. Birth complications including asphyxia are now estimated to account for about 6 percent of congenital cerebral palsy cases.

- **Stroke.** Coagulation disorders in mothers or infants can produce stroke in the fetus or newborn baby. Bleeding in the brain has several causes—including broken blood vessels in the brain, clogged blood vessels, or abnormal blood cells—and is one form of stroke. Although strokes are better known for their effects on older adults, they can also occur in the fetus during pregnancy or the newborn around the time of birth, damaging brain tissue and causing neurological problems. Ongoing research is testing potential treatments that may one day help prevent stroke in fetuses and newborns.

What are the risk factors?

Research scientists have examined thousands of expectant mothers, followed them through childbirth, and monitored their children's early neurological development. As a result, they have uncovered certain characteristics, called risk factors, that increase the possibility that a child will later be diagnosed with cerebral palsy:

- **Breech presentation.** Babies with cerebral palsy are more likely to present feet first, instead of head first, at the beginning of labor.

- **Complicated labor and delivery.** Vascular or respiratory problems of the baby during labor and delivery may sometimes be the first sign that a baby has suffered brain damage or that a baby's brain has not developed normally. Such complications can cause permanent brain damage.

- **Low Apgar score.** The Apgar score (named for anesthesiologist Virginia Apgar) is a numbered rating that reflects a newborn's condition. To determine an Apgar score, doctors periodically check the baby's heart rate, breathing, muscle tone, reflexes, and skin color in the first minutes after birth. They then assign points; the higher the score, the more normal the baby's condition. A low score at ten to twenty minutes after delivery is often considered an important sign of potential problems.

- **Low birth weight and premature birth.** The risk of cerebral palsy is higher among babies who weigh less than 2,500 grams (5 lbs., 7 1/2 oz.) at birth and among babies who are born less than thirty-seven weeks into pregnancy. This risk increases as birth weight falls.

- **Multiple births.** Twins, triplets, and other multiple births are linked to an increased risk of cerebral palsy.

- **Nervous system malformations.** Some babies born with cerebral palsy have visible signs of nervous system malformation, such as an abnormally small head (microcephaly). This suggests that problems occurred in the development of the nervous system while the baby was in the womb.

- **Maternal bleeding or severe proteinuria late in pregnancy.** Vaginal bleeding during the sixth to ninth months of pregnancy and severe proteinuria (the presence of excess proteins in the urine) are linked to a higher risk of having a baby with cerebral palsy.

- **Maternal hyperthyroidism, mental retardation, or seizures.** Mothers with any of these conditions are slightly more likely to have a child with cerebral palsy.

- **Seizures in the newborn.** An infant who has seizures faces a higher risk of being diagnosed, later in childhood, with cerebral palsy.

Knowing these warning signs helps doctors keep a close eye on children who face a higher risk for long-term problems in the nervous system. However, parents should not become too alarmed if their child has one or more of these factors. Most such children do not have and do not develop cerebral palsy.

Can cerebral palsy be prevented?

Several of the causes of cerebral palsy that have been identified through research are preventable or treatable:

- Head injury can be prevented by regular use of child safety seats when driving in a car and helmets during bicycle rides, and elimination of child abuse. In addition, common sense measures around the household—like close supervision during bathing and keeping poisons out of reach—can reduce the risk of accidental injury.

- Jaundice of newborn infants can be treated with phototherapy. In phototherapy, babies are exposed to special blue lights that break down bile pigments, preventing them from building up and threatening the brain. In the few cases in which this treatment is not enough, physicians can correct the condition with a special form of blood transfusion.

- Rh incompatibility is easily identified by a simple blood test routinely performed on expectant mothers and, if indicated, expectant fathers. This incompatibility in blood types does not usually cause problems during a woman's first pregnancy, since the mother's body generally does not produce the unwanted antibodies until after delivery. In most cases, a special serum given after each childbirth can prevent the unwanted production of antibodies. In unusual cases, such as when a pregnant woman develops the antibodies during her first pregnancy or antibody production is not prevented, doctors can help minimize problems by closely watching the developing baby and, when needed, performing a transfusion to the baby while in the womb or an exchange transfusion (in which a large volume of the baby's blood is removed and replaced) after birth.

- Rubella, or German measles, can be prevented if women are vaccinated against this disease before becoming pregnant.

In addition, it is always good to work toward a healthy pregnancy through regular prenatal care and good nutrition and by eliminating smoking, alcohol consumption, and drug abuse. Despite the best efforts of parents and physicians, however, children will still be born with cerebral palsy. Since in most cases the cause of cerebral palsy is unknown, little can currently be done to prevent it. As investigators learn more about the causes of cerebral palsy through basic and clinical research, doctors and parents will be better equipped to help prevent this disorder.

What are the early signs?

Early signs of cerebral palsy usually appear before three years of age, and parents are often the first to suspect that their infant is not developing motor skills normally. Infants with cerebral palsy are frequently slow to reach developmental milestones, such as learning to roll over, sit, crawl, smile, or walk. This is sometimes called developmental delay.

Some affected children have abnormal muscle tone. Decreased muscle tone is called hypotonia; the baby may seem flaccid and relaxed, even floppy. Increased muscle tone is called hypertonia, and the baby may seem stiff or rigid. In some cases, the baby has an early period of hypotonia that progresses to hypertonia after the first two to three months of life. Affected children may also have unusual posture or favor one side of their body.

Parents who are concerned about their baby's development for any reason should contact their physician, who can help distinguish normal variation in development from a developmental disorder.

How is cerebral palsy diagnosed?

Doctors diagnose cerebral palsy by testing an infant's motor skills and looking carefully at the infant's medical history. In addition to checking for those symptoms described previously—slow development, abnormal muscle tone, and unusual posture—a physician also tests the infant's reflexes and looks for early development of hand preference.

Reflexes are movements that the body makes automatically in response to a specific cue. For example, if a newborn baby is held on its back and tilted so the legs are above its head, the baby will automatically extend its arms in a gesture, called the Moro reflex, that looks like an embrace. Babies normally lose this reflex after they reach six months, but those with cerebral palsy may retain it for abnormally long periods. This is just one of several reflexes that a physician can check.

Doctors can also look for hand preference—a tendency to use either the right or the left hand more often. When the doctor holds an object in front and to the side of the infant, an infant with hand preference will use the favored hand to reach for the object, even when it is held closer to the opposite hand. During the first twelve months of life, babies do not usually show hand preference. But infants with spastic hemiplegia, in particular, may develop a preference much earlier, since the hand on the unaffected side of their body is stronger and more useful.

The next step in diagnosing cerebral palsy is to rule out other disorders that can cause movement problems. Most important, doctors must determine that the child's condition is not getting worse. Although its symptoms may change over time, cerebral palsy by definition is not progressive. If a child is continuously losing motor skills, the problem more likely springs from elsewhere—including genetic diseases, muscle diseases, disorders of metabolism, or tumors in the nervous system. The child's medical history, special diagnostic tests, and, in some cases, repeated check-ups can help confirm that other disorders are not at fault.

The doctor may also order specialized tests to learn more about the possible cause of cerebral palsy. One such test is computed tomography, or CT, a sophisticated imaging technique that uses x-rays and a computer to create an anatomical picture of the brain's tissues and structures. A CT scan may reveal brain areas that are underdeveloped, abnormal cysts (sacs that are often filled with liquid) in the brain, or other physical problems. With the information from CT scans, doctors may be better equipped to judge the long-term outlook for an affected child.

Magnetic resonance imaging, or MRI, is a relatively new brain imaging technique that is rapidly gaining widespread use for identifying brain disorders. This technique uses a magnetic field and radio waves, rather than x-rays. MRI gives better pictures of structures or abnormal areas located near bone than does CT.

A third test that can expose problems in brain tissues is ultrasonography. This technique bounces sound waves off the brain and uses the pattern of echoes to form a picture, or sonogram, of its structures. Ultrasonography can be used in infants before the bones of the skull harden and close. Although it is less precise than CT and MRI scanning, this technique can detect cysts and structures in the brain, is less expensive, and does not require long periods of immobility.

Finally, physicians may want to look for other conditions that are linked to cerebral palsy, including seizure disorders, mental impairment, and vision or hearing problems.

When the doctor suspects a seizure disorder, an electroencephalogram, or EEG, may be ordered. An EEG uses special patches called electrodes placed on the scalp to record the natural electrical currents inside the brain. This recording can help the doctor see telltale patterns in the brain's electrical activity that suggest a seizure disorder.

Intelligence tests are often used to determine if a child with cerebral palsy is mentally impaired. Sometimes, however, a child's intelligence may be underestimated because problems with movement, sensation, or speech due to cerebral palsy make it difficult for him or her to perform well on these tests.

If problems with vision are suspected, the doctor may refer the patient to an ophthalmologist for examination; if hearing impairment seems likely, an otologist may be called in.

Identifying these accompanying conditions is important and is becoming more accurate as ongoing research yields advances that make diagnosis easier. Many of these conditions can then be addressed through specific treatments, improving the long-term outlook for those with cerebral palsy.

How is cerebral palsy managed?

Cerebral palsy cannot be cured, but treatment can often improve a child's capabilities. In fact, progress due to medical research now means that many patients can enjoy near-normal lives if their neurological problems are properly managed. There is no standard therapy that works for all patients. Instead, the physician must work with a team of health care professionals first to identify a child's unique needs and impairments and then to create an individual treatment plan that addresses them.

Some approaches that can be included in this plan are drugs to control seizures and muscle spasms, special braces to compensate for muscle imbalance, surgery, mechanical aids to help overcome impairments, counseling for emotional and psychological needs, and physical, occupational, speech, and behavioral therapy. In general, the earlier treatment begins, the better chance a child has of overcoming developmental disabilities or learning new ways to accomplish difficult tasks.

The members of the treatment team for a child with cerebral palsy should be knowledgeable professionals with a wide range of specialties. A typical treatment team might include:

- a physician, such as a pediatrician, a pediatric neurologist, or a pediatric physiatrist, trained to help developmentally disabled children. This physician, often the leader of the treatment team, works to synthesize the professional advice of all team members into a comprehensive treatment plan, implements treatments, and follows the patient's progress over a number of years.

- an orthopedist, a surgeon who specializes in treating the bones, muscles, tendons, and other parts of the body's skeletal system. An orthopedist might be called on to predict, diagnose, or treat muscle problems associated with cerebral palsy.

- a physical therapist, who designs and implements special exercise programs to improve movement and strength.

- an occupational therapist, who can help patients learn skills for day-to-day living, school, and work.

- a speech and language pathologist, who specializes in diagnosing and treating communication problems.

- a social worker, who can help patients and their families locate community assistance and education programs.

- a psychologist, who helps patients and their families cope with the special stresses and demands of cerebral palsy. In some cases, psychologists may also oversee therapy to modify unhelpful or destructive behaviors or habits.

- an educator, who may play an especially important role when mental impairment or learning disabilities present a challenge to education.

Individuals who have cerebral palsy and their family or caregivers are also key members of the treatment team, and they should be intimately involved in all steps of planning, making decisions, and applying treatments. Studies have shown that family support and personal determination are two of the most important predictors of which individuals who have cerebral palsy will achieve long-term goals.

Too often, however, physicians and parents may focus primarily on an individual symptom—especially the inability to walk. While mastering specific skills is an important focus of treatment on a day-to-day basis, the ultimate goal is to help individuals grow to adulthood and have maximum independence in society. In the words of one physician, "After all, the real point of walking is to get from point A to point B. Even if a child needs a wheelchair, what's important is that they're able to achieve this goal."

What specific treatments are available?

Physical, behavioral, and other therapies. Therapy—whether for movement, speech, or practical tasks—is a cornerstone of cerebral palsy treatment. The skills a two-year-old needs to explore the world are very different from those that a child needs in the classroom or a young adult needs to become independent. Cerebral palsy therapy should be tailored to reflect these changing demands.

Physical therapy usually begins in the first few years of life, soon after the diagnosis is made. Physical therapy programs use specific sets of exercises to work toward two important goals: preventing the weakening or deterioration of muscles that can follow lack of use (called disuse atrophy) and avoiding contracture, in which muscles become fixed in a rigid, abnormal position.

Contracture is one of the most common and serious complications of cerebral palsy. Normally, a child whose bones are growing stretches the body's muscles and tendons through running and walking and other daily activities. This ensures that muscles will grow at the same rate. But in children with cerebral palsy, spasticity prevents this stretching and, as a result, muscles do not grow fast enough to keep up with lengthening bones. The resulting contracture can disrupt balance and trigger loss of previous abilities. Physical therapy alone, or in combination with special braces (sometimes called orthotic devices), works to prevent this complication by stretching spastic muscles. For example, if a child has spastic hamstrings (tendons located behind the knee), the therapist and parents should encourage the child to sit with the legs extended to stretch them.

A third goal of some physical therapy programs is to improve the child's motor development. A widespread program of physical therapy that works toward this goal is the Bobath technique, named for a husband and wife team who pioneered this approach in England. This program is based on the idea that the primitive reflexes retained by many children with cerebral palsy present major roadblocks to learning voluntary control. A therapist using the Bobath technique tries to counteract these reflexes by positioning the child in an opposing movement. So, for example, if a child with cerebral palsy normally keeps his arm flexed, the therapist would repeatedly extend it.

A second such approach to physical therapy is "patterning," which is based on the principle that motor skills should be taught in more or less the same sequence that they develop normally. In this controversial approach, the therapist guides the child with movement problems along the path of normal motor development. For example, the child is first taught elementary movements like pulling himself to a standing position and crawling before he is taught to walk—regardless of his age. Some experts and organizations, including the American Academy of Pediatrics, have expressed strong reservations about the patterning approach, because studies have not documented its value.

Physical therapy is usually just one element of an infant development program that also includes efforts to provide a varied and stimulating environment. Like all children, the child with cerebral palsy needs new experiences and interactions with the world around him in order to learn. Stimulation programs can bring this valuable experience to the child who is physically unable to explore.

As the child with cerebral palsy approaches school age, the emphasis of therapy shifts away from early motor development. Efforts now focus on preparing the child for the classroom, helping the child master activities of daily living, and maximizing the child's ability to communicate.

Physical therapy can now help the child with cerebral palsy prepare for the classroom by improving his or her ability to sit, move independently or in a wheelchair, or perform precise tasks, such as writing. In occupational therapy, the therapist works with the child to develop such skills as feeding, dressing, or using the bathroom. This can help reduce demands on caregivers and boost self-reliance and self-esteem. For the many children who have difficulty communicating, speech therapy works to identify specific difficulties and overcome them through a program of exercises. For example, if a child has difficulty saying words that begin with "b," the therapist may suggest daily practice with a list of "b" words, increasing their difficulty as each list is mastered. Speech therapy can also work to help the child learn to use special communication devices, such as a computer with voice synthesizers.

Behavioral therapy provides yet another avenue to increase a child's abilities. This therapy, which uses psychological theory and techniques, can complement physical, speech, or occupational therapy. For example, behavioral therapy might include hiding a toy inside a box to reward a child for learning to reach into the box with his weaker hand. Likewise, a child learning to say his "b" words might be given a balloon for mastering the word. In other cases, therapists may try to discourage unhelpful or destructive behaviors, such as hair pulling or biting, by selectively presenting a child with rewards and praise during other, more positive activities.

As a child with cerebral palsy grows older, the need for and types of therapy and other support services will continue to change. Continuing physical therapy addresses movement problems and is supplemented by vocational training, recreation and leisure programs, and special education when necessary. Counseling for emotional and psychological challenges may be needed at any age, but is often most critical during adolescence. Depending on their physical and intellectual abilities, adults may need attendant care, living accommodations, transportation, or employment opportunities.

Regardless of the patient's age and which forms of therapy are used, treatment does not end when the patient leaves the office or treatment center. In fact, most of the work is often done at home. The therapist functions as a coach, providing parents and patients with the strategy and drills that can help improve performance at home, at school, and in the world. As research continues, doctors and parents can expect new forms of therapy and better information about which forms of therapy are most effective for individuals with cerebral palsy.

Drug therapy. Physicians usually prescribe drugs for those who have seizures associated with cerebral palsy, and these medications are very effective in preventing seizures in many patients. In general, the drugs given to individual patients are chosen based on the type of seizures, since no one drug controls all types. However, different people with the same type of seizure may do better on different drugs, and some individuals may need a combination of two or more drugs to achieve good seizure control.

Drugs are also sometimes used to control spasticity, particularly following surgery. The three medications that are used most often are diazepam, which acts as a general relaxant of the brain and body; baclofen, which blocks signals sent from the spinal cord to contract the muscles; and dantrolene, which interferes with the process of muscle contraction. Given by mouth, these drugs can reduce spasticity for short periods, but their value for long-term control of spasticity has not been clearly demonstrated. They may also trigger significant side effects, such as drowsiness, and their long-term effects on the developing nervous system are largely unknown. One possible solution to avoid such side effects may lie in current research to explore new routes for delivering these drugs.

Patients with athetoid cerebral palsy may sometimes be given drugs that help reduce abnormal movements. Most often, the prescribed drug belongs to a group of chemicals called anticholinergics that work by reducing the activity of acetylcholine. Acetylcholine is a chemical messenger that helps some brain cells communicate and that triggers muscle contraction. Anticholinergic drugs include trihexyphenidyl, benztropine, and procyclidine hydrochloride.

Occasionally, physicians may use alcohol "washes"—or injections of alcohol into a muscle—to reduce spasticity for a short period. This technique is most often used when physicians want to correct a developing contracture. Injecting alcohol into a muscle that is too short weakens the muscle for several weeks and gives physicians time to work on lengthening the muscle through bracing, therapy, or casts. In some cases, if the contracture is detected early enough, this technique may avert the need for surgery.

Surgery. Surgery is often recommended when contractures are severe enough to cause movement problems. In the operating room, surgeons can lengthen muscles and tendons that are proportionately too short. First, however, they must determine the exact muscles at fault, since lengthening the wrong muscle could make the problem worse.

Finding problem muscles that need correction can be a difficult task. To walk two strides with a normal gait, it takes more than thirty major muscles working at exactly the right time and exactly the right force. A problem in any one muscle can cause abnormal gait. Furthermore, the natural adjustments the body makes to compensate for muscle problems can be misleading. A new tool that enables doctors to spot gait abnormalities, pinpoint problem muscles, and separate real problems from compensation is called gait analysis. Gait analysis combines cameras that record the patient while walking, computers that analyze each portion of the patient's gait, force plates that detect when feet touch the ground, and a special recording technique that detects muscle activity (known as electromyography). Using these data, doctors are better equipped to intervene and correct significant problems. They can also use gait analysis to check surgical results.

Because lengthening a muscle makes it weaker, surgery for contractures is usually followed by months of recovery. For this reason, doctors try to fix all of the affected muscles at once when it is possible or, if more than one surgical procedure is unavoidable, they may try to schedule operations close together.

A second surgical technique, known as selective dorsal root rhizotomy, aims to reduce spasticity in the legs by reducing the amount of stimulation that reaches leg muscles via nerves. In the procedure, doctors try to locate and selectively sever overactivated nerves controlling leg muscles. Although there is scientific controversy over how selective this technique actually is, recent research results suggest it can reduce spasticity in some patients, particularly those who have spastic diplegia. Ongoing research is evaluating this surgery's effectiveness.

Experimental surgical techniques include chronic cerebellar stimulation and stereotaxic thalamotomy. In chronic cerebellar stimulation, electrodes are implanted on the surface of the cerebellum—the part of the brain responsible for coordinating movement—and are used to stimulate certain cerebellar nerves. While it was hoped that this technique would decrease spasticity and improve motor function, results of this invasive procedure have been mixed. Some studies have reported improvements in spasticity and function, others have not.

377

Stereotaxic thalamotomy involves precise cutting of parts of the thalamus, which serves as the brain's relay station for messages from the muscles and sensory organs. This has been shown effective only for reducing hemiparetic tremors.

Mechanical aids. Whether they are as humble as Velcro shoes or as advanced as computerized communication devices, special machines and gadgets in the home, school, and workplace can help the child or adult with cerebral palsy overcome limitations.

The computer is probably the most dramatic example of a new device that can make a difference in the lives of those with cerebral palsy. For example, a child who is unable to speak or write but can make head movements may be able to learn to control a computer using a special light pointer that attaches to a headband. Equipped with a computer and voice synthesizer, this child could communicate with others. In other cases, technology has led to new versions of old devices, such as the traditional wheelchair and its modern offspring that runs on electricity.

Many such devices are products of engineering research supported by private foundations and other groups.

What other major problems are associated with cerebral palsy?

Poor control of the muscles of the throat, mouth, and tongue sometimes leads to drooling. Drooling can cause severe skin irritation and, because it is socially unacceptable, can lead to further isolation of affected children from their peers. Although numerous treatments for drooling have been tested over the years, there is no one treatment that always helps. Drugs called anticholinergics can reduce the flow of saliva but may cause significant side effects, such as mouth dryness and poor digestion. Surgery, while sometimes effective, carries the risk of complications, including worsening of swallowing problems. Some patients benefit from a technique called biofeedback that can tell them when they are drooling or having difficulty controlling muscles that close the mouth. This kind of therapy is most likely to work if the patient has a mental age of more than two or three years, is motivated to control drooling, and understands that drooling is not socially acceptable.

Difficulty with eating and swallowing—also triggered by motor problems in the mouth—can cause poor nutrition. Poor nutrition, in turn, may make the individual more vulnerable to infections and cause or aggravate "failure to thrive"—a lag in growth and development that is common among those with cerebral palsy. To make swallowing easier, the caregiver may want to prepare semisolid food, such as strained vegetables and fruits. Proper position, such as sitting up while eating or drinking and extending the individual's neck away from the body to reduce the risk of choking, is also helpful. In severe cases of swallowing problems and malnutrition, physicians may recommend tube feeding, in which a tube delivers food and nutrients down the throat and into the stomach, or gastrostomy, in which a surgical opening allows a tube to be placed directly into the stomach.

A common complication is incontinence, caused by faulty control over the muscles that keep the bladder closed. Incontinence can take the form of bed-wetting (also known as enuresis), uncontrolled urination during physical activities (or stress incontinence), or slow leaking of urine from the bladder. Possible medical treatments for incontinence include special exercises, biofeedback, prescription drugs, surgery, or surgically implanted devices to replace or aid muscles. Specially designed undergarments are also available.

What research is being done?

Investigators from many arenas of medicine and health are using their expertise to help improve treatment and prevention of cerebral palsy. Much of their work is supported through the National Institute of Neurological Disorders and Stroke (NINDS), the National Institute of Child Health and Human Development, other agencies within the federal government, nonprofit groups such as the United Cerebral Palsy Research Foundation, and private institutions.

The ultimate hope for overcoming cerebral palsy lies with prevention. In order to prevent cerebral palsy, however, scientists must first understand the complex process of normal brain development and what can make this process go awry.

Between early pregnancy and the first months of life, one cell divides to form first a handful of cells, and then hundreds, millions, and, eventually, billions of cells. Some of these cells specialize to become brain cells. These brain cells specialize into different types and migrate to their appropriate site in the brain. They send out branches to form crucial connections with other brain cells. Ultimately, the most complex entity known to us is created: a human brain with its billions of interconnected neurons.

Mounting evidence is pointing investigators toward this intricate process in the womb for clues about cerebral palsy. For example, a group of researchers has recently observed that more than one-third of children who have cerebral palsy also have missing enamel on certain teeth. This tooth defect can be traced to problems in the early months of fetal development, suggesting that a disruption at this period in development might be linked both to this tooth defect and to cerebral palsy.

As a result of this and other research, many scientists now believe that a significant number of children develop cerebral palsy because of mishaps early in brain development. They are examining how brain cells specialize, how they know where to migrate, how they form the right connections—and they are looking for preventable factors that can disrupt this process before or after birth.

Scientists are also scrutinizing other events—such as bleeding in the brain, seizures, and breathing and circulation problems—that threaten the brain of the newborn baby. Through this research, they hope to learn how these hazards can damage the newborn's brain and to develop new methods for prevention.

Some newborn infants, for example, have life-threatening problems with breathing and blood circulation. A recently introduced treatment to help these infants is extracorporeal membrane oxygenation, in which blood is routed from the patient to a special machine that takes over the lungs' task of removing carbon dioxide and adding oxygen. Although this technique can dramatically help many such infants, some scientists have observed that a substantial fraction of treated children later experience long-term neurological problems, including developmental delay and cerebral palsy. Investigators are studying infants through pregnancy, delivery, birth, and infancy, and are tracking those who undergo this treatment. By observing them at all stages of development, scientists can learn whether their problems developed before birth, result from the same breathing problems that made them candidates for the treatment, or spring from errors in the treatment itself. Once this is determined, they may be able to correct any existing problems or develop new treatment methods to prevent brain damage.

Other scientists are exploring how brain insults like hypoxic-ischemic encephalopathy (brain damage from a shortage of oxygen or blood flow), bleeding in the brain, and seizures can cause the abnormal release of brain chemicals and trigger brain damage. For example, research has shown that bleeding in the brain unleashes dangerously high amounts of a brain chemical called glutamate. While glutamate is normally used in the brain for communication, too much glutamate overstimulates the brain's cells and causes a cycle of destruction. Scientists are now looking closely at glutamate to detect how its release harms brain tissue and spreads the damage from stroke. By learning how such brain chemicals that normally help us function can hurt the brain, scientists may be equipped to develop new drugs that block their harmful effects.

In related research, some investigators are already conducting studies to learn if certain drugs can help prevent neonatal stroke. Several of these drugs seem promising because they appear to reduce the excess production of potentially dangerous chemicals in the brain and may help control brain blood flow and volume. Earlier research has linked sudden changes in blood flow and volume to stroke in the newborn.

Low birth weight itself is also the subject of extensive research. In spite of improvements in health care for some pregnant women, the incidence of low birth weight babies born each year in the United States remains at about 7.5 percent. Some scientists currently investigating this serious health problem are working to understand how infections, hormonal problems, and genetic factors may increase a woman's chances of giving birth prematurely. They are also conducting more applied research that could yield: 1) new drugs that can safely delay labor, 2) new devices to further improve medical care for premature infants, and 3) new insight into how smoking and alcohol consumption can disrupt fetal development.

While this research offers hope for preventing cerebral palsy in the future, ongoing research to improve treatment brightens the outlook for those who must face the challenges of cerebral palsy today. An important thrust of such research is the evaluation of treatments already in use so that physicians and parents have the information they need to choose the best therapy. A good example of this effort is an ongoing NINDS-supported study that promises to yield new information about which patients are most likely to benefit from selective dorsal root rhizotomy, a recently introduced surgery that is becoming increasingly in demand for reduction of spasticity.

Similarly, although physical therapy programs are a popular and widespread approach to managing cerebral palsy, little scientific evidence exists to help physicians, other health professionals, and parents determine how well physical therapy works or to choose the best approach among many. Current research on cerebral palsy aims to provide this information through careful studies that compare the abilities of children who have had physical and other therapy with those who have not.

As part of this effort, scientists are working to create new measures to judge the effectiveness of treatment, and ongoing research to precisely identify the specific brain areas responsible for movement may yield one such approach. Using magnetic pulses, researchers can locate brain areas that control specific actions, such as raising an arm or lifting a leg, and construct detailed maps. By comparing charts made before and after therapy among children who have cerebral palsy, researchers may gain new insights into how therapy affects the brain's organization and new data about its effectiveness.

Investigators are also working to develop new drugs—and new ways of using existing drugs—to help relieve cerebral palsy's symptoms. In one such set of studies, early research results suggest that doctors may improve the effectiveness of the anti-spasticity drug called baclofen by giving the drug through spinal injections, rather than by mouth. In addition, scientists are also exploring the use of tiny implanted pumps that deliver a constant supply of anti-spasticity drugs into the fluid around the spinal cord, in the hope of improving these drugs' effectiveness and reducing side effects, such as drowsiness.

Other experimental drug development efforts are exploring the use of minute amounts of the familiar toxin called botulinum. Ingested in large amounts, this toxin is responsible for botulism poisoning, in which the body's muscles become paralyzed. Injected in tiny amounts, however, this toxin has shown early promise in reducing spasticity in specific muscles.

A large research effort is also directed at producing more effective, nontoxic drugs to control seizures. Through its Antiepileptic Drug Development Program, the NINDS screens new compounds developed by industrial and university laboratories around the world for toxicity and anticonvulsant activity and coordinates clinical studies of efficacy and safety. To date, this program has screened more than thirteen thousand compounds and, as a result, five new antiepileptic drugs—carbamazepine, clonazepam, valproate, clorazepate, and felbamate—have been approved for marketing. A new project within the program is exploring how the structure of a given antiseizure medication relates to its effectiveness. If successful, this project may enable scientists to design better antiseizure medications more quickly and cheaply.

As researchers continue to explore new treatments for cerebral palsy and to expand our knowledge of brain development, we can expect significant medical advances to prevent cerebral palsy and many other disorders that strike in early life.

Research update: June 2000. Research conducted and supported by the National Institute of Neurological Disorders and Stroke (NINDS) continuously seeks to uncover new clues about cerebral palsy (CP). Investigators from the NINDS and the California Birth Defects Monitoring Program (CBDMP) presented data suggesting that very low birth weight babies have a decreased incidence of CP when their mothers are treated with magnesium sulfate soon before giving birth. The results of this study, which were based on observations of a group of children born in four Northern California counties, were published in the February 1995 issue of *Pediatrics*.

Low birth weight babies are one hundred times more likely to develop CP than normal birth weight infants. If further research confirms the study's findings, use of magnesium sulfate may prevent 25 percent of the cases of CP in the approximately fifty-two thousand low birth weight babies born each year in the United States.

Magnesium is a natural compound that is responsible for numerous chemical processes within the body and brain. Obstetricians in the United States often administer magnesium sulfate, an inexpensive form of the compound, to pregnant women to prevent preterm labor and high blood pressure brought on by pregnancy. The drug, administered intravenously in the hospital, is considered safe when given under medical supervision.

Scientists speculate that magnesium may play a role in brain development and possibly prevent bleeding inside the brains of preterm infants. Previous research has shown that magnesium may protect against brain bleeding in very premature infants. Animal studies have demonstrated that magnesium given after a traumatic brain injury can reduce the severity of brain damage.

Despite these encouraging research findings, pregnant women should not change their magnesium intake because the effects of high doses have not yet been studied and the possible risks and benefits are not known.

Researchers caution that more research will be required to establish a definitive relationship between the drug and prevention of the disorder. Clinical trials now underway, one of them a collaboration between the NINDS and the National Institute of Child Health and Human Development, are evaluating magnesium for the prevention of cerebral palsy in prematurely born babies.

Section 24.2

Botox in the Management of Children with Cerebral Palsy

Summary

Botulinum toxin injections have been found to be effective in the treatment of spasticity associated with cerebral palsy when used as one element of a multidisciplinary physical therapy program.

Botulinum toxin-A is a potent agent for inhibiting transmission between nerve cells and the muscles they innervate. As the name indicates, taken in sufficient amounts (usually by eating spoiled canned products), it can cause serious systemic effects including widespread muscle weakness and paralysis. Injected in small amounts into spastic or overactive muscles, it can reduce muscle pain and improve function. First used in the early 1980s for the treatment of imbalance in eye muscles, it is now used for an increasing number of neuromuscular abnormalities including cerebral palsy. Botox is the brand name of the injectable product.

Morton and his associates[1] have reviewed the available evidence for using Botox in children and adults with cerebral palsy. They cite well-conducted experiments to show that botulinum toxin is better than placebo in management of spastic calf muscles, improving gait. Injection into appropriate thigh muscles reduces hip pain. They cite many studies demonstrating the effectiveness of other specific injections for hemiplegic, diplegic, and quadriplegic children. Botox has been less effective in dealing with arm movement, in part because it weakens the patient's grip.

The effects are transient, usually wearing off in three to four months and often requiring re-injection. It should be used in concert with a multidisciplinary team and carefully defined goals. In the authors' view, it works best in younger children in combination with stretching exercises, gait training, and often splinting. They have treated children with Botox for more than seven years and believe it to be safe in the amounts recommended by the manufacturer.

Comment

In the United States, the Food and Drug Administration (FDA) has approved Botox only for strabismus (eye squint), blepharospasm (forced eye blinking), and dystonia (muscle spasms) of the neck. However, it is widely used for other conditions both in the United States and elsewhere. Such "off use" of medication is a widespread practice. When Botox is offered, parents should be convinced that the physician administering the agent is trained and experienced in its use in children and that it has been adequately studied for the specific indication for which it is being offered. Participation in future studies should be encouraged.

References

1. Morton, R.E., Hankinson, J., Nicholson, J., Botulinum toxin for cerebral palsy; where are we now? *Archives of Diseases of Childhood*, 2004 Dec; 89(12):1133–37.

Section 24.3

Hyperbaric Oxygen Therapy for Cerebral Palsy

Excerpted from "Hyperbaric Oxygen Therapy for Brain Injury, Cerebral Palsy, and Stroke," Summary, Evidence Report/Technology Assessment: Number 85, AHRQ Publication Number 03-E049, Agency for Healthcare Research and Quality, September 2003.

Overview

Hyperbaric oxygen therapy (HBOT) is the inhalation of 100 percent oxygen inside a hyperbaric chamber that is pressurized to greater than 1 atmosphere (atm). HBOT causes both mechanical and physiologic effects by inducing a state of increased pressure and hyperoxia. HBOT is typically administered at 1 to 3 atm. While the duration of an HBOT session is typically 90 to 120 minutes, the duration, frequency, and cumulative number of sessions have not been standardized.

HBOT is administered in two primary ways, using a monoplace chamber or a multiplace chamber. The monoplace chamber is the less costly option for initial setup and operation but provides less opportunity for patient interaction while in the chamber. Multiplace chambers allow medical personnel to work in the chamber and care for acute patients to some extent. The entire multiplace chamber is pressurized, so medical personnel may require a controlled decompression, depending on how long they were exposed to the hyperbaric air environment.

The purpose of this section is to provide a guide to the strengths and limitations of the evidence about the use of HBOT to treat patients who have cerebral palsy. Cerebral palsy refers to a motor deficit that usually manifests itself by two years of age and is secondary to an abnormality of at least the part of the brain that relates to motor function.

Predicting the outcome of cerebral palsy is difficult. Prognostic instruments are not precise enough to reliably predict an individual patient's mortality and long-term functional status. Various prognostic criteria for the cerebral palsy patient's function have been developed over the years. For example, if a patient is not sitting independently when placed by age two, then one can predict with approximately 95 percent confidence that he or she never will be able to walk. However, it is not possible to predict precisely when an individual patient is likely to acquire a particular ability, such as smiling, recognizing other individuals, or saying or understanding a new word.

This section focuses on the quality and consistency of studies reporting clinical outcomes of the use of HBOT in humans who have cerebral palsy. The information can be used to help providers counsel patients who use this therapy and to identify future research needs.

Research Questions

This section addresses the following questions:

1. Does HBOT improve functional outcomes in patients who have cerebral palsy? (Examples of improved functional outcomes are decreased spasticity, improved speech, increased alertness, increased cognitive abilities, and improved visual functioning.)

2. What are the adverse effects of using HBOT in these conditions?

Findings

There is insufficient evidence to determine whether the use of HBOT improves functional outcomes in children with cerebral palsy. The results of the only truly randomized trial were difficult to interpret because of the use of pressurized room air in the control group. As both groups improved, the benefit of pressurized air and of HBOT at 1.3 to 1.5 atm should both be examined in future studies.

The only other controlled study compared HBOT treatments with 1.5 atm to delaying treatment for six months. As in the placebo-controlled study, significant improvements were seen, but there was not a significant difference between groups.

Two fair-quality uncontrolled studies (one time-series, one before-after) found improvements in functional status comparable to the degree of improvement seen in both groups in the controlled trial.

Although none of the studies adequately measured caregiver burden, study participants often noted meaningful reductions in caregiver burden as an outcome of treatment.

Adverse Events

Evidence about the type, frequency, and severity of adverse events in actual practice is inadequate. Reporting of adverse effects was limited, and no study was designed specifically to assess adverse effects.

No study of HBOT for cerebral palsy has been designed to identify the chronic neurologic complications.

Pulmonary complications were relatively common in the trials of brain-injured patients. There are no reliable data on the incidence of aspiration in children treated for cerebral palsy with hyperbaric oxygen.

Ear problems are a known potential adverse effect of HBOT. While ear problems were reported in cerebral palsy studies, the incidence, severity, and effect on outcome are not clear. However, the rates reported among cerebral palsy patients were higher (up to 47 percent experiencing a problem) than reported with brain injury or stroke. However, the data in brain injury are limited by the use of prophylactic myringotomies.

Supplemental Qualitative Analysis

Opinions about the frequency and severity of risks of HBOT vary widely.

Several participants emphasized the importance of continued treatments to maximize results.

Patients and caregivers value any degree of benefit from HBOT highly. An improvement that may appear small on a standard measure of motor, language, or cognitive function can have a very large impact on caregiver burden and quality of life.

Future Research

We identified several barriers to conducting controlled clinical trials of HBOT for brain injury, particularly cerebral palsy:

- Lack of agreement on the dosage and the duration of treatment
- Need for better measures of relevant outcome measures, such as caregiver burden
- Lack of independent, reliable data on the frequency and severity of adverse events
- Patients' unwillingness to be assigned to a placebo or sham treatment group

As described in the following, strategies can be developed to conduct good-quality studies to overcome each of these barriers.

Dose and duration of treatment. Oxygen, the "active ingredient" in HBOT, is fundamentally a drug. As for any drug, dose and duration of treatment must be determined in carefully designed dose-ranging studies before definitive studies demonstrating clinical efficacy can be started. Good-quality dose-ranging studies of HBOT for brain injury can be done, based on the model used by pharmaceutical manufacturers and the FDA. It is likely that the dosage of HBOT needs to be individualized based on the patient's age, clinical condition, and other factors. This is the case for many other drugs and does not pose an insurmountable barrier to designing dose-finding trials. In fact, the need to individualize therapy makes it essential to base the design of long-term studies of clinical outcomes on the results of dose-ranging studies.

Better outcome measures. In describing the course of their patients, experienced clinicians who use HBOT to treat patients with brain injury, cerebral palsy, and stroke refer to improvements that may be ignored in standardized measures of motor and neuro-cognitive dysfunction. These measures do not seem to capture the impact of the changes that clinicians and parents perceive. Caregivers' perceptions should be given more weight in evaluating the significance of objective improvements in a patient's function. Unfortunately, studies have not consistently measured caregiver burden, or have assessed it only by self-report. Studies in which the caregivers' burden was directly observed would provide much stronger evidence than is currently available about treatment outcome.

Adverse events. Uncertainty about the frequency and severity of serious adverse events underlies much of the controversy about HBOT. The case against HBOT is based on the reasoning that, because HBOT may be harmful, it must be held to the highest standard of proof. A corollary is that, if HBOT can be shown to be as safe as its supporters believe it to be, the standard of proof of its efficacy can be lowered.

Good-quality studies of adverse effects are designed to assess harms that may not be known or even suspected. The most common strategy is to use a standard template of several dozen potential adverse effects affecting each organ system. Other characteristics of a good study of adverse events are a clear description of patient selection factors, independent assessment of events by a neutral observer, and the use of measures for the severity (rather than just the occurrence) of each event.

Unwillingness to be in a placebo group. The issue of placebo groups has been the subject of a great deal of debate. Participants on both sides make the assumption that an "evidence-based" approach implies devotion to double blind, placebo-controlled trials without regard to practical or ethical considerations. This assumption is false. Double blind, placebo-controlled trials are the "gold standard" for government regulators overseeing the approval of new pharmaceuticals, but not for clinical decision making or for insurance coverage decisions. Evidence-based clinical decisions rely more heavily on comparisons of a treatment to other potentially effective therapies than to placebos.

Several alternatives to the double blind, placebo-controlled trial can be used to examine effectiveness. One approach is to compare immediate to delayed treatment with HBOT, as was done in the Cornell trial. Another is to design a trial in which patients are randomly assigned to several alternative HBOT regimens. Because of uncertainty about the dosage and duration of treatment, such a trial would be preferable to a trial that offered a choice between one particular regimen and no treatment at all. It is also easier to incorporate a sham therapy arm in such a trial: patients may be more willing to enter a trial if they have a 10 percent or 20 percent chance of being assigned to sham treatment instead of a 50 percent chance. Other alternatives to a placebo include conventional physical, occupational, and recreational therapy, or another alternative therapy, such as patterning.

The Canadian trial of HBOT for cerebral palsy has important implications for the design of future research. In the trial there was a clinically significant benefit in the control group. Debate about the trial centers largely on how the response in the control group should be interpreted. The trial investigators believe that the beneficial effect was the result of the psychological effect of participating in the trial and extra attention paid the children in and out of the hyperbaric chamber. Alternatively, the slightly pressurized air (that is, "mild" hyperbaric oxygen) may have caused the improvement. A third possibility is that the slightly increased oxygen concentration, not the pressure per se, was responsible for the benefit.

A trial that could sort out which of these explanations was true would have a major impact on clinical practice. Such a trial might compare (1) room air under slightly elevated pressure, delivered in a hyperbaric chamber, to (2) elevated oxygen concentration alone, delivered in a hyperbaric chamber, and to (3) an equal amount of time in a hyperbaric chamber, with room air at atmospheric pressure. From the perspective of a neutral observer, the third group is not a "sham" but rather an attempt to isolate the effect of the social and psychological intervention cited by the Canadian investigators.

In addition to needing improved design, future trials of HBOT need better reporting. This would aid interpretation and the application of the research results. Two types of information are essential: a clear description of the research design, particularly of the control and comparison groups, and a detailed description of the patient sample. It is frequently difficult to tell from published studies how comparable the patient populations are, not only demographically but also clinically, in order to interpret the diagnosis and prognosis.

Section 24.4

Hypothermia in the Prevention of Cerebral Palsy among Newborn Infants

Summary

Three articles are reviewed that lend support to the usefulness of one or more techniques of hypothermia in the prevention of death and cerebral palsy among term babies born with evidence of hypoxic-ischemic encephalopathy. The study conducted under the auspices of the National Institute of Child Health and Human Development contains the most significant data.

Previous research fact sheets (April 1998 and February 2003) have commented on the potential role of hypothermia in preventing cerebral palsy and have reported on encouraging animal research models. Cooling inhibits a number of potentially damaging chemical reactions in the hypoxic brain and is ready for human trials. Two approaches are under evaluation: whole body cooling and selective cooling of the head using a device called the Cool-Cap®.

Seetha Shrankaran and her many colleagues report on a multi-center study on whole body infant cooling financed by the National Institute of Child Health and Human Development.[1] They studied newborn infants with evidence of hypoxic-ischemic brain injury randomized within six hours of birth to either traditional care plus whole body hypothermia for seventy-two hours (hypothermia group) or traditional care without hypothermia (control group). One hundred and two infants were assigned to the hypothermia group and 106 to the control group. The authors followed the surviving babies in both groups out to eighteen to twenty-two months of age. Follow-up was available on all the babies treated with hypothermia and all but five of the babies in the control group.

Their statistics clearly showed that fewer babies in the hypothermia group died or survived with severe disabilities. The difference was statistically significant, although individual outcome measures showed only trends. However, the trends within the study were very encouraging. Seventy-six percent of the hypothermia-treated babies survived compared to 63 percent of the controls. Concerns that the increased survival rate might translate into increased numbers of severely handicapped children proved to be unfounded. In the control group 30 percent of surviving children had disabling cerebral palsy, compared to only 19 percent of the hypothermic babies. Only 55 percent of the control babies had IQ's of 85 or better compared to 62 percent of the hypothermic babies. Similar reductions were seen in severe vision and hearing impairment.

Some months earlier, Gluckman and his associates[2] reported a similar study cooling only the heads of the babies using the Cool-Cap®. They applied EEG criteria to divide infants into those with moderate and those with severe brain injury. Sixty-six percent of babies in the control group died or had severe disabilities compared to 55 percent in the hypothermic group. Among the survivors, 31 percent of controls have severe neurosensory deficits compared to 19 percent of the babies treated with head cooling. Although these numbers did not reach statistical significance, their findings reinforce those of the whole body cooling study. The trend is encouraging.

In a smaller study, Inder and her group[3] demonstrated that among twenty-six infants randomized to control and hypothermic treatment, the hypothermic babies had much less abnormality in the cortical grey mater than did the controls.

Comment

Term babies with hypoxic-ischemic encephalopathy are at risk for spastic hemiplegic cerebral palsy as well as other forms. Although statistically significant results are most convincing, the trends reported in these three studies are certainly encouraging. Historically, one would hope we would soon see additional studies showing improved outcomes after technical fine-tuning. It is just possible that we are on our way to a management strategy capable of preventing cerebral palsy in a significant number of children.

References

1. Whole body hypothermia for neonates with hypoxic-ischemic encephalopathy. *New England Journal of Medicine* 2005; Vol 353: Pg. 1574–84.

2. Gluckman PD et al. Selective head cooling with mild systemic hypothermia after neonatal encephalopathy: multicenter, randomized trial. *The Lancet* 2005; Vol 365: Pg. 632–34.

3. Inder, TE et al. Randomized trial of systemic hypothermia selectively protects the cortex on MRI in term hypoxic-ischemic encephalopathy. *J. Pediatrics* 2004; Vol 145:Pg 835–37.

Chapter 25

Spina Bifida

Chapter Contents

Section 25.1—What You Should Know about Spina Bifida 396
Section 25.2—Urinary Tract Concerns in Spina Bifida 403
Section 25.3—Latex Allergy in Spina Bifida 405
Section 25.4—Fetal Surgery for Spina Bifida 407
Section 25.5—Tethering Spinal Cord 409

Section 25.1

What You Should Know about Spina Bifida

Reprinted from "Spina Bifida Fact Sheet," National Institute of Neurological Disorders and Stroke, National Institutes of Health, NIH Publication No. 05-309, January 25, 2006.

The human nervous system develops from a small, specialized plate of cells along the back of an embryo. Early in development, the edges of this plate begin to curl up toward each other, creating the neural tube—a narrow sheath that closes to form the brain and spinal cord of the embryo. As development progresses, the top of the tube becomes the brain and the remainder becomes the spinal cord. This process is usually complete by the twenty-eighth day of pregnancy. But if problems occur during this process, the result can be brain disorders called neural tube defects, including spina bifida.

What is spina bifida?

Spina bifida, which literally means "cleft spine," is characterized by the incomplete development of the brain, spinal cord, and/or meninges (the protective covering around the brain and spinal cord). It is the most common neural tube defect in the United States—affecting 1,500 to 2,000 of the more than 4 million babies born in the country each year.

What are the different types of spina bifida?

There are four types of spina bifida: occulta, closed neural tube defects, meningocele, and myelomeningocele.

Occulta is the mildest and most common form, in which one or more vertebrae are malformed. The name "occulta," which means "hidden," indicates that the malformation, or opening in the spine, is covered by a layer of skin. This form of spina bifida rarely causes disability or symptoms.

Closed neural tube defects make up the second type of spina bifida. This form consists of a diverse group of spinal defects in which the spinal cord is marked by a malformation of fat, bone, or membranes.

In some patients there are few or no symptoms; in others the malformation causes incomplete paralysis with urinary and bowel dysfunction.

In the third type, **meningocele**, the meninges protrude from the spinal opening, and the malformation may or may not be covered by a layer of skin. Some patients with meningocele may have few or no symptoms while others may experience symptoms similar to closed neural tube defects.

Myelomeningocele, the fourth form, is the most severe and occurs when the spinal cord is exposed through the opening in the spine, resulting in partial or complete paralysis of the parts of the body below the spinal opening. The paralysis may be so severe that the affected individual is unable to walk and may have urinary and bowel dysfunction.

What causes spina bifida?

The exact cause of spina bifida remains a mystery. No one knows what disrupts complete closure of the neural tube, causing a malformation to develop. Scientists suspect genetic, nutritional, and environmental factors play a role. Research studies indicate that insufficient intake of folic acid—a common B vitamin—in the mother's diet is a key factor in causing spina bifida and other neural tube defects. Prenatal vitamins that are prescribed for the pregnant mother typically contain folic acid as well as other vitamins.

What are the signs and symptoms of spina bifida?

The symptoms of spina bifida vary from person to person, depending on the type. Often, individuals with occulta have no outward signs of the disorder. Closed neural tube defects are often recognized early in life due to an abnormal tuft or clump of hair or a small dimple or birthmark on the skin at the site of the spinal malformation.

Meningocele and myelomeningocele generally involve a fluid-filled sac—visible on the back—protruding from the spinal cord. In meningocele, the sac may be covered by a thin layer of skin, whereas in most cases of myelomeningocele, there is no layer of skin covering the sac and a section of spinal cord tissue usually is exposed.

What are the complications of spina bifida?

Complications of spina bifida can range from minor physical problems to severe physical and mental disabilities. It is important to note, however, that most people with spina bifida are of normal intelligence. Severity is determined by the size and location of the malformation, whether or not skin covers it, whether or not spinal nerves protrude from it, and which spinal nerves are involved. Generally all nerves located below the malformation are affected. Therefore, the higher the malformation occurs on the back, the greater the amount of nerve damage and loss of muscle function and sensation.

In addition to loss of sensation and paralysis, another neurological complication associated with spina bifida is Chiari II malformation—a rare condition (but common in children with myelomeningocele) in which the brainstem and the cerebellum, or rear portion of the brain, protrude downward into the spinal canal or neck area. This condition can lead to compression of the spinal cord and cause a variety of symptoms including difficulties with feeding, swallowing, and breathing; choking; and arm stiffness.

Chiari II malformation may also result in a blockage of cerebrospinal fluid, causing a condition called hydrocephalus, which is an abnormal buildup of cerebrospinal fluid in the brain. Cerebrospinal fluid is a clear liquid that surrounds the brain and spinal cord. The buildup of fluid puts damaging pressure on the brain. Hydrocephalus is commonly treated by surgically implanting a shunt—a hollow tube—in the brain to drain the excess fluid into the abdomen.

Some newborns with myelomeningocele may develop meningitis, an infection in the meninges. Meningitis may cause brain injury and can be life-threatening.

Children with both myelomeningocele and hydrocephalus may have learning disabilities, including difficulty paying attention, problems with language and reading comprehension, and trouble learning math.

Additional problems such as latex allergies, skin problems, gastrointestinal conditions, and depression may occur as children with spina bifida get older.

How is it diagnosed?

In most cases, spina bifida is diagnosed prenatally, or before birth. However, some mild cases may go unnoticed until after birth, or postnatally. Very mild cases, in which there are no symptoms, may never be detected.

Prenatal diagnosis. The most common screening methods used to look for spina bifida during pregnancy are second trimester maternal serum alpha fetoprotein (MSAFP) screening and fetal ultrasound. The MSAFP screen measures the level of a protein called alpha-fetoprotein (AFP), which is made naturally by the fetus and placenta. During pregnancy, a small amount of AFP normally crosses the placenta and enters the mother's bloodstream. But if abnormally high levels of this protein appear in the mother's bloodstream it may indicate that the fetus has a neural tube defect. The MSAFP test, however, is not specific for spina bifida, and the test cannot definitively determine that there is a problem with the fetus. If a high level of AFP is detected, the doctor may request additional testing, such as an ultrasound or amniocentesis to help determine the cause.

The second trimester MSAFP screen described previously may be performed alone or as part of a larger, multiple-marker screen. Multiple-marker screens look not only for neural tube defects, but also for other birth defects, including Down syndrome and other chromosomal abnormalities. First trimester screens for chromosomal abnormalities also exist but signs of spina bifida are not evident until the second trimester when the MSAFP screening is performed.

Amniocentesis—an exam in which the doctor removes samples of fluid from the amniotic sac that surrounds the fetus—may also be used to diagnose spina bifida. Although amniocentesis cannot reveal the severity of spina bifida, finding high levels of AFP may indicate that the disorder is present.

Postnatal diagnosis. Mild cases of spina bifida not diagnosed during prenatal testing may be detected postnatally by x-ray during a routine examination. Doctors may use magnetic resonance imaging (MRI) or a computed tomography (CT) scan to get a clearer view of the spine and vertebrae. Individuals with the more severe forms of spina bifida often have muscle weakness in their feet, hips, and legs. If hydrocephalus is suspected, the doctor may request a CT scan and/or x-ray of the skull to look for extra fluid inside the brain.

How is spina bifida treated?

There is no cure for spina bifida. The nerve tissue that is damaged or lost cannot be repaired or replaced, nor can function be restored to the damaged nerves. Treatment depends on the type and severity of the disorder. Generally, children with the mild form need no treatment, although some may require surgery as they grow.

The key priorities for treating myelomeningocele are to prevent infection from developing through the exposed nerves and tissue of the defect on the spine, and to protect the exposed nerves and structures from additional trauma. Typically, a child born with spina bifida will have surgery to close the defect and prevent infection or further trauma within the first few days of life.

Doctors have recently begun performing fetal surgery for treatment of myelomeningocele. Fetal surgery—which is performed in utero (within the uterus)—involves opening the mother's abdomen and uterus and sewing shut the opening over the developing baby's spinal cord. Some doctors believe the earlier the defect is corrected, the better the outcome is for the baby. Although the procedure cannot restore lost neurological function, it may prevent additional loss from occurring. However, the surgery is considered experimental and there are risks to the fetus as well as to the mother.

The major risks to the fetus are those that might occur if the surgery stimulates premature delivery such as organ immaturity, brain hemorrhage, and death. Risks to the mother include infection, blood loss leading to the need for transfusion, gestational diabetes, and weight gain due to bed rest.

Still, the benefits of fetal surgery are promising, and include less exposure of the vulnerable spinal nerve tissue and bones to the intrauterine environment, in particular the amniotic fluid, which is considered toxic. As an added benefit, doctors have discovered that the procedure affects the way the brain develops in the uterus, allowing certain complications—such as Chiari II with associated hydrocephalus—to correct themselves, thus, reducing or, in some cases, eliminating the need for surgery to implant a shunt.

Many children with myelomeningocele develop a condition called progressive tethering, or tethered cord syndrome, in which their spinal cords become fastened to an immovable structure—such as overlying membranes and vertebrae—causing the spinal cord to become abnormally stretched and the vertebrae elongated with growth and movement. This condition can cause loss of muscle function to the legs, bowel, and bladder. Early surgery on the spinal cord may allow the child to regain a normal level of functioning and prevent further neurological deterioration.

Some children will need subsequent surgeries to manage problems with the feet, hips, or spine. Individuals with hydrocephalus generally will require additional surgeries to replace the shunt, which can be outgrown or become clogged.

Some individuals with spina bifida require assistive devices such as braces, crutches, or wheelchairs. The location of the malformation on the spine often indicates the type of assistive devices needed. Children with a defect high on the spine and more extensive paralysis will often require a wheelchair, while those with a defect lower on the spine may be able to use crutches, bladder catheterizations, leg braces, or walkers.

Treatment for paralysis and bladder and bowel problems typically begins soon after birth, and may include special exercises for the legs and feet to help prepare the child for walking with braces or crutches when he or she is older.

Can the disorder be prevented?

Folic acid, also called folate, is an important vitamin in the development of a healthy fetus. Although taking this vitamin cannot guarantee having a healthy baby, it can help. Recent studies have shown that by adding folic acid to their diets, women of childbearing age significantly reduce the risk of having a child with a neural tube defect, such as spina bifida. Therefore, it is recommended that all women of childbearing age consume 400 micrograms of folic acid daily. Foods high in folic acid include dark green vegetables, egg yolks, and some fruits. Many foods—such as some breakfast cereals, enriched breads, flours, pastas, rice, and other grain products—are now fortified with folic acid. A lot of multivitamins contain the recommended dosage of folic acid as well.

Women who have a child with spina bifida, have spina bifida themselves, or have already had a pregnancy affected by any neural tube defect are at greater risk of having a child with spina bifida or another neural tube defect. These women may require more folic acid before they become pregnant.

What is the prognosis?

Children with spina bifida can lead relatively active lives. Prognosis depends on the number and severity of abnormalities and associated complications. Most children with the disorder have normal intelligence and can walk, usually with assistive devices. If learning problems develop, early educational intervention is helpful.

What research is being done?

Within the federal government, the National Institute of Neurological Disorders and Stroke (NINDS), a component of the National Institutes of Health (NIH), supports and conducts research on brain and nervous system disorders, including spina bifida. NINDS conducts research in its laboratories at the NIH in Bethesda, Maryland, and supports research through grants to major medical institutions across the country.

In one study supported by NINDS, scientists are looking at the hereditary basis of neural tube defects. The goal of this research is to find the genetic factors that make some children more susceptible to neural tube defects than others. Lessons learned from this research will fill in gaps of knowledge about the causes of neural tube defects and may lead to ways to prevent these disorders. These researchers are also studying gene expression during the process of neural tube closure, which will provide information on the human nervous system during development.

In addition, NINDS-supported scientists are working to identify, characterize, and evaluate genes for neural tube defects. The goal is to understand the genetics of neural tube closure, and to develop information that will translate into improved clinical care, treatment, and genetic counseling.

Other scientists are studying genetic risk factors for spina bifida, especially those that diminish or lessen the function of folic acid in the mother during pregnancy, possibly leading to spina bifida in the fetus. This study will shed light on how folic acid prevents spina bifida and may lead to improved forms of folate supplements.

NINDS also supports and conducts a wide range of basic research studies to understand how the brain and nervous system develop. These studies contribute to a greater understanding of neural tube defects, such as spina bifida, and offer hope for new avenues of treatment for and prevention of these disorders as well as other birth defects.

Another component of the NIH, the National Institute of Child Health and Human Development (NICHD), is conducting a large five-year study to determine if fetal surgery to correct spina bifida in the womb is safer and more effective than the traditional surgery—which takes place a few days after birth. Researchers hope this study, called the Management of Myelomeningocele Study, or MOMS, will better establish which procedure, prenatal or postnatal, is best for the baby.

Section 25.2

Urinary Tract Concerns in Spina Bifida

Reprinted from "Spina Bifida: Urinary Tract Concerns," © Texas Pediatric Surgical Associates (www.pedisurg.com). Reprinted with permission. The text of this document is available online at http://www.pedisurg.com/PtEduc/Spina_Bifida_(Urinary_Tract_Concerns).htm; accessed February 17, 2006.

What is spina bifida?

Spina bifida (myelomeningocele) is a condition in which the lower part of the spinal cord does not form normally. Infants with this condition are born with remnants of the abnormal spinal cord enclosed in a sac on their back. These infants can have a number of problems, but this section will focus on problems in their urinary tract.

What is the urinary tract?

The urinary tract consists of the kidneys, ureters, bladder, and urethra. The kidneys are the organs that are responsible for filtering waste products from the bloodstream and produce urine continuously. The urine drains down tubes called ureters to the bladder, which normally stores urine and empties intermittently by muscular contraction. The urine exits the bladder through the urethra in a process is called voiding or urination.

Why evaluate the urinary tract in children with spina bifida?

Children who are born with spina bifida can have abnormalities of the urinary tract. Therefore, we obtain a renal ultrasound of the kidneys soon after birth to diagnose any congenital abnormalities of the kidneys. This test also provides an initial assessment of the kidneys so that we can later determine if there has been any damage to them from the abnormal bladder function. We also will obtain an x-ray of the bladder called a voiding cystourethrogram (VCUG) to assess for reflux (or backing up) of urine into the kidneys.

What is normal urination and what can happen in children with spina bifida?

Control over urination requires functional nerves in the lower spine (sacral spinal cord). These nerves sense bladder fullness and transmit this message to the brain. In an older child or adult who has normal urinary control, the brain is able to inhibit the bladder from contracting until it is socially acceptable. In many children with spina bifida the nerves to the bladder that control this reflex voiding are damaged. Only about 5 to 10 percent of children with spina bifida have normal urinary control and are able to toilet train and void spontaneously. This means that the majority of children with spina bifida are at risk for poor urinary control and incontinence as well as damage to the kidneys and bladder.

How is urinary control evaluated in children with spina bifida?

Urodynamic studies or cystometrograms are done in children with spina bifida to evaluate bladder function. These studies involve placing a catheter into the bladder and filling the bladder with water. While this is done, the pressure in the bladder is continuously monitored. Normally, when the bladder pressure reaches a certain level, urine begins to leak around the catheter. Some children with spina bifida, however, tolerate very high pressures in their bladder without any urine leakage, with the result that urine can reflux up the ureters and damage the kidneys. These children are often managed with intermittent catheterization, antibiotics for infection, and occasionally other medications and/or surgery.

Section 25.3

Latex Allergy in Spina Bifida

The first allergic reactions to natural latex rubber in people with spina bifida were reported in the late 1980s, one hundred years after latex was first used to make surgical rubber gloves. Since that time, research studies have shown that up to 73 percent of children and adolescents with spina bifida are sensitive to latex as measured by blood test or by a history of an allergic reaction.

Although the cause of latex allergy in individuals with spina bifida is not known, it is theorized that sensitization has developed because of the early, intense, and constant exposure to rubber products through repeated surgeries, diagnostic tests and examinations, and bladder and bowel programs. People with spina bifida who have shunts for hydrocephalus, other allergies, and multiple surgeries may be at highest risk for latex reactions. Latex allergy is also a problem for people who don't have spina bifida but who have had multiple latex exposures because of their occupation (health care workers) or their medical condition (asthma or other allergic disease, congenital bladder anomalies, frequent surgery or surgery in infancy).

Latex, a milky fluid harvested from the *Hevea brasiliensis* tree, is found in many common items, including medical and surgical gloves, urinary catheters, elastic bandages, Band-Aids, balloons, pacifiers, and condoms. Allergic reactions to latex proteins in these items can include watery and itchy eyes, sneezing and coughing, rash or hives, swelling of the windpipe, wheezing, difficulty breathing, and the life-threatening collapse of circulation called anaphylactic shock.

Exposure to latex can occur when products containing rubber come in contact with a person's skin or mucous membranes such as the mouth, eyes, genitals, bladder, or rectum. Serious reactions can also occur when latex enters the bloodstream, injected through the latex ports on intravenous tubing. The powder from balloon or gloves can absorb latex proteins and become airborne, causing reactions when breathed or touched by a latex-sensitive person. Food that has been handled by someone wearing latex gloves may also be contaminated by this glove powder. (People who have allergic reactions to latex may also be allergic to certain foods, including: bananas, tomatoes, potatoes, avocados, and kiwi fruit.) The only way to prevent allergic reactions to latex is by avoiding contact with items containing latex and the latex-contaminated powder.

Latex is often a hidden ingredient in medical and consumer products, and it is difficult to know if a product does or does not contain the substance. For this reason, the Food and Drug Administration now requires labeling of natural latex rubber in all medical devices. Consumer products are not yet covered by a labeling mandate, however. Research is currently focused on identifying all the proteins causing the allergy, standardizing reagents for improved testing, developing rubber products that do not cause allergy, and possibly learning how to desensitize people with severe latex allergy.

Latex allergy is not fully understood at this time. Current knowledge and available evidence indicate that people that people with spina bifida are at significant risk of becoming allergic to natural latex rubber, with possible life-threatening reactions. Individuals with spina bifida and their families are urged to consider the following recommendations and to and to discuss them with members of their health care team:

- All individuals with spina bifida should be considered at high risk for having an allergic reaction to rubber and should avoid contact with latex products in all settings from birth. Alternative products, usually made of silicone, plastic, nitrile, or vinyl, can usually be safely substituted.

- Individuals who have had an allergic reaction to latex should:

  - wear a medic-alert bracelet or necklace;

  - carry auto-injectable epinephrine;

  - carry sterile non-latex gloves and other necessary non-latex equipment for emergency use.

- Latex allergy and latex avoidance should be discussed with all health care and community providers including school, day care, and camp.

- Consultation with health care providers familiar with the latex allergy is recommended before hospitalization or surgery to prevent inadvertent exposure and plan for latex-safe care.

Commonly encountered items may contain latex and may pose a risk to the latex-sensitive individual.

Healthcare items that may contain latex: gloves, catheters, tourniquets, elastic bandages, ace wraps, IV tubing injection ports, medication vials, adhesive tape, dental dams, Band-Aids.

Home and community items that may contain latex: balloons, pacifiers, rubber bands, elastic in clothing, beach toys, Koosh balls, baby bottle nipples, condoms, diaphragms, diapers, art supplies.

Please note that this is only a partial list and it is strongly recommended that individuals with spina bifida and their families ask about the composition of products used in their case.

Section 25.4

Fetal Surgery for Spina Bifida

Reprinted from "Fetal Surgery for Spina Bifida Shows Early Benefits in Leg Function, Fewer Shunts," © 2003 The Children's Hospital of Philadelphia. All rights reserved. Reprinted with permission.

Physicians at the Children's Hospital of Philadelphia have reported encouraging short-term outcomes in fetal surgery for the birth defect spina bifida. Among the benefits were a reduced need for a shunt to divert excess fluid from the brain, the reversal of a potentially devastating neurologic condition called hindbrain herniation, and better-than-expected neurologic function in the infants' legs.

Mark Johnson, M.D., and colleagues from Children's Hospital's Center for Fetal Diagnosis and Treatment reported on the outcomes of fifty fetal surgeries for spina bifida in the September 2003 issue of the *American Journal of Obstetrics and Gynecology.*

The fetal surgeries were performed at Children's Hospital between 1998 and 2002. The mean gestational age of the fetuses undergoing the surgery was twenty-three weeks, and their mean gestational age at birth was thirty-four weeks.

Of the fifty fetuses, three died from complications following premature delivery. Of the remaining forty-seven infants, all had reversal of the hindbrain herniation, and twenty infants (43 percent) required a shunt—compared to an 85 percent rate of shunting, found in another study, for infants with spina bifida who had surgery after birth. Twenty-four of the infants (57 percent of the surviving forty-seven) had better neurologic leg function than predicted, based on the level of the spina bifida lesion.

Hindbrain herniation occurs when a portion of the brain protrudes through the base of the skull into the spinal column. If the tissue blocks the flow of cerebrospinal fluid within the brain, excess fluid may accumulate and cause increased pressure within the brain. The protruding hindbrain tissue may also injure nerves in the spinal cord. In all the fetuses, hindbrain herniation was present before the surgery, but resolved after the surgery.

However, the authors caution that long-term studies are needed to further evaluate leg function, bladder and bowel function, and neurodevelopment beyond the infant period.

Spina bifida is the most common birth defect of the central nervous system, affecting one in two thousand live births. A developmental failure early in pregnancy leaves an opening in part of the bone and tissue covering the fetus's spinal cord. The most common and most severe form of spina bifida is myelomeningocele, which may cause the child to suffer leg paralysis, lack of bowel and bladder control, and fluid pressure on the brain (hydrocephaly).

Surgery currently performed on newborns with open spina bifida lesions requires closing tissue over the defect to protect the spinal tissue. However, previous studies have suggested that neurological injury may occur before or during birth. To prevent that injury, physicians at Children's Hospital have performed surgery for spina bifida on the fetus prior to birth.

Performing the surgical closure of the spina bifida lesion in midpregnancy, between twenty and twenty-five weeks' gestation, may prevent the progressive neurological injury which occurs during the later part of pregnancy, according to the authors. They added that the potential benefits must be balanced against the risk of preterm delivery, and the surgical risks to the mother. "Following the fetal surgery, mothers remain in the Philadelphia area so we can monitor them closely until they deliver," said Dr. Johnson.

Dr. Johnson and his co-authors note in the study that they followed a "highly selected" population. The team did not operate on fetuses in whom fetal ultrasound detected irreversible neurologic damage, nor on fetuses in which the spina bifida defect occurred at a spinal level that would not be expected to cause neurological damage.

Because the current study reports only on short-term outcomes, longer-term studies are important in evaluating fetal surgery for spina bifida. The Children's Hospital of Philadelphia is currently participating in a multicenter, randomized clinical trial of the procedure, sponsored by the National Institutes of Health. That trial, which runs from 2002 through 2006, will compare the long-term outcomes of prenatal versus postnatal spina bifida repair.

Section 25.5

Tethering Spinal Cord

Spinal cord tethering is a common cause of deterioration in a child with spina bifida. Although the exact frequency with which it occurs isn't entirely known, it is estimated that from 20 to 50 percent of children with spina bifida will, at some time, require surgery to untether the spinal cord, making this operation the second most common operation (behind shunt operations) in these children. This section will address some of the common questions that have been raised about spinal cord tethering.

What is spinal cord tethering, and why is it bad?

During the early stages of a pregnancy, the spinal cord of the fetus extends from the brain all the way down to the coccygeal (tailbone) region of the spine. As the pregnancy progresses, the bony spine grows faster than the spinal cord, so the end of the spinal cord appears to rise, or ascend, relative to the adjacent bony spine. By the time a child is born, the spinal cord is normally located opposite the disc between the first and second lumbar vertebrae, in about the upper part of the lower back. In a baby with spina bifida, the spinal cord is still attached to the surrounding skin, and is prevented from ascending normally; the spinal cord at birth is therefore low-lying, or tethered. Although the myelomeningocele is separated from the skin and closed at birth, the spinal cord, which has grown in this position, stays in roughly the same location after the closure, and usually quickly scars to the site of the surgical closure. As the child (and the bony spine) continues to grow, the spinal cord can become stretched; this damages the spinal cord both by directly stretching it and by interfering with the blood supply to the spinal cord. The result can be progressive neurological, urological, or orthopedic deterioration.

What are the symptoms and signs of spinal cord tethering?

Children with spinal cord tethering may develop many different symptoms and signs. Conversely, many of the symptoms and signs of tethering can be caused by other problems, and the neurosurgeon needs to sort out the likely causes of the signs and symptoms in each case. Back pain, typically brought on or worsened by activity and relieved with rest, can be a sign of tethering. Sometimes the back pain is also associated with leg pain, even in areas that are numb. Changes in leg strength, or deterioration in gait (walking) can be signs of tethering. Manual muscle testing (MMT) of muscle strength is usually performed by physical therapists experienced in performing these tests, and can detect muscle weakness; these tests should ideally be performed on at least an annual basis, or whenever there is a change, to document changes before they become severe. The MMT has been shown to be a very reliable test of muscle strength if performed by experienced therapists. Progressive or repeated muscle contractures or orthopedic deformities of the legs, and scoliosis, may be signs of tethering as well. Finally, changes in bowel or bladder function can be signs of tethering; urodynamic studies, which provide an objective test of bladder function, can be very helpful in determining whether the changes are significant, and can sometimes detect bladder changes before they become apparent clinically.

How is a tethered cord diagnosed?

If a child with myelomeningocele and shunted hydrocephalus presents with clinical worsening, the first issue is to determine whether or not the shunt is working. As shunt malfunction can cause any of the signs or symptoms discussed previously, one should therefore always check the shunt first! Accordingly, the first test is usually a computed tomography (CT) or magnetic resonance imaging (MRI) scan of the brain. Although an increase in the size of the ventricles of the brain (that contain the cerebrospinal fluid) suggests a shunt malfunction, it is important to know that as many as 10 to 15 percent of children with shunt malfunction may have little or no change in the size of the ventricles. In some cases, the shunt is tapped (by inserting a needle through the skin into a "tapping chamber" for this purpose) and the flow of cerebrospinal fluid from the shunt, and the shunt pressures, are measured as another means of assessing shunt function. If there is any question about shunt function, the neurosurgeon may explore or revise the shunt at surgery before considering an untethering operation.

Once the shunt is found to be working, an MRI of the spine is performed. It is important to know that virtually every child with spina bifida has evidence of tethering on the MRI for the reasons discussed previously; untethering is therefore generally performed only if there are clinical signs or symptoms of deterioration. The MRI is obtained both to show the neurosurgeon the anatomy of the tethering and to exclude other abnormalities such as a syringomyelia, or syrinx for short (a fluid-filled cavity within the spinal cord); diastematomyelia, or split cord malformation (in which the spinal cord is split into two halves over a part of its length, with a bony spur between the two halves of the spinal cord); or a dermoid cyst (in which a small tag of skin is enclosed within the area around or within the spinal cord). Although MRI is the imaging study most commonly used, additional studies may include spine x-rays or CT scans of the spine, to look for various other bony abnormalities, or to follow the progress of scoliosis. Again, other functional studies may be done, including MMT and urodynamics, both to compare with previous studies to document a change and to give a baseline against which to compare after the surgery.

When and how is surgery performed?

After all of the diagnostic studies have been performed, the neurosurgeon may want to untether the spinal cord. The decision to untether requires some clinical judgment on the part of the neurosurgeon, who must take into account both the patient's symptoms and signs and the results of the preoperative studies. Unfortunately, since the MRI almost always shows tethering radiographically, the decision usually relies on the neurosurgeon's judgment as to what is causing the patient's symptoms and signs. A child with mild back pain who is otherwise stable might reasonably be watched or managed without surgery as long as he or she remains stable and the pain is manageable.

On the other hand, progressive or severe pain, loss of muscle function or deterioration in gait, or changes in bladder or bowel function usually require an operation to prevent further deterioration. Timing of surgery is important, as the longer deterioration is allowed to continue, the less likely function will be to return to its baseline with surgery; the timing depends upon the magnitude and rapidity of the changes.

The untethering procedure usually involves opening the scar from the prior closure; occasionally, an incision may be made perpendicular to the original scar, particularly if the original closure was horizontal on the back. The scar is dissected down to the covering (dura) over the myelomeningocele; often the dissection includes the more normal covering just above the scarred area to obtain landmarks and orientation. Sometimes a small portion of the bony vertebrae (the laminae) is removed to obtain better exposure or to decompress the spinal cord. The dura is then opened, and the spinal cord and myelomeningocele are gently dissected away from the scarred attachments to the surrounding dura. There are many methods for doing this, including scissors, scalpels, and various lasers; one way is not necessarily better than the others, and the surgeon usually has his or her own preference based upon personal experience. Once the myelomeningocele is freed from all of its scarred attachments, the dura and the wound are closed.

Recovery in the hospital is generally about two to five days; some surgeons require that the child remain flat in bed for a couple of days to minimize the risk of spinal fluid leakage from the wound. Pain is usually not severe, as the child usually has some degree of numbness in that area anyway. The child is usually back to fairly normal activities within a few weeks. Recovery of lost muscle and bladder function is variable, and again depends upon both the degree and length of the preoperative losses. Although we hope for improvements, it is important to understand that untethering is designed primarily to prevent further deterioration, rather than to improve deterioration that has already occurred.

What are the complications of untethering?

Untethering is generally a very safe procedure in experienced hands; however, the scar can make dissection difficult and the abnormal anatomy can be confusing at times, even to the experienced neurosurgeon. Complications are few, but include infection, bleeding, and damage to the spinal cord and myelomeningocele resulting in worsening muscle, bladder, or bowel function. The combined complication rate of surgery is usually only 1 to 2 percent. Although some have suggested that shunt malfunction may occur secondary to untethering surgery, it is probably more likely that an occult or unrecognized shunt malfunction was the original cause of the deterioration in the first place.

Is repeat untethering necessary?

Symptomatic tethering can occur at any time in the child's life, although the most common time is in the early preadolescent period (seven to twelve years) and extending into mid-adolescence. Symptoms from tethering can often occur during periods of growth, as might be expected, or during growth hormone treatments for short stature. Since all children grow, it is puzzling as to why some children develop symptoms and signs of tethering, while others don't; perhaps some children's spinal cords are more lax early in life, or tolerate a greater degree of stretching than others.

Although most children require only one untethering procedure, a minority (perhaps 10 to 20 percent) require repeated untethering operations as the children continue to grow. Those who undergo untethering very early in life (as toddlers or young children) may more frequently require additional untethering procedures later, as they continue to grow. Fortunately, once the child stops growing, and the "adult" height is reached, clinical deterioration from tethering becomes much less frequent (although it can still occur).

Can anything be done to prevent tethering?

Many techniques have been tried to prevent or minimize tethering, but none has met with unqualified success in long-term studies. Surgeons have placed grafts of various substances such as Dacron, Teflon, and other materials around the myelomeningocele, hoping to prevent scarring to the surrounding dura. Some of these have actually produced more scarring. Others have cut off the myelomeningocele (cordectomy) if the child has no leg function, hoping to eliminate the scar from the myelomeningocele (however, this technique carries a risk of worsening bladder function and obviously eliminates any hope of recovering any functions if something in the future were to allow this). Most neurosurgeons now bring the edges of the flat myelomeningocele "placode" together during the initial closure, and sew the edges together to re-create the spinal cord in order to minimize

413

formation of scar. Although this makes subsequent untethering easier and less risky should it need to be done, neither this nor any other technique has been proven to reduce the frequency of subsequent tethering in the long run. Research continues into this important area.

In conclusion, although the tethered cord is a common condition requiring surgery, it is also very treatable. Modern microsurgical techniques and the availability of such techniques as the operating microscope and lasers have made this a relatively routine surgical procedure in the hands of an experienced neurosurgeon. With close observation, it should be possible to diagnose this condition early and untether the cord before progressive and permanent damage occurs.

Chapter 26

Congenital Lung Lesions

What are congenital lung lesions?

There are three broad categories of congenital lung lesions: Cystic adenomatoid malformations (also called CCAM), bronchopulmonary sequestrations (or sequestrations, for short), and bronchogenic cysts. All three types represent the abnormal development of lung tissue, which may occur during normal fetal development. Why these lesions form is not really known; how they differ from each other may have to do with the timing and location of their development.

In the embryo, the lungs develop as an outpouching of what will become the esophagus: a "bud" develops, which elongates to become the trachea, then divides to become the left and right main stem bronchi. Further division of each bronchus will, like the branches of a growing tree, form the "tracheobronchial" tree of airways. At the same time, the lung parenchyma (the actual lung tissue responsible for exchange of oxygen and gases into and out of the bloodstream) develops around each of those airway branches.

A bronchogenic cyst is nothing more than an airway branch that buds off, loses all connections with the rest of the tracheobronchial tree, and does not connect with actual tissue. As a result, a cyst forms, which is lined by the same cells one finds in the trachea or the bronchi.

A sequestration represents a portion of lung (with a bronchus and some lung tissue) that has completely separated from the rest of the lung. If this separation occurs relatively early in embryonic life (before the sixth week of pregnancy), this "mini-lung" is usually fully developed and separate from the rest of the organ. It also contains its own blood supply: an artery that is directly connected to the aorta, for example. However, because it is separate from the rest of the lung, no air goes in or out of this "extralobar" sequestration.

If the separation from the rest of the lung occurs later (between the eighth and the twelfth week of pregnancy), it usually remains within the normal lung (but may still have separate blood vessels). Even though it is not connected to the rest of the tracheobronchial tree by a normal bronchus, there may be microscopic communications with the rest of the lung: in this type, the "intralobar" sequestration, some air (and bacteria) may get trapped in the lesion after birth, which may cause recurrent infections.

The congenital cystic adenomatoid malformation (CCAM) is less easily explained, but consists of some or all types of lung and bronchial cells and structures, arranged in a disorderly fashion. It is not a tumor, however: the cells themselves are not malignant and do not grow, invade other organs, or spread to other parts of the body; rather, it is a "clumsily put together" part of lung that doesn't function properly. Because a CCAM tends to develop within the normal lung, microscopic communications with that lung also place the child at risk for infections, from trapped air and bacteria.

While the preceding classification is helpful, it is not always clear-cut, and many "hybrid" forms exist: lesions that have characteristics of more than one type. In addition, in up to 50 percent of sequestrations, part of the otherwise normal lung tissue is replaced by a CCAM.

Congenital lobar emphysema is one more form of congenital lung lesions, but it is much less common than the ones mentioned previously. In congenital lobar emphysema, or CLE, one of the bronchi of a lung may be partially and/or intermittently blocked, causing accumulation of fluid and distension of the lung tissue connected to that bronchus. While the cause of this condition is different, its course and treatment is remarkably similar to that of the lesions described above.

How common is it?

Congenital lung lesions are seen in approximately one of every three thousand live births. They are most often isolated findings, not associated with chromosomal or genetic disorders. CCAMs and sequestrations are sometimes seen in fetuses with a congenital diaphragmatic hernia, and can be an incidental finding (i.e., discovered by chance) in otherwise healthy children or children with unrelated anomalies.

What can happen before birth?

Most congenital lung lesions do not become visible until early in the second trimester. They often grow, sometimes fast, causing the lung on the same side to be compressed. In addition, the heart may be pushed to the other side, and even the lung on the other side may be compressed. If the lesion becomes very large, it may start to affect the well-being of the fetus: extreme compression of the heart and the large blood vessels of the chest may impair the heart's function, and this could lead to hydrops (heart failure) and death. If compression of organs in the chest is severe and continues for a long time during pregnancy, the baby's lungs may not function well at birth (pulmonary hypoplasia).

In most cases, however, growth of these lesions is limited, and they tend to become smaller toward the end of the second trimester. In approximately 75 percent of the cases, the lesion regresses either partially or completely by the time the baby is born; not uncommonly, the lesion is not visible by prenatal ultrasound anymore.

Of course, premature birth can affect the outcome, particularly if it occurs as the lesion is still large and compressing the lungs. However, the presence of a congenital lung lesion does not in itself increase the risk of prematurity.

It is important to realize that the accuracy of the diagnosis, although very good, is not 100 percent perfect. The condition most resembling a congenital lung lesion is congenital diaphragmatic hernia. In this condition, a hole in the diaphragm allows intestines and other abdominal organs to move into the chest cavity, thereby compressing the lungs. The effect of a diaphragmatic hernia on the lungs of the fetus is similar to that of a congenital lung lesion. However, a diaphragmatic hernia does not get better during pregnancy, and many of these infants are born with hypoplastic lungs. With current imaging techniques (ultrasound and magnetic resonance imaging, or MRI), the diagnosis of a diaphragmatic hernia can almost always be differentiated from a lung lesion (bronchogenic cyst, CCAM, or sequestration).

What can be done before birth?

In most cases, the lesion will eventually regress without causing any permanent damage. If this can be predicted to occur, there is of course no reason to intervene before birth. It will be important, though, to follow the lesion closely, usually with weekly ultrasounds, until it is clear that the lesion is getting smaller. In addition, it may be helpful to obtain a fetal MRI: this test may give more information than the ultrasound about the exact appearance of the lesion, possible feeding blood vessels, and the condition of the surrounding normal lung. It can help differentiate cystic lung lesions from congenital lobar emphysema or diaphragmatic hernia.

If the lesion seems to grow too much, and early signs of heart failure are seen, something may have to be done. If this occurs after twenty-five to twenty-six weeks of pregnancy, it may be safer to think about early delivery, rather than to continue the pregnancy or even to intervene directly on the fetus. This is recommended only if the life of the fetus is believed to be at risk, since such extreme prematurity carries an important risk of complications.

If signs of heart failure occur earlier in pregnancy (before twenty-three to twenty-four weeks), early delivery is not an option, since infants of that gestational age cannot survive outside the womb. Intervention on the fetus may be possible, although this is obviously an invasive and risky procedure. If the lesion consists mainly of one or two large cysts, it may be possible to remove the fluid inside those cysts, thereby collapsing the lesion and allowing heart and lungs to function better. This procedure, called thoracentesis, is usually performed under local anesthesia and constant ultrasound guidance. A long, thin needle is introduced directly into the womb, and into the fetus's chest. Fluid is aspirated from the lesion, and the needle is withdrawn, or a "double pigtail" catheter is left behind. This will then continue to drain fluid from the cyst into the amniotic cavity.

In rare cases, the lesion continues to grow and threatens the well-being of the fetus, but no single large cyst can be identified. In these cases, when the lesion is mostly solid, the only option may be to remove the lesion surgically. This type of fetal surgery is the most invasive and riskiest form of intervention on the fetus, and can be performed only in specialized centers. Although this can be life saving, not all babies can be saved, and the procedure carries some risks to the mother as well.

If the lesion does regress, as is seen in the majority of cases, no prenatal intervention is needed. It may be important to plan for the delivery, however:

Mode and timing of delivery. While cesarean section can sometimes be indicated for certain conditions of the fetus, there is no need for it in the case of a congenital lung lesion. Of course, a cesarean section may still be performed for obstetrical reasons.

As mentioned before, prematurity may increase the risk of complications for the newborn baby. Since the lesions usually regress toward the end of the second trimester or the beginning of the third trimester, preterm delivery is usually not indicated, unless there are signs that the fetus is in trouble.

Place of delivery. Because of the risks of lung failure in the newborn infant and the possibility of early hydrops in the fetus, it is recommended that the baby be born in a hospital that has immediate access to a tertiary neonatal intensive care unit. In some cases, the lesion is still sufficiently large at birth (particularly if the baby is born prematurely) that immediate surgical intervention is necessary. For that reason, presence of pediatric surgical specialists is also advisable.

What will happen at birth?

If everything goes as planned, you will deliver at a tertiary care center with direct access to a neonatal intensive care unit. The neonatologists will be present at delivery, so that they can immediately assess your baby and start treatment, if necessary. At the same time, the pediatric surgeons will be alerted. In many cases, however, you will be able to see (and hold) your baby after delivery.

Your baby will be "stabilized" in the intensive care unit. An intravenous line will be placed in an arm or a leg, so that fluids can be given. If you baby shows signs of distress, it is possible that he or she will be intubated, so that we can help him or her breathe better.

If it is clear that there are no other major problems, your baby will undergo imaging tests to look for the lesion. If your baby is stable and breathing well, a chest x-ray and/or an ultrasound will be obtained, usually within one or two days. Even if the lesion had "disappeared" by prenatal ultrasound, it can usually be found by ultrasound or chest x-ray after birth, since imaging the baby directly can show more details than when the fetus is still in the womb.

Babies who breathe well and show no other signs of distress don't need immediate intervention. Typically, your baby will be allowed to go home, and plans will be made for him or her to be seen by a pediatric surgeon. Even if there are no symptoms, surgical intervention may be recommended later in infancy (typically, between six and eighteen months), to avoid long-term complications of the lesion. In some cases, this can be done using minimally invasive techniques (thoracoscopy); in others, the operation will be performed using a thoracotomy.

If the infant has breathing difficulties and it is felt that this is due to the lesion, more urgent intervention may be necessary. This can be done immediately after birth, or later in the newborn period. The results of the operation and the outcome for your baby depend primarily on the severity of the condition and the degree of prematurity. Surgical removal of part of a lung is an invasive procedure, but one that can be performed safely in even the smallest of patients. Even if a portion of normal lung has to be removed or if the lesion has prevented full development of the normal lung, full recovery is likely: normally, lungs continue to grow until a child is several years old.

What complications are likely, and what is the long-term outlook?

The overall outcome of congenital lung lesions (CCAM, bronchogenic cyst, sequestration) is generally excellent if the lesion has substantially shrunk by the time of birth. As mentioned before, CCAM and intralobar sequestrations are at a significant risk of recurrent infections (pneumonia). The infected cysts may look like lung abscesses—the knowledge of an underlying cystic lesion greatly facilitates the diagnosis. Pneumonia and other lung infections are treated with antibiotics, but recurrence of infections can be avoided by surgically removing the lesion.

In a small number of patients, the lung lesion (usually a CCAM) may harbor a malignant tumor later in life. This is another reason to recommend surgical removal of the lesion in early childhood, even if your child has never shown any symptoms.

Chapter 27

Defects of the
Liver and Pancreas

Chapter Contents

Section 27.1—Annular Pancreas 422
Section 27.2—Pancreas Divisum 424
Section 27.3—Biliary Atresia 425

Section 27.1

Annular Pancreas

Definition: An annular pancreas is a ring or collar of pancreatic tissue that abnormally encircles the duodenum (the part of the small intestine that connects to the stomach).

Causes, Incidence, and Risk Factors: Annular pancreas is thought to be caused by a malformation during the development of the pancreas, before birth. This condition may result in a narrowing of the duodenum due to constriction by the ring of pancreas.

Complete obstruction of the duodenum is often seen in newborns with this condition. However, half of the cases occur in adults. There are probably many cases that go undetected due to mild symptoms.

There is an increased incidence of peptic ulcer associated with this condition. Annular pancreas affects approximately one in seven thousand people.

Symptoms:

- Fullness after eating
- Nausea
- Vomiting
- Feeding intolerance in newborns

Signs and Tests:

Signs that may indicate annular pancreas include the following:

- Polyhydramnios (excessive amniotic fluid during pregnancy);
- Pancreatitis;
- Down syndrome;
- Other congenital gut anomalies.

Tests include:

- Abdominal x-ray;
- Computed tomography (CT) scan;
- Upper gastrointestinal (GI) and small bowel series;
- Abdominal ultrasound.

Treatment: Surgical bypass of the obstructing segment of the duodenum is the usual treatment for this disorder.

Expectations (Prognosis): There is a good prognosis with surgery.

Complications:

- Peptic ulcer
- Perforation of the intestine due to obstruction
- Peritonitis

Calling Your Health Care Provider: Call for an appointment with your health care provider if you or your child develop any symptoms of annular pancreas.

Section 27.2

Pancreas Divisum

Definition: Pancreas divisum is a congenital (present from birth) defect in which parts of the pancreas to fail to fuse together.

Causes, Incidence, and Risk Factors: In this condition, the ducts of the pancreas are affected. In many cases this defect goes undetected. The cause of the defect is unknown. However, if the pancreatic ducts become obstructed, symptoms similar to pancreatitis may develop. Pancreas divisum affects about 5 percent of the general population.

Symptoms:

- Abdominal pain
- Nausea or vomiting
- Abdominal distention

Note: There may be no symptoms.

Signs and Tests:

- An ERCP (endoscopic retrograde cholangiopancreatography)
- Elevated blood amylase and lipase
- Abdominal computed tomography (CT) scan

Treatment: If a person has symptoms of this condition or has had recurrent pancreatitis, surgical bypass or reconstruction of the malformed pancreatic ducts may be indicated to relieve obstruction.

Expectations (Prognosis): The probable outcome is good with treatment.

Complications: The main complication of pancreas divisum is pancreatitis.

Calling Your Health Care Provider: Call for an appointment with your health care provider if symptoms of this disorder develop.

Prevention: Because this condition is present at birth, there is no known prevention.

Section 27.3

Biliary Atresia

From the *Gale Encyclopedia of Medicine*,
by J. Ricker Polsdorfer, 3, Gale Group, © 2002, Gale Group.
Reprinted by permission of The Gale Group.

Definition: Biliary atresia is the failure of a fetus to develop an adequate pathway for bile to drain from the liver to the intestine.

Description: Biliary atresia is the most common lethal liver disease in children, occurring once in every ten thousand to fifteen thousand live births. Half of all liver transplants are done for this reason.

The normal anatomy of the bile system begins within the liver, where thousands of tiny bile ducts collect bile from liver cells. These ducts merge into larger and larger channels, like streams flowing into rivers, until they all pour into a single duct that empties into the duodenum (first part of the small intestine). Between the liver and the duodenum this duct has a side channel connected to the gall bladder. The gall bladder stores bile and concentrates it, removing much of its water content. Then, when a meal hits the stomach, the gall bladder contracts and empties its contents.

Bile is a mixture of waste chemicals that the liver removes from the circulation and excretes through the biliary system into the intestine. On its way out, bile assists in the digestion of certain nutrients. If bile cannot get out because the channels are absent or blocked, it backs up into the liver and eventually into the rest of the body. The major pigment in bile is a chemical called bilirubin, which is yellow. Bilirubin is a breakdown product of hemoglobin (the red chemical in blood that carries oxygen). If the body accumulates an excess of bilirubin, it turns yellow (jaundiced). Bile also turns the stool brown. Without it, stools are the color of clay.

Causes and Symptoms: It is possible that a viral infection is responsible for this disease, but evidence is not yet convincing. The cause remains unknown.

The affected infant will appear normal at birth and during the newborn period. After two weeks the normal jaundice of the newborn will not disappear, and the stools will probably be clay-colored. At this point, the condition will come to the attention of a physician. If not, the child's abdomen will begin to swell, and the infant will get progressively more ill. Nearly all untreated children will die of liver failure within two years.

Diagnosis: The persistence of jaundice beyond the second week in a newborn with clay-colored stools is a sure sign of obstruction to the flow of bile. An immediate evaluation that includes blood tests and imaging of the biliary system will confirm the diagnosis.

Treatment: Surgery is the only treatment. Somehow the surgeon must create an adequate pathway for bile to escape the liver into the intestine. The altered anatomy of the biliary system is different in every case, calling upon the surgeon's skill and experience to select and execute the most effective among several options. If the obstruction is only between the gall bladder and the intestine, it is possible to attach a piece of intestine directly to the gall bladder. More likely, the upper biliary system will also be inadequate, and the surgeon will attach a piece of intestine directly to the liver—the Kasai procedure. In its wisdom, the body will discover that the tiny bile ducts in that part of the liver are discharging their bile directly into the intestine. Bile will begin to flow in that direction, and the channels will gradually enlarge. Survival rates for the Kasai procedure are commonly 50 percent at five years and 15 percent at ten years. Persistent disease in the liver gradually destroys the organ.

Liver transplantation must be anticipated in all but the few patients who continue to do well after a Kasai procedure. Accumulating experience and newer techniques of liver transplantation are producing very gratifying early results.

Prognosis: Before liver transplants became available, even prompt and effective surgery did not cure the whole problem. Biliary drainage can usually be established, but the patients still have a defective biliary system that develops progressive disease and commonly leads to an early death. Transplantation now achieves up to 90 percent one-year survival rates and promises to prevent the chronic disease that used to accompany earlier procedures.

Prevention: The specific cause of this birth defect is unknown, so all that women can do is to practice the many general preventive measures, even before they conceive.

Chapter 28

Defects of the Upper Gastrointestinal Tract

Chapter Contents

Section 28.1—Esophageal Atresia and Tracheoesophageal
    Fistula 430
Section 28.2—Congenital Diaphragmatic Hernia 432
Section 28.3—Fetal Surgery for Congenital Diaphragmatic
    Hernia 435
Section 28.4—Gastroschisis 437
Section 28.5—Omphalocele 441

Section 28.1

Esophageal Atresia and Tracheoesophageal Fistula

© Texas Pediatric Surgical Associates. Reprinted with permission. The text of this document is available online at http://www.pedisurg.com/PtEduc/ TEF-Esophageal_Atresia.htm; accessed February 17, 2006.

What are the esophagus and trachea?

- Esophagus: tube that connects the mouth to the stomach

- Trachea: "windpipe"

- Atresia: absence of a normal opening

- Congenital: found at birth

- Fistula: abnormal passage from a body organ to the body surface or between two internal body organs

Congenital esophageal atresia (EA) represents a failure of the esophagus to develop as a continuous passage. Instead, it ends as a blind pouch. Tracheoesophageal fistula (TEF) represents an abnormal opening between the trachea and esophagus. EA and TEF can occur separately or together. EA and TEF are diagnosed in the intensive care unit at birth and treated immediately.

How are esophageal atresia and tracheoesophageal fistula diagnosed and treated?

The presence of EA is suspected in an infant with excessive salivation (drooling) and in a newborn with drooling that is frequently accompanied by choking, coughing, and sneezing. When fed, these infants swallow normally but begin to cough and struggle as the fluid returns through the nose and mouth. The infant may become cyanotic (turn bluish due to lack of oxygen) and may stop breathing as the overflow of fluid from the blind pouch is aspirated (sucked into) the trachea. The cyanosis is a result of laryngospasm (a protective mechanism that the body has to prevent aspiration into the trachea). Over time respiratory distress will develop.

If any of the above signs or symptoms are noticed, a catheter is gently passed into the esophagus to check for resistance. If resistance is noted, other studies will be done to confirm the diagnosis. A catheter can be inserted and will show up as white on a regular x-ray film to demonstrate the blind pouch ending. Sometimes a small amount of barium (chalk-like liquid) is placed through the mouth to diagnose the problems.

Treatment of EA and TEF is surgery to repair the defect. If EA or TEF is suspected, all oral feedings are stopped and intravenous fluids are started. The infant will be positioned to help drain secretions and decrease the likelihood of aspiration. Babies with EA may sometimes have other problems. Studies will be done to look at the heart and spine. Sometimes studies are done to look at the kidneys.

Surgery to fix EA is rarely an emergency. Once the baby is in condition for surgery, an incision is made on the side of the chest. The esophagus can usually be sewn together. Following surgery, the baby may be hospitalized for a variable length of time. Care for each infant is individualized.

Section 28.2

Congenital Diaphragmatic Hernia

What is congenital diaphragmatic hernia?

The wide, flat muscle that separates the chest and abdominal cavities is called the diaphragm. The diaphragm forms when a fetus is at eight weeks' gestation. When it does not form completely, a defect, called a congenital diaphragmatic hernia (CDH), is created. This is a hole in the muscle between the chest and the abdomen.

The majority of CDHs occur on the left side. The hole allows the contents of the abdomen (stomach, intestine, liver, spleen, and kidneys) to go up into the fetal chest. The herniation of these abdominal organs into the chest occupies that space and prevents the lungs from growing to normal size. The growth of both lungs can be affected. This is called pulmonary hypoplasia.

While in the uterus, a fetus does not need its lungs to breathe, because the placenta performs this function. However, if the lungs are too small after the baby is born, the baby will not be able to provide itself with enough oxygen to survive.

What is the outcome for a fetus with CDH?

There is a wide range of severity and outcomes for CDH. In the best cases, some infants do very well with routine treatment after birth. In the worst cases, some will not survive no matter how hard we try. And in the middle, some will live normally while others will have a difficult time and have to deal with some handicaps ranging from mild learning problems to breathing and growth problems. How the baby does after birth is determined by how well the lung grows before birth.

Fetuses on the best end of the spectrum have an excellent chance to lead a perfectly normal life. They do not require special prenatal management in terms of the timing or type of delivery, but should be delivered in a perinatal center with a Level III intensive care nursery with good neonatal and pediatric surgery support. The place of delivery is very important because transporting these babies after birth can be dangerous for the infant. Many babies still have to have the defect repaired after birth and will be in the intensive care nursery for several weeks. Even though the lung isn't of normal size at birth, it has the capacity to grow and adapt for many years, so these kids will lead normal active lives without restriction.

On the other end of the spectrum, babies with severe CDH and very small lungs are guaranteed to have a difficult struggle after birth, and some will not survive. These babies require very skilled intensive care to stay alive—things like high-frequency or oscillatory ventilation, inhaled nitric oxide and, in some cases, extracorporeal membrane oxygenation (ECMO). ECMO provides temporary support for lung failure by circulating the baby's blood through a heart-lung type machine. It can be life saving, but can be used for only a limited time before complications become excessive.

These babies must be delivered in a very experienced tertiary perinatal center with ECMO capability. The surgery to repair diaphragmatic hernia after birth is not an extreme emergency and is usually performed when the baby has stabilized in the first week of life. After repair, these babies will need intensive support for many weeks or even months. Even when the CDH is severe, greater than 70 percent of affected babies can be saved with intensive support. However, there will be long-term health issues related to breathing, feeding, growth, and development problems.

Most fetuses with CDH fall between these extremes of severity.

How serious is my fetus's diaphragmatic hernia?

For you to make the best decision, you must have accurate and complete information about your fetus's condition. This includes:

- The type of defect—distinguishing it from other similar-appearing problems;
- The severity of the defect—whether your fetus's defect is mild or severe;
- Associated defects—whether there is another problem or a cluster of problems (syndrome).

Amniocentesis may be necessary for chromosome testing. Sonography is the best imaging tool, but is dependent on the experience and expertise of the operator. Magnetic resonance imaging may be necessary in some cases. Many problems are first detected during routine screening procedures performed in your doctor's office (amniocentesis, maternal serum screening, routine sonography), but assessment of complex problems usually requires a tertiary perinatal/neonatal center with experience managing complex and rare fetal problems.

Fortunately, we can now predict before birth how good or bad your fetus's CDH is. Careful and accurate prenatal assessment [level II sonogram, echocardiogram, sometimes magnetic resonance imaging (MRI)] is critical for your decision-making and planning. One of the most important issues is to make sure there are no other birth defects (like heart problems) that will affect outcome. When CDH is the only problem, we have learned that severity and, thus, outcome is determined by two factors: 1) liver position, and 2) lung-to-head ratio or LHR. Liver position refers to whether or not any portion of the liver has herniated, or gone up into the chest of the fetus. Fetuses with the liver up in the chest have a more severe form of CDH and a low survival rate. About 75 percent of all CDH patients have some portion of the liver herniated into the chest. The lung-to-head ratio, or LHR, is a numeric estimate of the size of the fetal lungs, based on measurement of the amount of visible lung. High LHR values are associated with a good outcome.

Fetuses on the best end of the spectrum do not have liver herniated into the chest (liver down) and have a high lung-to-head ratio greater than 1.4, indicating a relatively large lung. In our experience evaluating many hundreds of CDH patients, about 25 percent are on the best end of the spectrum (liver down and/or high LHR greater than 1.4), and they all do well after birth. We are, of course, delighted when we can confidently predict a good outcome. We recommend these babies be delivered normally near term in a center with a very good intensive care nursery and good pediatric surgery.

Fetuses with liver herniated into the chest and a lung-to-head ratio less than 1.0 are on the worst end of the spectrum. We can be sure that they will have a very difficult time after birth. Most can be helped with very high level intensive care, including ECMO. However, the very intensive care required for the most severe cases can lead to complications and long-term problems, including breathing and feeding difficulties for many years. In our experience, about 25 percent of fetuses have this severe form of CDH, and about 70 percent of these survive with very intensive management, but often with some handicap.

About half of all fetuses with CDH are neither very good nor very bad, but are somewhere in the middle of this spectrum. With good intensive care and surgery at an experienced medical center, most (more than 90 percent) will survive and do quite well.

Section 28.3

Fetal Surgery for Congenital Diaphragmatic Hernia

For those families who choose to continue the pregnancy after a diagnosis of congenital diaphragmatic hernia (CDH) the most important next step is the accurate prenatal diagnosis about the severity of the condition which determines the choices available for prenatal management. If your fetus is on the better end of the spectrum, the most important choice is where to deliver the baby. The timing and type of delivery will not greatly affect outcome, but the place of delivery certainly will. These families will want to work out a plan for delivery and postnatal care with their obstetrician/perinatologist, the neonatologist, and pediatric surgeons so the baby can be stabilized and treated in the same center.

For fetuses in the middle of the spectrum, the place of delivery becomes even more important. These babies will need very intensive support after birth and should be delivered in highly experienced centers with extracorporeal membrane oxygenation (ECMO) capability. ECMO is a heart-lung machine that provides oxygen to the baby when the lungs are not capable of doing this. It is a medical therapy that can be used for a limited time, usually up to two weeks. Careful planning and coordination of the timing of delivery is necessary to avoid high-risk situations such as delivering in one hospital and transporting a critically ill baby to another center.

Fetuses on the most severe end of the spectrum with liver up and lung-to-head ratio (LHR) less than 1.0 are candidates for prenatal intervention. For more than two decades, we have been working on ways to improve the outcome for these fetuses by getting the lung to grow before birth, so that it will be adequate at the time of birth. The most promising uses Fetendo fetal surgery, specifically a fetoscopic temporary tracheal occlusion to enlarge the lung. While in the uterus, the fetal lung constantly makes fluid that escapes through its mouth and into the amniotic fluid. When the trachea is blocked, this fluid stays in the lungs. As it builds up, the lung fluid expands the lungs, stimulates their growth, and pushes the abdominal contents (liver, intestine) out of the chest and into the abdomen. The goal of this treatment is to have a baby born with lungs that are big enough that the child can breathe and provide itself enough oxygen to breath on its own.

Temporary tracheal occlusion of the fetal trachea can now be accomplished at twenty-two to twenty-eight weeks' gestation using a very small telescope (the size of a straw) placed through the mother's skin. A tiny detachable balloon is placed in the fetal trachea. Once the fetal lung has grown, the balloon can be removed or deflated so the baby can be born normally. This deflation procedure is usually done before birth. Again, fetal intervention is offered only when the diaphragmatic hernia is on the bad end of the spectrum with the liver up and an LHR less than 1.0.

What will happen after birth?

All babies with CDH should be delivered at a tertiary perinatal center with a high-level intensive care nursery and pediatric surgery. Although some babies with a very favorable outlook (LHR greater than 1.4) will not need very high level intensive care, most should be cared for by neonatologists and surgeons in an intensive care nursery (ICN) experienced in high frequency and oscillation ventilation, nitric oxide inhalation, and particularly extracorporeal membrane oxygenation (ECMO). It is not possible to tell before birth how much support any baby will need after birth. Babies with CDH known before birth should never be delivered in an institution incapable of providing all the support needed: transporting a sick baby is dangerous.

All babies with CDH should be delivered into a "set-up" where the neonatologists take the baby from the obstetricians and immediately provide life support—breathing, oxygen, IV fluids, and so on, as needed. The baby's response will determine the amount of breathing support that is needed, ranging from a little oxygen to a breathing machine to ECMO.

The severity of the lung problem will also determine the course in the intensive care nursery—again, ranging from surgical repair in the first day and home in a few weeks, to full support including ECMO for weeks, surgical repair (sometimes done while the baby is on ECMO), and then months of very intensive support before going home.

The long-term outcome depends on this need for very intensive support.

Section 28.4

Gastroschisis

What is gastroschisis?

Gastroschisis (sometimes called "laparoschisis") means the presence of a hole in the abdominal wall of the fetus, through which loops of intestines (and sometimes stomach, liver, and other organs) protrude. The term applies to only those conditions where the hole is located to the side of the umbilicus (umbilical cord); practically speaking, this hole is almost always to the left of the umbilical cord. Gastroschisis is not the same as omphalocele, which refers to a hole in the abdominal wall in the belly button. Although both conditions appear the same (intestines protruding outside the abdomen), each condition has its own features. Abdominal wall defects can be detected by ultrasound from the third month of pregnancy on (fourteen to fifteen weeks). As the pregnancy progresses, diagnosis becomes more accurate: loops of intestine can then be seen outside the abdomen, "floating" into the amniotic cavity.

How common is it?

Gastroschisis occurs in approximately one of every two thousand live births, making it a relatively "common" congenital anomaly. In fact, its incidence seems to be increasing in recent years, for reasons unknown. There seems to be a relationship with young maternal age, although it can occur at any age.

What can be done before birth?

Gastroschisis can be diagnosed with fairly good accuracy from the fourteenth week of gestation (three months). It is now possible to intervene during pregnancy for a number of anomalies. It would be tempting, therefore, to try and treat the fetus with gastroschisis before birth. However, extensive research has shown that patients with gastroschisis (and omphalocele) are best treated after they are born, and that most in utero interventions would be too risky for mother and child.

We can intervene in other ways, though: with advance knowledge of an abdominal wall defect, it is possible to change the plans for delivery of the baby. One can change the mode, place, and time of delivery.

Mode of delivery. If intestines and other organs are outside the abdomen, it would seem logical that they would be at an increased risk of being damaged during normal delivery. Some have therefore advocated cesarean section ("C-section") for all cases of gastroschisis and omphalocele. In fact, the risk of injury is only theoretical, and vaginal delivery does not put the baby at an increased risk of complications. For that reason, most (although not all) physicians now recommend normal delivery, even for gastroschisis, unless there are obstetrical reasons to proceed with a C-section.

Place of delivery. As long as he or she is inside the womb, the fetus with a gastroschisis is relatively well shielded from trauma and complications. After birth, however, the exposed intestines have to be protected from direct trauma, dehydration, and infection. The baby can be safely transported to a treatment center, as long as certain precautions are taken. However, if the diagnosis of gastroschisis has been made beforehand, it would seem logical to have the baby be born directly in such a treatment center (i.e., a center with a neonatal intensive care unit and immediate access to a pediatric surgery service). Therefore, we generally recommend that, if you are pregnant with a fetus with gastroschisis or omphalocele, you plan to deliver in such a tertiary institution. Your care will likely be transferred to a maternal-fetal medicine specialist, to facilitate the transition to peri- and postnatal care.

Time of delivery. One of the concerns with gastroschisis is that the exposed bowel becomes so damaged that function is impaired and the baby may end up staying in intensive care for a long time. It is known that many infants with gastroschisis have what appears to be damaged bowel, with very thick, rigid loops of intestines containing a "peel." One of the theories for this peel and thickened intestinal wall in gastroschisis (and for the fact that some babies have little or no peel at all) is that prolonged exposure of the bowel to the amniotic fluid causes progressive damage. In other words, limiting the amount of time that the bowel is floating in this fluid (or even diluting that fluid by infusing sterile saline water inside the womb) could theoretically decrease the amount of peel and intestinal damage.

Many centers have therefore recommended early delivery (between thirty-five and thirty-seven weeks of gestation, instead of the normal forty weeks). Unfortunately, there are no good scientific studies proving the benefits of this. In fact, at our institution, we have reviewed all babies born with gastroschisis in the last ten years, and have found no benefit at all of early delivery. For that reason, we recommend that your baby be born as close to term as possible.

What will happen at birth?

If everything goes as planned, you will deliver at a tertiary care center with direct access to a neonatal intensive care unit. The neonatologists will be present at delivery, so that they can immediately assess your baby and start treatment, if necessary. At the same time, the pediatric surgeons will be alerted, so that surgical correction can be performed as soon as possible. In most cases, however, you will be able to see (and hold) your baby after delivery.

Your baby will be "stabilized" in the intensive care unit. An intravenous line will be placed in an arm or a leg, so that fluids can be given. Because of the exposed intestines, your baby is likely to lose a lot of fluid by evaporation, and is likely to cool off more rapidly as well. Your baby will therefore be placed under a warmer, and the loops of bowel will be carefully wrapped to protect them from the outside. If your baby shows signs of distress, it is possible that he or she will be intubated, so that we can help him or her breathe better.

Once it is clear that there are no other major problems, your baby will be ready to undergo surgical repair of the defect. How this is done will depend on how much of the intestines and other organs are exposed, and how big your baby is. In many cases all the intestines can safely be placed back in the abdomen (so-called primary repair) and the abdominal wall can be closed. Of course, this is done in the operating room with your baby under anesthesia. Often, however, there is so much out that this cannot be safely replaced all at once. In that case, we try at least to protect the intestines until they are ready to be put back in the abdomen. For this, we place a "silo" (a clear plastic or silicone pouch) over the intestines, so that they are now shielded from trauma, infection, and dehydration. This can be done at the bedside, in the intensive care unit, or in the operating room.

Once the swelling has gone down and the abdomen has become used to the presence of more bowel, the silo can be removed and the abdomen closed over the intestines. This typically takes a few days to a week.

What happens next?

As mentioned before, the intestines have suffered somewhat during pregnancy, and they will need some time to recover. On average, it may take two to three weeks before the intestinal tract functions properly again. During that time, your baby will be fed through the veins only, by "total parenteral nutrition," or TPN. He or she will get all the calories necessary to grow, until he or she can be fed by mouth again. Once gut function returns, it will likely take a while before your baby can tolerate full feeds and nutrition through the veins can be stopped. Your baby is likely to stay in the hospital for at least one month. Sometimes this can be much longer, depending on the degree of prematurity and the condition of the bowel.

What complications may arise, and what is the long-term outlook?

The overall outcome of gastroschisis is usually excellent: some infants may have minor intestinal problems in the first few months, but will recover from that and lead a completely normal life. Although the belly button may not look perfectly normal, there should be minimal scarring.

In some rare cases, however, there may be some complications. While gastroschisis is usually not associated with other anomalies, there may be intestinal defects in 5 to 10 percent of cases. These represent in utero "accidents," where a piece of intestine becomes necrotic and disappears. As a result, there may be a missing portion of intestine (intestinal atresia), which will have to be fixed. Often, this is not discovered until a few weeks after birth. An additional operation will then be necessary. Very rarely, a large portion of intestine suffers and dies off. In those rare instances, bowel function may suffer.

Section 28.5

Omphalocele

What is omphalocele?

Omphalocele (sometimes called "exomphalos") refers to a condition in the fetus whereby some abdominal contents (small and/or large intestine, stomach, and even liver) protrude through a hole in the abdominal wall. Unlike in gastroschisis, the hole is in the middle of the abdomen, right where the belly button would be. Instead, there is a variable size defect (hole) covered by a membrane (which somewhat protects the exteriorized organs). The umbilical cord of the fetus inserts at the top of this membrane, rather than on the abdomen itself. Although both omphalocele and gastroschisis appear the same (intestines protruding outside the abdomen), each condition has its own features. Abdominal wall defects can be detected by ultrasound from the third month of pregnancy on (fourteen to fifteen weeks). As the pregnancy progresses, diagnosis becomes more accurate: loops of intestine can then be seen outside the abdomen, "floating" into the amniotic cavity.

How common is it?

Omphalocele occurs somewhat less often than gastroschisis, and is estimated to be present in one of every five thousand live births. It can be an isolated finding, but omphalocele is also seen in a number of chromosomal anomalies and other syndromes. The most common associated anomaly is a heart defect; others include the pentalogy of

Cantrell (which includes heart, diaphragm, and other defects) and cloacal exstrophy (a severe anomaly involving the intestines, the bladder, and the pelvic organs). Omphaloceles are also seen in trisomy 13 and trisomy 18, two severe chromosomal anomalies. In all these cases, the omphalocele is only a small component of the fetal condition, and the outcome will largely depend on the other anomalies, not on the omphalocele itself.

Because of the relatively common association of omphalocele with other, vaster syndromes, many have, in the past, painted a grim picture for all omphaloceles. However, isolated omphaloceles have a prognosis similar to gastroschisis: once the extruded organs can be replaced in the abdomen and the defect closed, most of these children will have a normal life.

What can be done before birth?

There is no reason to treat omphaloceles before birth (i.e., try to operate on the fetus). However, some measures can be taken once an omphalocele, or gastroschisis, has been diagnosed by ultrasound. Additional diagnostic tests may be necessary, particularly with omphalocele: an amniocentesis may be indicated, with chromosomal analysis; and efforts should be made to detect heart anomalies. The course of the pregnancy can be altered in three ways:

Mode of delivery. If intestines and other organs are outside the abdomen, it would seem logical that they would be at an increased risk of being damaged during normal delivery. Some have therefore advocated cesarean section ("C-section") for all cases of gastroschisis and omphalocele. In fact, the risk of injury is only theoretical, and vaginal delivery does not put the baby at an increased risk of complications. For that reason, most (although not all) physicians now recommend normal delivery, even for gastroschisis, unless there are obstetrical reasons to proceed with a C-section. The main exception may be cases of "giant" omphalocele, where a large portion of the liver is exposed as well: here, there may be an increased risk of liver trauma with vaginal delivery.

Place of delivery. As long as he or she is inside the womb, the fetus with an omphalocele is relatively well shielded from trauma and complications. After birth, however, the exposed intestines and/or liver have to be protected from direct trauma and infection. The baby can be safely transported to a treatment center, as long as certain precautions are taken. However, if the diagnosis of omphalocele has been made beforehand, it would seem logical to have the baby be born directly in such a treatment center (i.e., a center with a neonatal intensive care unit and immediate access to a pediatric surgery service). Therefore, we generally recommend that, if you are pregnant with a fetus with gastroschisis or omphalocele, you plan to deliver in such a tertiary institution. Your care will likely be transferred to a maternal-fetal medicine specialist, to facilitate the transition to peri- and postnatal care.

Time of delivery. One of the concerns with gastroschisis is that the exposed bowel becomes so damaged that function is impaired and the baby may end up staying in intensive care for a long time. It is known that many infants with gastroschisis have what appears to be damaged bowel, with very thick, rigid loops of intestines containing a "peel." One of the theories for this peel (and for the fact that some babies have little or no peel at all) is that prolonged exposure of the bowel to the amniotic fluid causes progressive damage. In other words, limiting the amount of time that the bowel is floating in this fluid (or even diluting that fluid by infusing sterile saline water inside the womb) could theoretically decrease the amount of peel and intestinal damage.

In omphaloceles this is rarely a problem, because a membrane envelops the organs and shields them from exposure. However, that membrane can have ruptured (so-called ruptured omphalocele), exposing the intestines to the same potential trauma as with gastroschisis.

What will happen at birth?

If everything goes as planned, you will deliver at a tertiary care center with direct access to a neonatal intensive care unit. The neonatologists will be present at delivery, so that they can immediately assess your baby and start treatment, if necessary. At the same time, the pediatric surgeons will be alerted, so that surgical correction can be performed as soon as possible. In most cases, however, you will be able to see (and hold) your baby after delivery.

Your baby will be "stabilized" in the intensive care unit. An intravenous line will be placed in an arm or a leg, so that fluids can be given. Because of the exposed intestines, your baby is likely to lose a lot of fluid by evaporation, and is likely to cool off more rapidly as well. Your baby will therefore be placed under a warmer, and if the omphalocele membrane is ruptured, the loops of bowel will be carefully wrapped to protect them from the outside. If your baby shows signs of distress, it is possible that he or she will be intubated, so that we can help him or her breathe better.

If it is clear that there are no other major problems, your baby will be ready to undergo surgical repair of the defect. How this is done will depend on how much of intestines and other organs are exposed, and how big your baby is. In many cases, all the intestines can safely be placed back in the abdomen (so-called primary repair) and the abdominal wall can be closed. Of course, this is done in the operating room with your baby under anesthesia. Often, however, there is so much out that this cannot be safely replaced all at once. In that case, we try at least to protect the intestines until they are ready to be put back in the abdomen. For this, we place a "silo" (a clear plastic or silicone pouch) over the intestines, so that they are now shielded from trauma, infection, and dehydration. This can be done at the bedside, in the intensive care unit, or in the operating room.

Once the swelling has gone down and the abdomen has become used to the presence of more bowel, the silo can be removed and the abdomen closed over the intestines. This typically takes a few days to a week.

If the membrane around the omphalocele is intact, it acts as a silo, and surgical intervention can be delayed somewhat. Small omphaloceles can be treated as described previously. With giant omphaloceles, where a large portion of the liver is exposed, surgical intervention may be more difficult. If complete correction cannot rapidly be achieved, the first goal is to close the skin over the abdominal organs, so that they can be protected. Repair of the muscle defect may have to occur later.

Of course, associated anomalies may have to be addressed as well; as discussed, these anomalies (chromosomal or other) may be the determining factor for the baby's outcome.

What happens next?

On average, it may take two to three weeks before the intestinal tract functions properly again. During that time, your baby will be fed through the veins only, by "total parenteral nutrition," or TPN. He or she will get all the calories necessary to grow, until he or she can be fed by mouth again. Once gut function returns, it will likely take a while before your baby can tolerate full feeds and nutrition through the veins can be stopped. Your baby is likely to stay in the hospital for at least one month. Sometimes, this can be much longer, depending on the degree of prematurity and the associated anomalies.

What complications may arise, and what is the long-term outlook?

The overall outcome of isolated omphalocele is excellent: some infants may have minor intestinal problems in the first few months, but will recover from that and lead a completely normal life. Although the belly button may not look perfectly normal, there should be minimal scarring.

As mentioned, omphaloceles can be associated with other conditions. This happens in approximately 50 percent of patients with an omphalocele. If there are associated anomalies, these may have to be addressed as well. Trisomy 13 and trisomy 18 are severe chromosomal anomalies with a generally poor prognosis; cloacal exstrophy is not an immediately life-threatening condition, but is a complex anomaly that will require multiple surgical interventions and the input of many specialists. The prognosis of children with pentalogy of Cantrell depends mostly on the degree of heart anomaly and whether the heart is exposed or not.

Beckwith-Wiedemann syndrome, which may present at birth with pancreas anomalies (too much insulin secretion, resulting in a very low blood sugar), is important because of its associated risk of childhood tumors. While most of these tumors can be treated effectively today, early detection is important. Therefore, babies with Beckwith-Wiedemann syndrome need to be screened (usually by ultrasound) on a regular basis for the first few years of life.

Chapter 29

Defects of the Lower Gastrointestinal Tract

Chapter Contents

Section 29.1—Bowel Obstruction 448
Section 29.2—Intestinal Malrotation 450
Section 29.3—Hirschsprung Disease 454
Section 29.4—Imperforate Anus 462

Section 29.1

Bowel Obstruction

Reprinted from "Overview of Bowel Obstruction," © 2006 Fetal Treatment Center, University of California, San Francisco. All rights reserved. Reprinted with permission. For additional information, visit http://fetus.ucsfmedicalcenter.org.

What is a bowel obstruction?

A baby's gastrointestinal tract is divided into two segments: the small intestine and the large intestine. The small intestine is made up of three parts: the duodenum (the segment connected to the stomach), the jejunum (where most of the liquid in food is absorbed), and the ileum (which empties into the large intestine). The large intestine is also called the colon. There are many causes of bowel obstruction in the fetus. Most are caused by an atresia, a narrowing at some point in the small intestine. A bowel obstruction is named by the place in the small intestine where it occurs: duodenal atresia, jejunal atresia, ileal atresia, or colon atresia.

What is the outcome for a fetus with a bowel obstruction?

Your fetus's bowel obstruction may have been discovered one of two ways. You may have undergone a routine ultrasound that showed a segment of bowel that was dilated, or larger than normal. This is a clue to your doctor that there is a problem with the intestine. This dilation happens because while in the uterus the fetus constantly swallows amniotic fluid. This narrowing can slow down or stop the flow of amniotic fluid in the intestine, causing it to swell, so that it appears too large in an ultrasound. The second way a bowel obstruction can be discovered is by the development of polyhydramnios, the buildup of too much amniotic fluid. Because of the blockage in the intestine, the normal flow of amniotic fluid is stopped. It accumulates on the outside of the baby—inside your uterus. Your uterus size may suddenly grow very large, alerting your doctor to a possible problem. Your doctor may then order an ultrasound study. The ultrasound study can confirm a problem in the intestine.

What will happen after birth?

Your baby should be born at a hospital with an intensive care nursery and a pediatric surgeon. Soon after birth your child will have surgery to repair the abnormal piece of intestine. The pediatric surgeon will repair your baby's intestine in one of two ways. If the stricture, or narrowing, is small the surgeon may be able to remove the damaged segment, taper the dilated portion, and sew the two ends of the intestine together. If the narrowing is long, or if the surgeon believes the intestine is damaged and cannot be used for a period of time, a temporary stoma may be placed. A stoma is a surgically created opening in the abdomen in which the small bowel is brought out through the abdominal wall. It is through this opening, or stoma, that stool will pass. It is not possible before birth to known which surgical repair will be performed. The surgeon will make that decision in the operating room after looking at the intestine. Babies with bowel obstruction can stay in the hospital from one week to one month, depending on the amount of intestine involved in the defect. The return of the function of the gastrointestinal tract and the baby's ability to tolerate feedings are two things that determine length of stay in the hospital. Babies are discharged from the hospital when they are taking all their feedings by mouth and gaining weight. Most babies with bowel obstruction do not have long-term problems.

Section 29.2

Intestinal Malrotation

Any blockage of the digestive tract that prevents the proper passage of food is known as an intestinal obstruction. Some causes of intestinal obstruction include a congenital (present at birth) malformation of the digestive tract, hernias, abnormal scar tissue growth after an abdominal operation, and inflammatory bowel disease. These blockages are also called mechanical obstructions because they physically block a portion of the intestine or another part of the digestive tract.

Malrotation is a type of mechanical obstruction caused by abnormal development of the intestines while a fetus is in the mother's womb. It occurs in one out of every five hundred births in the United States and accounts for approximately 5 percent of all intestinal obstructions. Some children with malrotation have other congenital malformations including:

- defects of the digestive system;

- heart defects;

- abnormalities of other organs, including the spleen or liver.

Some people who have malrotation never experience complications and are never diagnosed. But most children with this condition develop symptoms during infancy, often during the first month of life, and the majority are diagnosed by the time they reach one year of age. Although surgery is required to repair malrotation, most children experience normal growth and development once the condition and any problems associated with it are treated and corrected.

What Is Malrotation?

The small and large intestines are the longest part of the digestive system. If stretched out to their full length, they would measure more than twenty feet long by adulthood, but because they are coiled up, they fit into the relatively small space of the abdominal cavity. Malrotation occurs when the intestines don't "coil" properly during fetal development. The exact cause is unknown.

When a fetus is developing in the womb, the intestines start out as a small, straight tube between the stomach and the rectum. As this tube develops into separate organs, the intestines move for a time into the umbilical cord, which supplies nutrients to the developing embryo.

Around the tenth week of pregnancy, the intestine moves from the umbilical cord into the abdomen. It fits in by making two turns that allow it to lie in a specific position within the abdomen. When the intestine does not make these turns properly, malrotation has occurred.

Malrotation in itself may not cause any problems. However, it may be accompanied by additional complications:

- Bands of tissue called Ladd bands may form, obstructing the first part of the small intestine (the duodenum).

- After birth, volvulus may occur. This is when the intestine twists on itself, causing a lack of blood flow to the tissue and leading to tissue death. Malrotation is often diagnosed when volvulus occurs, frequently during the first weeks of life.

Obstruction caused by volvulus or Ladd bands are both life-threatening problems. The intestines can stop functioning and intestinal tissue can die from lack of blood supply if an obstruction isn't recognized and treated.

Signs and Symptoms

One of the earliest signs of malrotation and volvulus is abdominal pain and cramping caused by the inability of the bowel to push food past the obstruction. Infants cannot tell you when their stomachs hurt, but you may notice the following pattern of behavior:

- pulling up the legs and crying
- stopping crying suddenly

- behaving normally for fifteen to thirty minutes

- repeating this behavior when the next cramp happens

Infants may also be irritable, lethargic, or have irregular stools. Vomiting is another symptom of malrotation, and it can help your child's doctor determine where the obstruction is located. Vomiting that happens soon after your baby starts to cry often means the obstruction is in the small intestine; if it's delayed, it's usually in the large intestine. The vomit may be bilious (this means it contains bile, which is yellow or green in color) or may resemble your child's feces.

Additional symptoms of malrotation and volvulus may include:

- a swollen abdomen that's tender to the touch;

- diarrhea and/or bloody stools (or sometimes no stools at all);

- irritability or crying in pain, with nothing seeming to help;

- rapid heart rate and breathing;

- little or no urine because of fluid loss;

- fever.

Diagnosis and Treatment

If your child's doctor suspects volvulus or another intestinal blockage, he or she will order x-rays, a computed tomography (CT) scan, or an ultrasound of the abdominal area.

Your doctor may use barium to see the x-ray or scan more clearly. Barium provides a contrast that can show if the intestine has a malformation and can usually determine where a blockage is located. Adults and older children usually drink barium in a liquid form. Infants may need to be given barium through a tube inserted from their nose into the stomach, or sometimes are given a barium enema, in which the liquid barium is inserted through the rectum.

The specific treatment of malrotation will depend on your child's age and other health problems. Because malrotation is usually only recognized after a blockage occurs because of volvulus or Ladd bands, your child's doctor will order corrective treatment immediately.

Any child with bowel obstruction will need to be hospitalized. A tube called a nasogastric (NG) tube is usually inserted through the nose and down into the stomach to remove the contents of the stomach and upper intestines. This keeps fluid and gas from building up in the abdomen. Your child may also be given intravenous (IV) fluids to help prevent dehydration and antibiotics to prevent infection.

Surgery to correct bowel obstruction from malrotation is always necessary and is often performed as an emergency procedure to prevent irreversible, life-threatening injury to the bowel. During surgery, which is called a Ladd procedure, the intestine is straightened out, the Ladd bands are divided, the small intestine is coiled on the right side of the abdomen, and the colon is placed on the left side. Because the appendix is usually found on the left side of the abdomen in cases of malrotation (it is normally found on the right), it is removed. Its altered position would make symptoms of appendicitis difficult to determine in the future.

If the doctor suspects that blood may still not be flowing properly to the intestines (because they don't look pink and healthy after being untwisted), he or she may perform a second surgery within forty-eight hours of the first. If the intestine still looks unhealthy at this time, the damaged portion may be removed.

If the baby is seriously ill at the time of surgery, an ileostomy or colostomy will usually be performed. In this procedure, the diseased bowel is completely removed, and the end of the normal, healthy intestine is brought out through an opening on the skin of the abdomen (called a stoma). Fecal matter passes through this opening and into a bag that is taped or attached with adhesive to the child's belly. In young children, depending on how much bowel was removed, ileostomy or colostomy is often a temporary condition that can later be reversed with another operation.

The doctor will monitor your child's progress after surgery to make sure she's developing normally. The majority of these surgeries are successful, although some children have recurring problems after surgery. Recurrent volvulus is rare, but a second bowel obstruction due to adhesions (scar tissue build-up after any type of abdominal surgery) could occur later.

Children who require removal of a large portion of the small intestine can have too little bowel to maintain adequate nutrition (a condition known as short bowel syndrome). They may be dependent on intravenous nutrition for a time after surgery and may require a special diet afterward. Most children in whom the volvulus and malrotation are identified early, before permanent injury to the bowel has occurred, do well and develop normally.

When to Call the Doctor

If you suspect any kind of intestinal obstruction because your child has bilious vomiting, a swollen abdomen, or bloody stools, take her to the emergency room immediately.

Section 29.3

Hirschsprung Disease

Reprinted from "What I Need to Know about Hirschsprung Disease," National Institute of Diabetes and Digestive and Kidney Diseases, NIH Publication No. 05-4384, October 2004.

What is Hirschsprung disease?

Hirschsprung disease, or HD, is a disease of the large intestine. The large intestine is also sometimes called the colon. The word *bowel* can refer to the large and small intestines. HD usually occurs in children. It causes constipation, which means that bowel movements are difficult. Some children with HD can't have bowel movements at all. The stool creates a blockage in the intestine.

If HD is not treated, stool can fill up the large intestine. This can cause serious problems like infection, bursting of the colon, and even death.

Most parents feel frightened when they learn that their child has a serious disease. This section will help you understand HD and how you and the doctor can help your child.

Why does HD cause constipation?

Normally, muscles in the intestine push stool to the anus, where stool leaves the body. Special nerve cells in the intestine, called ganglion cells, make the muscles push. A person with HD does not have these nerve cells in the last part of the large intestine.

In a person with HD, the healthy muscles of the intestine push the stool until it reaches the part without the nerve cells. At this point, the stool stops moving. New stool then begins to stack up behind it.

454

Sometimes the ganglion cells are missing from the whole large intestine and even parts of the small intestine before it. When the diseased section reaches to or includes the small intestine, it is called long-segment disease. When the diseased section includes only part of the large intestine, it is called short-segment disease.

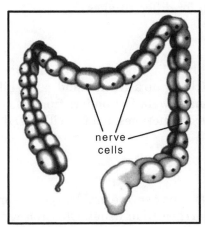 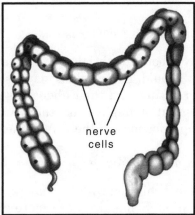

Figure 29.1. Left: Healthy large intestine; nerve cells are found through-out the intestine. Right: HD large intestine; Nerve cells are missing from the last part of the intestine.

What causes HD?

HD develops before a child is born. Normally, nerve cells grow in the baby's intestine soon after the baby begins to grow in the womb. These nerve cells grow down from the top of the intestine all the way to the anus. With HD, the nerve cells stop growing before they reach the end.

No one knows why the nerve cells stop growing. But we do know that it's not the mother's fault. HD isn't caused by anything the mother did while she was pregnant.

Some children with HD have other health problems, such as Down syndrome and other rare disorders.

If I have more children, will they have HD too?

In some cases, HD is hereditary, which means mothers and fathers could pass it to their children. This can happen even if the parents don't have HD. If you have one child with HD, you could have more children with the disease. Talk to your doctor about the risk.

What are the symptoms?

Symptoms of HD usually show up in very young children, but sometimes they don't appear until the person is a teenager or an adult. The symptoms are a little different for different ages.

Symptoms in Newborns

Newborns with HD don't have their first bowel movement when they should. These babies may also throw up a green liquid called bile after eating, and their abdomens may swell. Discomfort from gas or constipation might make them fussy. Sometimes, babies with HD develop infections in their intestines.

Symptoms in Young Children

Most children with HD have always had severe problems with constipation. Some also have more diarrhea than usual. Children with HD might also have anemia, a shortage of red blood cells, because blood is lost in the stool. Also, many babies with HD grow and develop more slowly than they should.

Symptoms in Teenagers and Adults

Like younger children, teenagers and adults with HD usually have had severe constipation all their lives. They might also have anemia.

How does the doctor find out if HD is the problem?

To find out if a person has HD, the doctor will do one or more tests:

- barium enema x-ray
- manometry
- biopsy

Barium Enema X-ray

An x-ray is a black-and-white picture of the inside of the body. The picture is taken with a special machine that uses a small amount of radiation. For a barium enema x-ray, the doctor puts barium through the anus into the intestine before taking the picture. Barium is a liquid that makes the intestine show up better on the x-ray.

In some cases, instead of barium another liquid, called Gastrografin, may be used. Gastrografin is also sometimes used in newborns to help remove a hard first stool. Gastrografin causes water to be pulled into the intestine, and the extra water softens the stool.

In places where the nerve cells are missing, the intestine looks too narrow. If a narrow large intestine shows on the x-ray, the doctor knows HD might be the problem. More tests will help the doctor know for sure.

Other tests used to diagnose HD are manometry and biopsy.

Manometry

The doctor inflates a small balloon inside the rectum. Normally, the anal muscle will relax. If it doesn't, HD may be the problem. This test is most often done in older children and adults.

Biopsy

This is the most accurate test for HD. The doctor removes and looks at a tiny piece of the intestine under a microscope. If the nerve cells are missing, HD is the problem.

The doctor may do one or all of these tests. It depends on the child.

What is the treatment?

Pull-through Surgery

HD is treated with surgery. The surgery is called a pull-through operation. There are three common ways to do a pull-through, and they are called the Swenson, the Soave, and the Duhamel procedures. Each is done a little differently, but all involve taking out the part of the intestine that doesn't work and connecting the healthy part that's left to the anus. After pull-through surgery, the child has a working intestine.

Colostomy and Ileostomy

Often, the pull-through can be done right after the diagnosis. However, children who have been very sick may first need surgery called an ostomy. This surgery helps the child get healthy before having the pull-through. Some doctors do an ostomy in every child before doing the pull-through.

In an ostomy, the doctor takes out the diseased part of the intestine. Then the doctor cuts a small hole in the baby's abdomen. The hole is called a stoma. The doctor connects the top part of the intestine to the stoma. Stool leaves the body through the stoma while the bottom part of the intestine heals. Stool goes into a bag attached to

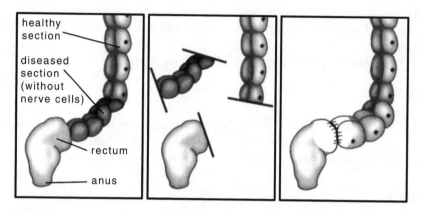

healthy section

diseased section (without nerve cells)

rectum

anus

Figure 29.2. Pull-through Surgery. Left: Before surgery—the diseased section is the part of the intestine that doesn't work. Middle: Step 1—the doctor removes the diseased section. Right: Step 2—the healthy section is attached to the rectum or anus.

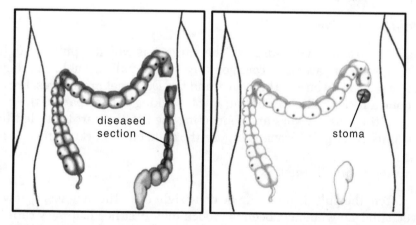

diseased section

stoma

Figure 29.3. Ostomy surgery. Left: Step 1—the doctor takes out most of the diseased part of the intestine. Right: Step 2—the doctor attaches the healthy part of the intestine to the stoma (a hole in the abdomen).

the skin around the stoma. You will need to empty this bag several times a day.

If the doctor removes the entire large intestine and connects the small intestine to the stoma, the surgery is called an ileostomy. If the doctor leaves part of the large intestine and connects that to the stoma, the surgery is called a colostomy.

Later, the doctor will do the pull-through. The doctor disconnects the intestine from the stoma and attaches it just above the anus. The stoma isn't needed any more, so the doctor either sews it up during surgery or waits about six weeks to make sure that the pull-through worked.

What will my child's life be like after surgery?

Ostomy

Most babies are more comfortable after having an ostomy because they can pass gas more easily and aren't constipated anymore.

Older children will be more comfortable, too, but they may have some trouble getting used to an ostomy. They will need to learn how to take care of the stoma and how to change the bag that collects stool. They may be worried about being different from their friends. Most children can lead a normal life after surgery.

Adjusting after Pull-through

After a pull-through, nine out of ten children pass stool normally. Some children may have diarrhea for a while, and babies may develop a nasty diaper rash. Eventually the stool will become more solid and the child will need to go to the bathroom less often. Toilet training may be delayed, as the child learns how to use the bottom muscles only after pull-through surgery. Older children might stain their underwear for a while after the surgery. It is not their fault. They can't control this problem, but it improves with time.

Some children become constipated, because one in ten children with HD has difficulty moving stool through the part of the colon without nerve cells. A mild laxative may also be helpful. Ask your doctor for suggestions.

Diet and Nutrition

One job of the large intestine is to collect the water and salts the body needs. Since your child's intestine is shorter now, it absorbs less. Your child will need to drink more to make sure his body gets enough fluids.

An infant who has long-segment disease requiring an ileostomy may need special tube feedings. The shortened intestine does not allow the bloodstream enough time to absorb nutrients from food before it is pushed out of the body as stool. Tube feedings that deliver nutrients can make up for what is lost.

Eating high-fiber foods like cereal and bran muffins can help reduce constipation and diarrhea.

Infection

Infections can be very dangerous for a child with Hirschsprung disease. Infection of the large and small intestines is called enterocolitis. It can happen before or after surgery to treat Hirschsprung disease. Here are some of the signs to look for:

- fever
- swollen abdomen
- vomiting
- diarrhea
- bleeding from the rectum
- sluggishness

Call your doctor immediately if your child shows any of these signs. If the problem is enterocolitis, your child may be admitted to the hospital. In the hospital, an intravenous (I.V.) line may be needed to keep body fluids up and to deliver antibiotics to fight the infection. The large intestine will be rinsed regularly with a mild saltwater solution until all remaining stool has been removed. The rinse may also contain antibiotics to kill bacteria.

When the child has recovered from the infection, the doctor may advise surgery. If the child has not had the pull-through surgery yet, the doctor may prepare for it by doing a colostomy or ileostomy before the child leaves the hospital. If the child has already had a pull-through operation, the doctor may correct the obstruction with surgery.

Enterocolitis can be life threatening, so watch for the signs and call your doctor immediately if they occur.

Long-Segment HD

Sometimes HD affects most or all of the large intestine, plus some of the small intestine. Children with long-segment HD can be treated with pull-through surgery, but there is a risk of complications such as infection, diarrhea, and diaper rash afterward. Parents need to pay close attention to their child's health. Also, since some, most, or all of the intestine is removed, drinking a lot of fluid is important.

Points to Remember

- HD is a disease of the large intestine.

- HD develops in children before they are born. It is not caused by anything the mother did while pregnant.

- Symptoms of HD include
  - delayed first bowel movement in newborns
  - swollen abdomen and vomiting
  - constipation since birth
  - slow growth and development
  - anemia

- Children with HD may get an infection, called enterocolitis, which can cause fever and diarrhea.

- HD is a serious disease that needs to be treated right away. HD is treated with pull-through surgery or, sometimes, ostomy.

- After treatment, most children with HD lead normal lives.

Section 29.4

Imperforate Anus

What is imperforate anus?

Imperforate anus is the absence of a normal anal opening. The diagnosis is usually made shortly after birth by a routine physical examination. Imperforate anus occurs in about one in five thousand births and its cause is unknown.

Children who have imperforate anus may also have other congenital anomalies. The acronym VACTERL describes the associated problems that infants with imperforate anus may have: Vertebral defects, anal atresia, cardiac anomalies, tracheoesophageal fistula, esophageal atresia, renal anomalies, and limb anomalies. The incidence of kidney and bladder problems increases with the severity of the imperforate anus, ranging from 5 to 20 percent with low lesions up to 60 to 90 percent with high lesions. While some of these anomalies may be noted on physical examination, others require further diagnostic tests. Renal ultrasound is done shortly after birth on all infants to evaluate the kidneys. Chest x-ray, electrocardiogram (EKG), and cardiac ultrasound may be ordered to evaluate the heart. Other x-rays may be done to evaluate the trachea and esophagus and the spine.

How is imperforate anus evaluated?

Although the diagnosis of imperforate anus can be made by physical examination, it is often difficult to determine whether the infant has a high or low lesion. A plain radiograph of the abdomen can help locate the lesion. Ultrasound of the perineum (rectal and vaginal areas) is also useful: with ultrasound we can determine the distance between a meconium-filled distal rectum and a finger on the perineum; we can also determine if there are any anomalies of the urinary tract or the spinal cord.

How is imperforate anus treated?

Surgical treatment of infants with imperforate anus depends upon the severity of the condition. A low imperforate anus can be repaired in the newborn period by a procedure called a perineal anoplasty. With a high imperforate anus, a colostomy (to divert the path of stool) is usually done. The infant with a high lesion is therefore given time to grow until definitive repair can be done with a pull-through operation (in which the rectum is "pulled down" and sewn into a newly made anal opening in the perineum). After surgery, the newly formed anus needs to be dilated regularly for several months until a soft, mature scar is obtained. The colostomy can then be closed.

What is the long-term outlook for children after repair of imperforate anus?

The most important prognostic feature is the severity of the imperforate anus and the presence or absence of associated spinal abnormalities. Children with a low lesion, especially those who require only a perineal anoplasty, have a very good chance of having normal stool patterns. Children with spinal abnormalities of the lower sacrum and a high imperforate anus have a poorer chance of obtaining normal bowel function. Even this latter group, however, are helped by a bowel training program with diet changes and use of stimulant cathartics and regular enemas.

Chapter 30

Kidney Defects

Chapter Contents

Section 30.1—Ectopic Kidneys 466
Section 30.2—Hydronephrosis 468
Section 30.3—Multicystic Dysplastic Kidney 470
Section 30.4—Renal Fusion (Horseshoe Kidney)..................... 471
Section 30.5—Detecting Kidney and Urinary Tract
            Abnormalities before Birth 473

Section 30.1

Ectopic Kidneys

Most people are born with two kidneys, which are located in the back of the abdominal cavity on either side of the body, covered by the ribs. But factors can occasionally interfere with the development of the kidneys, as is the case for people with ectopic kidneys. The following information will help you talk to your urologist when your condition, or that of your child, belongs to this family of diseases.

What happens under normal conditions?

The kidney is the organ whose principal function is to filter toxins from the blood and maintain an appropriate chemical environment so that the body's other organ systems can function properly. Other functions that the kidneys serve include maintaining appropriate blood pressure and ensuring that enough red blood cells are produced by the bone marrow. As a child develops in its mother's uterus, the kidneys are formed lower in the abdomen and gradually ascend to their final position as they develop.

What is an ectopic kidney?

Renal ectopia or ectopic kidney describes a kidney that is not located in its usual position. Ectopic kidneys are thought to occur in approximately one in one thousand births, but only about one in ten of these are ever diagnosed. Some of these are discovered incidentally, such as when a child or adult is having surgery or an x-ray for a medical condition unrelated to the renal ectopia. Ectopic kidneys can be located anywhere along the path of their usual ascent from where they initially form to where normal kidneys lie in the upper abdomen. Simple renal ectopia refers to a kidney that is located on the proper side but is in an abnormal position. Crossed renal ectopia refers to a kidney that has crossed from the left to the right side (or vice versa) so that both kidneys are located on the same side of the body. These kidneys may or may not be fused. It is important to note that renal ectopia is frequently associated with congenital abnormalities of other organ systems.

What are the symptoms of an ectopic kidney?

The function of the kidney itself is generally not abnormal to begin with, but because of the change in the usual anatomic relationships, the kidney may have difficulty draining. Up to 50 percent of ectopic kidneys are at least partially blocked. Over time, obstruction can lead to serious complications, including urinary tract infections, kidney stones, and kidney failure. Ectopic kidneys are also associated with vesicoureteral reflux (VUR), a condition where urine backs up from the bladder through the ureters into the kidneys. Over time, VUR can lead to infections that also can destroy the kidney. Interestingly, the non-ectopic kidney can also have functional abnormalities such as obstruction or VUR.

The most common symptoms related to the ectopic kidney that lead to diagnosis include urinary tract infections, abdominal pain, or a lump that can be felt in the abdomen.

What are some treatment options for ectopic kidney?

Treatment for the ectopic kidney is necessary only if obstruction or vesicoureteral reflux (VUR) is present. If the kidney is not severely damaged by the time the abnormality is discovered, the obstruction can be relieved or the VUR corrected with an operation. However, if the kidney is badly scarred and not working well, removing it may be the best choice.

What can I expect after treatment for ectopic kidney?

It is possible to live a normal life after removal of a kidney provided that the remaining kidney functions well.

Section 30.2

Hydronephrosis

What is antenatal hydronephrosis?

Antenatal (before birth) hydronephrosis (fluid-filled enlargement of the kidney) can be detected in the fetus by ultrasound studies performed as early as the first trimester of pregnancy. In most instances this diagnosis will not change obstetric care, but will require careful follow-up and possible surgery during infancy and childhood.

What causes antenatal hydronephrosis?

Possible causes of antenatal hydronephrosis include the following:

- **Blockage:** This may occur at the kidney in the ureteropelvic junction (UPJ), at the bladder in the ureterovesical junction, or in the urethra (posterior urethral valve).

- **Reflux:** Vesicoureteral reflux occurs when the valve between the bladder and the ureter does not function properly, permitting urine to flow back up to the kidney when the bladder fills or empties. Most children (75 percent) outgrow this during childhood but need daily antibiotic prophylaxis to try to prevent kidney damage before they outgrow the reflux.

- **Duplications:** Perhaps 1 percent of all humans have two collecting tubes from a kidney. These may show up on fetal ultrasound. Occasionally patients with duplication have a ureterocele, which is a balloon-like obstruction at the end of one of the duplex tubes.

- **Multicystic kidney:** This is a nonfunctional cystic kidney.

- **No significant abnormality:** Many of these dilated kidneys prove to be normal after delivery.

How is antenatal hydronephrosis managed?

Most cases of hydronephrosis diagnosed during pregnancy are just followed with ultrasound, monitoring the growth of the fetus and the condition of the kidneys. In these cases, a routine, normal delivery can be performed. Rarely, in a fetus with severe obstruction of both kidneys and insufficient amniotic fluid, drainage of the kidneys or bladder by tube or operation may need to be done. In these babies, however, the kidneys are often very abnormal and do not function properly regardless of treatment.

What is done to evaluate the hydronephrosis after the baby is born?

Several studies may need to be performed to evaluate the kidneys:

- ultrasound (done during the newborn period)
- voiding cystourethrogram (to exclude vesicoureteral reflux, a cause of 25 to 30 percent of antenatal hydronephrosis)
- diuretic renal scan (to evaluate kidney function)

What can be done to treat the hydronephrosis?

The treatment of antenatal hydronephrosis depends on the underlying cause. Infants and children who have vesicoureteral reflux are managed with antibiotics and surveillance with periodic ultrasounds and voiding cystograms. Infants and children with an obstruction or blockage of the urinary tract may require surgical correction. Babies with hydronephrosis without reflux or obstruction are followed with periodic ultrasounds to monitor the hydronephrosis and the growth of the kidneys. The management of multicystic dysplastic kidneys is controversial: the multicystic dysplastic kidney doesn't work, but the opposite kidney is usually normal. Some urologists recommend removal, whereas others do not remove the dysplastic kidney unless its large size causes problems or unless there is a question of tumor or blockage.

Section 30.3

Multicystic Dysplastic Kidney

Fetal multicystic dysplastic kidney (MCDK) is a condition that results from the malformation of the kidney during fetal development. The kidney consists of irregular cysts of varying sizes that resemble a bunch of grapes. It has no function, and nothing can be done to save this kidney. This defect generally affects only one of the kidneys, so typically the other healthy kidney will grow larger to compensate for the diseased one. Occasionally the disease affects both kidneys, which is incompatible with life, causing the fetus to be stillborn or to die shortly after birth.

Incidence of the Condition

In the United States it is estimated that 1 in every 2,400 live births are affected by fetal MCDK. It generally occurs at the same rate in both females and males. In approximately 50 percent of babies diagnosed with this disease other urological defects are found. However, the other defects can generally be corrected with surgery or by observation alone.

Diagnosis of Fetal Multicystic Dysplastic Kidney

A fetal MCDK is generally diagnosed by ultrasound (sonogram) examination before birth. Evaluation of the kidneys is part of the routine ultrasound examination done by many obstetricians as part of their prenatal care around the twentieth week of pregnancy.

Treatment for MCDK

Nothing can be done to treat a fetal MCDK. However, after the baby is born, the progress of the MCDK is tracked through a series of ultrasound examinations every six months to a year. It is monitored to make sure that it does not grow or develop a tumor. Most often, the MCDK will regress and disappear eventually, leaving the child with one healthy kidney. In addition to tracking the MCDK, the healthy kidney is screened for any defects such as a blockage or reflux. If there is something wrong, this allows the physicians time to intervene quickly to in order to save the functioning kidney before it worsens.

Long-Term Outlook

The long-term outlook is generally very good for these children. It is rare for a child with MCDK to have symptoms later in life that stem from this problem.

Section 30.4

Renal Fusion (Horseshoe Kidney)

Most people are born with two kidneys, which are located in the back of the abdominal cavity on either side of the body, covered by the ribs. But factors can occasionally interfere with the development of the kidneys, as is the case for people with renal fusion abnormalities. The following information will help you talk to your urologist when your condition, or that of your child, belongs to this family of diseases.

What happens under normal conditions?

The kidney is the organ whose principal function is to filter toxins from the blood and maintain an appropriate chemical environment so that the body's other organ systems can function properly. Other functions that the kidneys serve include maintaining appropriate blood pressure and ensuring that enough red blood cells are produced by the bone marrow. As a child develops in its mother's uterus, the kidneys are formed lower in the abdomen and gradually ascend to their final position as they develop.

What is horseshoe kidney?

Horseshoe kidney occurs in about one in five hundred children. It occurs during fetal development as the kidneys move into their normal position. With horseshoe kidney, however, as the kidneys of the fetus rise from the pelvic area, they fuse together at the lower end or base. By fusing, they form a "U" shape, which gives it the name "horseshoe." It is believed that this condition exists more frequently in males.

What are the symptoms of a horseshoe kidney?

Horseshoe kidneys are much more frequently symptomatic than other varieties of fused and ectopic kidneys. Up to 70 percent of children and adults with this abnormality will have symptoms, which can include abdominal pain, nausea, kidney stones, and urinary tract infections. Although still rare, cancerous tumors are somewhat more likely to occur in horseshoe kidneys than in normal kidneys. Blood in the urine, a mass in the abdomen, and flank pain can be symptoms of a kidney tumor.

How is horseshoe kidney treated?

In a child without symptoms, treatment may not be necessary. If your child has complications, they may require supportive treatment, which means their symptoms will be treated, but there is no cure for the condition. As with ectopic kidneys, obstruction and vesicoureteral reflux are very common in these patients and may require surgical correction.

What can be expected after treatment for horseshoe kidney?

It is important to note that if the patient's only complaint from the horseshoe kidney is pain, surgery frequently will not relieve the pain.

Section 30.5

Detecting Kidney and Urinary Tract Abnormalities before Birth

Ultrasound examinations are often done as part of prenatal care. This test allows the doctor to examine babies before they are born. With ultrasound, the doctor can see the baby's internal organs, including the kidneys and urinary bladder. Occasionally, an abnormality is detected in the developing urinary tract. A doctor can then determine whether treatment is necessary. Parents should know that, in many cases, these abnormalities do not have a major impact on the child's overall health.

What causes urinary tract abnormalities to occur before birth?

In about one of five hundred births, some abnormality occurs in the development of the kidneys or urinary tract. It is not really known why this happens. The development of the urinary tract is a complex process that is not fully understood. Problems in the development of the urinary tract that occur before birth are called "congenital."

What kinds of abnormalities may occur?

In some cases, one or both kidneys may fail to develop. In other instances, an abnormality may be present that blocks the outflow of urine. This blockage may cause urine to back up into the kidney, a condition called hydronephrosis, which causes the kidney to appear enlarged on the ultrasound test. Another common abnormality is called reflux. This occurs when a valve-like mechanism at the point where the ureter joins the bladder does not work, allowing urine to wash back up into the kidney.

Are there different kinds of blockages?

Yes. Blockages may occur at the point where the ureter leaves the kidney pelvis, or at the point where the bladder empties into the urethra. These urinary tract abnormalities may be associated with urinary tract infections in children, which can result in kidney injury. However, when detected early and treated appropriately, kidney injury may be avoided in many cases.

Do these blockages always cause kidney damage?

No. Before birth, the mother's placenta performs most of the functions of the kidney. As a result, babies with urinary tract abnormalities generally develop normally before delivery. In addition, many kidney or urinary tract abnormalities detected before birth have no major impact on the overall health of the baby following delivery. Nevertheless, certain conditions may interfere with the baby's kidney function or growth after birth. For example, severely blocked flow of urine may damage the developing kidney and result in poor function after birth, a condition called dysplasia. If both kidneys are involved, the amount of urine may be seriously decreased. As a result, there may not be enough amniotic fluid surrounding the fetus, and the baby's lungs may also be affected.

What happens if the child has only one functioning kidney?

In cases where only one kidney is affected, the other kidney is usually capable of increasing in size and function to compensate for the abnormal kidney. Children with only one normal kidney still have enough kidney function to grow and develop normally.

Should urinary tract abnormalities be treated before birth?

In most infants with congenital urinary tract abnormalities, no treatment is needed until after delivery. However, your doctor may want to do repeated ultrasound examinations during pregnancy to monitor your baby's kidney development.

What will need to be done after the baby is born?

After delivery, your doctor will examine your baby carefully and request certain tests to find out more about your baby's condition. The baby's blood pressure will be measured using an infant blood pressure cuff. Often, ultrasound of the baby's kidneys and bladder will be done to get a closer look at your baby's kidneys and bladder than is possible before delivery.

Another test that is often done is called a voiding cystourethrogram. In this test, a thin tube called a catheter is inserted into your baby's bladder through the urethra, and the bladder is filled with x-ray dye. The catheter is then removed and x-rays are taken as the baby urinates. This test evaluates the baby's bladder and urethra, and also determines if reflux is present.

In babies who have hydronephrosis, a type of x-ray called a renal scan is often done. In this test, a small amount of radioactive tracer is injected into a vein. This tracer is removed from the blood and excreted by the kidneys. By measuring the time the kidneys take to remove this tracer, the doctor can tell how well the kidneys function and whether there is something preventing them from emptying properly. Renal scans are often done several weeks after birth so that the infant's kidneys have time to begin functioning outside the uterus.

What can I expect for my child?

Babies with urinary tract abnormalities detected by prenatal ultrasound often do very well. Nevertheless, babies with these conditions need careful evaluation following birth to see if treatment is necessary. Your baby may need only periodic visits to your doctor, or a specialist in the treatment of children with congenital urinary tract abnormalities. Sometimes, a dose of antibiotics at bedtime is prescribed. Occasionally, infants with urinary tract abnormalities may need an operation to correct the problem. Your doctor can provide you with further information regarding congenital urinary tract abnormalities.

Chapter 31

Defects of the Urinary Tract

Chapter Contents

Section 31.1—Urinary Tract Obstruction 478
Section 31.2—Fetal Surgery for Obstructive Uropathy 480
Section 31.3—Bladder Exstrophy 484
Section 31.4—Epispadias 487
Section 31.5—Ectopic Ureter 489
Section 31.6—Megaureter 494
Section 31.7—Ureterocele 498
Section 31.8—Vesicoureteral Reflux...................................... 502
Section 31.9—Urachal Anomalies 504

Section 31.1

Urinary Tract Obstruction

Reprinted from "Urinary Tract Obstruction: Learn More," © 2006 Fetal Treatment Center, University of California, San Francisco. All rights reserved. Reprinted with permission. For additional information, visit http:// fetus.ucsfmedicalcenter.org.

What is urinary tract obstruction?

The urinary tract consists of two kidneys (where urine is made), two ureters (tubes which lead the urine into the bladder), the bladder, and the urethra (the tube which leads the urine from the bladder to the outside of the body). The urine should flow from the kidney, through the ureter, to the bladder, and out of the fetus through the urethra to the amniotic fluid. There are many causes of urinary tract obstruction in the fetus. Most are caused by a narrowing at some point in the urinary tract. This narrowing can slow down or stop the flow of urine, and this in turn can interfere with the development of both the kidneys and the lungs.

Amniotic fluid (fetal urine) is crucial in the development of the fetal lungs. If there is not enough amniotic fluid, the lungs of the fetus do not grow. As a result, fetal urinary tract obstruction can produce pulmonary hypoplasia (small lungs) and renal dysplasia (destruction of the kidneys). A low amniotic fluid level, or no amniotic fluid, can signal a blockage at some point in the urinary tract to the flow of urine.

What is the outcome for a fetus with urinary tract obstruction?

Outcome is related to the type of obstruction (where it is in the urinary tract), the severity of the obstruction, and the affect on renal function and amniotic fluid volume. Fetuses who have an obstruction or abnormality in one kidney and have a normal kidney on the other side will do very well. One good kidney can support a normal life. On the other end of the spectrum are fetuses with severe obstruction to both kidneys. This can be at the level of the bladder outlet (urethra), the bladder inlet (ureterovesical junction), or the kidney outlet (ureteropelvic junction). If the obstruction prevents urine from getting out into the amniotic space around the fetus, and the amniotic fluid goes away (oligohydramnios), the fetus's lungs will not develop. The small lungs may prevent survival after birth. The obstruction also damages the kidneys, leading to kidney failure after birth. Many of these babies will not survive.

However, most fetuses with urinary tract obstruction fall between these two extremes and their outcome depends on the severity of the obstruction and how it progresses throughout the pregnancy. For all types of urinary tract obstruction, fetuses that lose all their amniotic fluid (oligohydramnios) before eighteen to twenty-four weeks will not have big enough lungs to survive. Fetuses who maintain amniotic fluid volume throughout pregnancy will have large enough lungs to survive at birth, but may still develop renal failure after birth due to the damage to kidney function before birth. In addition to urologic procedures to relieve obstruction and sometimes reconstruct the urinary drainage system, these babies may develop renal failure over months or years and sometimes require kidney transplantation. Fetuses who maintain normal amniotic fluid and have only minor damage to the kidney will do well and may not need anything done after birth.

How serious is my fetus's urinary tract obstruction?

Fortunately, the severity of damage to both the lungs and the kidneys can be accurately assessed by ultrasound and, sometimes, by sonographically guided aspiration of fetal urine. In most cases, serial sonographic observation is all that is needed. This applies to all unilateral lesions in which there is one normal kidney. These fetuses can be safely followed by serial ultrasounds to make sure they maintain amniotic fluid volume and to help plan the delivery. Fetuses with obstruction to both kidneys must be closely followed for changes in amniotic fluid volume, further dilation of the urinary tract, and the sonographic appearance of the kidneys themselves (increased echogenicity or brightness suggests ongoing damage to the kidney itself). If amniotic fluid volume is maintained, the kidney echogenicity does not deteriorate, and the system does not become more dilated, then these fetuses can be followed to normal delivery near term and urologic repair after birth. Some will require several surgeries after birth, but most will do well. Fetuses with obstruction to both kidneys, dilated bladder and ureters, and increasing echogenicity of the kidney itself are on the severe end of the spectrum and some will not survive.

Very severely affected fetuses, who lose amniotic fluid before eighteen weeks of gestation and have very echogenic, dysplastic, or multicystic kidneys often cannot be saved. When these symptoms take place fetal urine will show a salt content which demonstrates that the kidneys cannot function properly.

Fetuses with obstruction to both kidneys that has not caused increased echogenicity or dysplasia and who have maintained the kidneys' ability to extract salt from the urine may be saved by fetal intervention to relieve the urinary tract obstruction. These fetuses should be carefully studied for the degree of renal dysplasia or echogenicity, for the degree of dilation of the urinary tract and the anatomy of the obstruction, either at the bladder outlet or above the bladder, and for the amniotic fluid volume. Those who are candidates for fetal intervention can be accurately assessed for the degree of renal functional damage by serial sonographically guided aspiration of fetal urine every twenty-four hours to measure fetal urine electrolytes and beta-2-microglobulin. These tests are quite accurate in predicting fetal renal function, impairment, and the potential to recover.

Section 31.2

Fetal Surgery for Obstructive Uropathy

Most fetuses with urinary tract obstruction do not require treatment before birth, but should be followed by serial ultrasound. All single-sided lesions, even those where the kidney is destroyed (dysplasia), can be successfully managed after birth. Fetuses with mild partial obstruction to both kidneys who do not have cysts in their kidneys or abnormal urine electrolytes and maintain their amniotic fluid volume can also be successfully managed after birth. It is important to follow these fetuses with serial ultrasound to make sure they maintain enough amniotic fluid volume for lung development and do not develop signs of kidney damage. This is a good time to plan the time, type, and place of delivery. Although most babies will require some surgery after birth, it is usually not urgent. Most babies will not require intensive care and can be evaluated for surgery in the nursery or even later after they have left the hospital. However, fetuses with urinary tract obstruction that develop very dilated kidneys and have any degree of oligohydramnios and any risk of small lungs should be delivered in a tertiary center with an intensive care nursery.

When is fetal intervention an option?

In cases where the urinary obstruction affects both kidneys and there is low or absent amniotic fluid, a careful and thorough evaluation is necessary because fetal intervention may be an option. Prior to fetal intervention, it is essential to determine that the kidneys have not suffered damage that would make normal function impossible. There are two ways that kidneys can be assessed. The first is by ultrasound evaluation. The radiologist can determine on an ultrasound whether or not the kidney tissue looks normal. The presence of cysts or echogenic (bright white) tissue is usually not a favorable sign.

The second method of determining kidney function in a fetus is by taking a sample of fetal urine and analyzing the electrolytes and protein levels. This procedure is done exactly like an amniocentesis. A needle is placed through the mother's abdomen and into the fetus's bladder. A fetal urine sample is taken, the fetal bladder is completely drained of urine, and the urine sample is sent for testing. Determination of normal karyotype (chromosomes) can also be done on this urine sample of the fetus. This procedure should be repeated in twenty-four to forty-eight hours and the fetal urine should again be sent for electrolyte and protein testing. It may be necessary to take a third urine sample in another twenty-four to forty-eight hours. A fetal urine sample is taken three times in order to get the most accurate assessment of kidney function, as the first sample has been in the bladder for a long time and may not give the best information. The second sample may be urine which had been in the kidneys for a prolonged period of time and drained into the bladder after the first bladder tap. The results of the analysis on the third sample enable the medical team to give the most accurate prognosis and recommendations for treatment. Only fetuses with bilateral (both kidneys) urinary obstruction and evidence of good kidney function by ultrasound and electrolyte and protein levels are candidates for fetal intervention.

Fetuses with bilateral obstructions (usually males with posterior urethral valves) who lose amniotic fluid volume and develop signs of renal compromise before twenty-four weeks require intensive management before and after birth.

The most severe cases have evidence of progressive renal failure. The kidneys show cysts or increased "brightness" (echogenicity), urine electrolytes are abnormal, and amniotic fluid may decrease or disappear. These fetuses may require decompression before birth.

How is it done?

The goal of fetal intervention is to allow the urine to get past the obstruction and exit the fetus into the amniotic fluid. Restoring the normal flow of urine into the amniotic fluid will allow the lungs to grow and the kidneys to develop. Fetal intervention for urinary obstruction has improved dramatically over the past twenty-five years. The first fetal intervention for urinary obstruction involved open fetal surgery (an incision in the uterus to expose the fetus) and placement of a vesicostomy. A vesicostomy is an opening in the lower fetal abdomen that goes directly into the fetal bladder. The urine is able to exit the fetus through this opening and drain into the amniotic fluid. This method of treatment was successful, but the women who underwent this procedure experienced preterm labor from the incision made in the uterus. Then, a less invasive means of intervention was developed. This involved the placement of a specially designed tube, the Harrison catheter, into the fetal bladder. The procedure is similar to an amniocentesis. A small hollow needle is placed through the mother's abdomen into the fetal bladder, using the sonogram for visualization. One end of the tube is in the fetal bladder and the other end in the amniotic fluid. Urine escapes the fetal bladder through the tube. The problem with these catheters is that they become plugged or dislodged, sometimes requiring repeated procedures. This technique has proven effective and has been used thousands of times around the world with good success. However, it is difficult to keep these little tubes in place and functioning.

More recently, we have developed a technique (Fetendo fetal surgery) to directly relieve the obstruction at the bladder outlet by putting a very small (3 mm) fetoscope directly into the fetal bladder and disrupting the valves. This can now be done through a very small scope placed through a nick in the mother's skin rather than through open surgery. Relieving fetal urinary tract obstruction has proven very effective in restoring amniotic fluid volume and allowing the fetal lungs to grow. It is not yet proven that relieving the obstruction before birth will always preserve renal function and prevent long-term renal failure.

What will happen after birth?

We recommend that after consulting with your primary physician, your newborn be started on Amoxicillin, an antibiotic, immediately after birth. This will prevent any infection of the urinary tract. No testing is recommended until the baby is one month of age and the kidney function has matured. At this time we would recommend a renal (kidney) ultrasound and a diuretic renal scan, and an appointment with a surgeon for consultation. Both of these tests will help evaluate the anatomy and function of the kidneys. On occasion, the surgeon will request a third test, called a "voiding cystourethrogram" or VCUG, to examine the urinary system for reflux (or backup) of urine from the bladder into the kidneys. Based on the results of these studies, the surgeon will be able to identify the specific renal abnormality, assess the health of the kidney(s), and make recommendations for the treatment of your baby's condition. The recommendations for treatment range from periodic testing to operation intervention.

Section 31.3

Bladder Exstrophy

Sometimes factors can interfere with bladder development, as is the case for children with bladder exstrophy. If your newborn has been diagnosed with this condition, what can you expect? The following information should help you talk to your child's doctor.

What is bladder exstrophy?

Bladder exstrophy is an abnormality present at birth in which the bladder and associated structures are improperly formed. Rather than being its normal round shape, the bladder is flattened. The skin covering the lower part of the abdomen does not form properly so the inside of the bladder is exposed outside the abdomen. There are associated deficiencies of the abdominal muscles and pelvic bones also.

How often does it occur?

It is a rare occurrence. The incidence of bladder exstrophy varies in different parts of the world, but is approximately one in thirty thousand live births and is slightly more common in males than females. The risk of a family having more than one child with this condition is approximately one in one hundred, and children born to a parent with exstrophy have a risk of approximately one in seventy of having the condition. Recent published evidence suggests that the risk of bladder exstrophy in children born as a result of assisted fertility techniques is seven times greater than in children conceived naturally without assistance.

Why does it happen?

There is no known cause for this condition but there are many theories. Some experts believe during the eleventh week of pregnancy the embryo undergoes structural changes including growth of tissue in the lower abdominal wall, which stimulates development of muscles and pelvic bones. Up to this point the primitive bladder and rectum are contained within tissue called the cloacal membrane. The rectum then separates from the bladder, and if migration of tissue toward the midline over the primitive bladder fails the cloacal membrane may rupture, creating an exstrophied bladder. The exact timing of premature rupture of the membrane determines whether the child is born with isolated epispadias, classic bladder exstrophy, or cloacal exstrophy. Generally classic bladder exstrophy is an isolated birth defect but spinal cord abnormalities occur in about 13 percent of cases.

It is known, however, that it is not a result of anything that a parent did or did not do during pregnancy.

How is it diagnosed?

Frequently it can be detected before birth during a routine sonogram. Nonetheless, this condition will be obvious at birth.

What will happen when the child is born?

If this condition has been detected before birth, arrangements will usually be made for birth at a specialist unit where a pediatrician and surgeon can assess the baby immediately. Alternatively, if the condition is not detected until the time of birth, transfer to such a unit for assessment will need to be arranged for the first day of life. In either case, the bladder will be visible on the outside of the baby's abdomen, and assessment of bladder size and quality, the shape of the pelvis, and also the condition of the genitals will be made.

What treatments are available?

Bladder exstrophy is treated surgically. Several surgical treatment options are available but they depend upon the severity of the condition.

The primary treatment objectives are:

1. Securely closing the bladder and pelvis

2. Reconstructing a cosmetically pleasing and functioning penis in the male and external genitalia in the female

3. Achieving urinary continence while ensuring preservation of kidney function

One form of treatment is modern staged reconstruction that involves closure of the bladder and pelvis in the newborn period, early reconstruction of the epispadiac urethra at approximately six to twelve months of age, and bladder neck surgery to achieve continence when the bladder has reached sufficient capacity and the child is psychologically ready to be dry (often around four to five years of age). Often further operations are needed to improve continence. Additional surgical procedures to improve the external genitalia are almost always required. In select cases where the bladder is of good quality and the penis is of good size, closure of the bladder and reconstruction of the penis and urethra can be combined in one operation. This is very technically demanding surgery and should be performed by only an experienced exstrophy surgeon.

The results of staged reconstruction have been well documented, and given the development of a bladder with sufficient capacity, continence can be achieved in up to 90 percent of cases. The most important factors in achieving continence are the quality of the bladder template and a successful initial bladder closure in the newborn. Of course, there are instances when the bladder at birth is of poor quality and unsuitable for closure in the way described, and a different management is adopted. Using techniques of modern reconstructive surgery, it is exceptionally rare for a patient to reach late adolescence without achieving continence and cosmetically acceptable external genitalia.

Other methods of treatment involve urinary diversion where the normal flow of urine is re-routed.

What is the outlook for a baby born with this condition?

There is no doubt that in modern times, children with exstrophy can and do grow up to be robust individuals with a normal life expectancy and no real restriction on their lifestyle.

Are there other disorders associated with bladder exstrophy?

Yes, some of these may include: epispadias, vesicoureteral reflux, diastasis, small bladder capacity, or missing bladder neck and sphincter.

Section 31.4

Epispadias

Definition: Epispadias is a rare congenital (present from birth) defect in the location of the opening of the urethra.

In boys with epispadias, the urethra generally opens on the top or side (rather than the tip) of the penis, though it is possible for the urethra to be open the entire length of the penis. In girls, the opening is usually between the clitoris and the labia, but may be in the abdomen.

Causes, Incidence, and Risk Factors: The causes of epispadias are unknown at this time. It is believed to be related to improper development of the pubic bone. Epispadias is often associated with bladder exstrophy. However, it can also occur alone or with defects other than exstrophy.

Epispadias occurs in 1 in 117,000 newborn boys and 1 in 484,000 newborn girls. The condition is usually diagnosed at birth or shortly thereafter.

Symptoms:

In males:

- Abnormal opening from the pubic symphysis to the area above the tip of the penis;
- Bladder exstrophy (may or may not be present);
- Widened pubic bone;
- Short, widened penis with chordee (abnormal curvature of the penis);
- Urinary incontinence;
- Reflux nephropathy;
- Urinary tract infections.

In females:

- Abnormal opening from the bladder neck to the area above the normal urethral opening;
- Bladder exstrophy (may or may not be present);
- Widened pubic bone;
- Bifid clitoris, rudimentary labia;
- Urinary incontinence;
- Reflux nephropathy;
- Urinary tract infections.

Signs and Tests:

- Complete blood count (CBC)
- Serum electrolytes
- Pelvic x-ray
- Intravenous pyelogram (IVP)
- Ultrasound of the urogenital system

Treatment: Surgical repair of epispadias is recommended. Leakage of urine (incontinence) is not uncommon and may require a second operation.

Expectations (Prognosis): Surgical repairs generally produce both continence (the ability to control the flow of urine) and a good cosmetic outcome.

Complications: Persistent urinary incontinence can occur in some people even after multiple operations. Also upper urinary tract (ureter and kidney) damage as well as infertility may occur.

Calling Your Health Care Provider: Call your health care provider if you have any questions or concerns regarding your child's genitourinary tract appearance or function.

Section 31.5

Ectopic Ureter

Most of us are born with two ureters, one to drain the urine from each kidney into the bladder. But nature has given some of us more than the normal allotment. In most cases, a bonus ureter causes no problems. Yet what if one of these ureters it is not connected correctly—and drains incorrectly? That is the case for children with an ectopic ureter, a bonus that is not a plus. Luckily, medicine has given urologists a bevy of diagnostic tests and surgical techniques to deal with this abnormality. So read the following to see how your child's doctor might correct this condition.

What are the causes of ectopic ureter?

Normally, there is a single ureter draining the urine from each kidney to the bladder. The urine is then stored in the bladder until one voluntarily urinates. Occasionally, there may be two ureters draining a single kidney. One ureter drains the upper part of the kidney and the second ureter drains the lower portion. So long as they both enter the bladder normally, this "duplicated collecting system" is not a problem. Rarely a child may be born with an ectopic ureter. This is a ureter that fails to connect properly to the bladder and drains somewhere outside the bladder. In girls, the ectopic ureter usually drains into the urethra or even the vagina. In boys, it usually drains into the urethra near the prostate or into the genital duct system. An ectopic ureter can occur in a nonduplicated collecting system but is more common in a duplicated system.

What are the symptoms of ectopic ureter?

Blockage of the ureter or the inability to control urination (incontinence) can indicate an ectopic ureter. Poor drainage, accompanied by back pressure, can cause the ureter and portion of the kidney it services to become distended or swollen. This condition is called hydronephrosis and can be spotted easily on an ultrasound. For this reason, many babies with an ectopic ureter are detected when the pregnant mother undergoes a prenatal ultrasound. However, not all ectopic ureters are hydronephrotic so they may not be detected by an ultrasound.

Poor drainage from an ectopic ureter may make children more likely to have urinary tract infections. In addition to hydronephrosis, ectopic ureters in girls may cause incontinence since the ureter drains urine directly into or near the vagina. This problem becomes evident after toilet training. It is usually distinguished from other forms of incontinence in girls because the incontinence is a constant dripping moistness rather than episodes of loss of bladder control. Some girls will be treated with medication and other therapies for many years before the correct diagnosis of an ectopic ureter is made. Boys with ectopic ureters do not generally have incontinence since the ectopic ureter drains inside the body. However, they may still show symptoms of hydronephrosis or a urinary tract infection.

When an ectopic ureter is present, there may also be a slight flaw in the normal ureter's connection between the kidney and bladder. This flaw can result in vesicoureteral reflux, a disruption of the passage of urine from the kidney, through the ureter, to the bladder and finally out the urethra. With reflux, as the bladder fills or empties some urine flows backward into the kidney. Vesicoureteral reflux places patients at a higher risk for kidney infections and is another reason some children with ectopic ureters show signs of a urinary tract infection.

How is ectopic ureter diagnosed?

The evaluation of an ectopic ureter depends on the problem shown by the patient (usually a child). For instance, if hydronephrosis is detected on a prenatal ultrasound, then the ultrasound is usually repeated after the child is born. A bladder x-ray, called a voiding cystourethrogram (VCUG), is then taken to rule out vesicoureteral reflux as the cause for swelling of the kidney and ureter. The VCUG is also used to determine if there is reflux in a second ureter associated with the ectopic ureter. Usually with the combination of an ultrasound and a VCUG the doctor can determine if there is hydronephrosis. Sometimes other diagnostic studies such as renal flow scan or a formal kidney x-ray, called an intravenous pyelogram (IVP), may help to clarify the anatomy. The kidney or portion of the kidney drained by the ectopic ureter often functions poorly. This can be assessed with a renal flow scan. Both tests involve an injection of contrast dye picked up by the kidney and then seen either by standard x-ray pictures (for an IVP) or with a special camera for detecting small amounts of radioactivity in the dye (for the renal flow scan). This functional information may be important in selecting the form of treatment. Finally, a cystoscopy may be performed (often at the time of definitive treatment). In this test, usually performed under a general anesthesia, a small telescope is placed into the urethra and vagina and the openings of the ureters from both kidneys are identified. Unfortunately, the ectopic ureter's opening cannot always be identified. However, by identifying the number and location of the other ureter openings, the diagnosis can usually be confirmed.

When a child shows symptoms of urinary incontinence, the same sequence of tests is usually undertaken. However, if the ureter is not swollen and there is no associated reflux, the ultrasound and VCUG may be normal. If the symptoms suggest an ectopic ureter, then sometimes this can be seen on a renal flow scan or IVP. Occasionally, a computed tomography (CT) scan is needed to see the ectopic ureter and the portion of the kidney it drains. The diagnosis is not always easy to make and since other causes of incontinence are very common in children, some children may be incontinent for years before the diagnosis is made.

How is an ectopic ureter treated?

The treatment for ectopic ureter is surgery. To control the risk of infection, the patient may be placed on a low dose of antibiotics prior to surgery.

While there are three surgical techniques—nephrectomy, ureteropyelostomy, and ureteral reimplantation—to correct this problem, each has advantages and disadvantages.

Nephrectomy (upper pole heminephrectomy). In this surgery, the kidney or the portion of it drained by the ectopic ureter is removed. This stops the flow of urine into the ectopic ureter, thus curing the incontinence and reducing the chance of infection. Technically the simplest operation, this also has the lowest complication risk. It is particularly attractive when the kidney or portion of the kidney draining through the ectopic ureter is functioning poorly. It may also be used when that kidney portion is functioning properly if the opposite kidney is normal. This operation has been traditionally performed through an incision under the ribs but can now be done laparoscopically in some patients. The main disadvantages are that the potentially functioning kidney tissue may be removed and the bottom end of the ectopic ureter is left in place. While usually not a problem, the remaining part of the ectopic ureter can be a future source for infection.

Ureteropyelostomy. In this procedure, the ectopic ureter is divided near the kidney and sewn into the normal collecting system of the lower part of the kidney. This allows the urine from the upper part of the kidney to drain normally. It has the advantage of protecting all the kidney tissue but still leaves the bottom half of the ectopic ureter in place. It also has a slightly higher complication rate than the other operations.

Ureteral reimplantation. In this operation, the ectopic ureter is divided near the bottom and sewn into the bladder in such a way that urine drains well and does not flow backward. Usually performed through an incision above the pubic bone, this procedure has a slightly higher complication rate than the other two surgeries. It can also be technically difficult if performed in small infants. However, like ureteropyelostomy, this operation preserves all kidney tissue. Furthermore, it removes more of the abnormal ectopic ureter than the other two procedures and allows the surgeon to stop any vesicoureteral reflux.

What can be expected after treatment for ectopic ureter?

Recovery depends on the operation selected. However, infants and small children are usually hospitalized from one to five days after the surgery. A small catheter may be left at the time of surgery, which is removed painlessly and quickly before the child goes home or in the office at a follow-up visit. The small openings, where the catheter went in, heal on their own without the need for stitches.

Are boys or girls more likely to have an ectopic ureter?

This condition is more common in girls than boys, but can occur in either sex.

What is the optimal age for ectopic ureter surgery?

Nephrectomies and heminephrectomies can be performed anytime after an infant reaches one month. Some surgeons prefer to wait until a child is older, usually after a first birthday, to perform a ureteral reimplantation.

What are the risk factors for an ectopic pregnancy?

There are no known risk factors for an ectopic ureter. It is a congenital problem that probably occurs because of a failure in the development of the connection between the ureter and bladder.

Was this caused by something that happened during pregnancy?

There is also no evidence that this abnormality is caused by anything a mother does or was exposed to during pregnancy.

Does an ectopic ureter have any impact on my child's future sexual function?

Although an ectopic ureter drains to the genital tract, it does not affect sexual function and rarely impairs fertility. In boys, the genital tract on the same side of the ectopic ureter may be abnormal but if the other side is unaffected (which is usually the case), then fertility should still be normal.

If part or all of a kidney is functioning poorly or removed, will my child have life-long kidney problems?

No, not as long as the other kidney is normal. Most ectopic ureters affect just the upper part of one kidney, which provides only one-third of that kidney's function to the body. Even when an entire kidney is affected, long-term problems are unlikely. Children are frequently born with a single kidney and never know it and patients who donate a kidney also do fine. The only implication is that the patient no longer has a "spare" kidney. Therefore, in the unlikely event that the person was to injure their only kidney in an accident, then they would develop kidney failure if a complete nephrectomy were performed. If only a portion of the kidney was removed during the nephrectomy, the patient would do very well in the long term.

Section 31.6

Megaureter

The vast majority of children are born with urinary tracts that
function efficiently. But in some infants, megaureters, a widening or
swelling of the connecting tube between the kidneys and bladder, can
cause infections, obstructions, and even serious kidney damage if the
problem is not diagnosed and treated. But what are the symptoms?
The following information should give you a head start in learning
about this potentially serious health hazard.

What are megaureters?

The ureters are tube-like structures in the body that carry or pro-
pel urine from the kidneys to the bladder. While the normal width of
a child's ureter is three to five millimeters (mm.), megaureters are
greater than 10 mm. (three-eighths of an inch) in diameter, hence the
term "megaureter." Certain conditions produce this abnormal widening. It can result from an abnormality of the ureter itself or for a secondary reason.

What are the different types of megaureters?

Most megaureters are classified as one of the following:

- **Primary obstructed megaureter:** A distinct blockage where
  the ureter enters the bladder. The obstruction can produce damage to the kidney over time. Even though the problem may improve with time, diligent follow-up is necessary.

- **Refluxing megaureters:** Source of a backward flow of urine
  (vesicoureteral reflux). It is linked to megacystis megaureter, a
  condition where the bladder, instead of emptying completely, is

enlarged due to cycling of urine between it and the ureters via reflux.

- **Nonobstructive, nonrefluxing megaureters:** These are wide ureters not caused by obstruction or urine backflow. Many of these improve with time.

- **Obstructed, refluxing megaureters:** An obstructed ureter that also suffers from reflux. A dangerous combination since the ureters get bigger and more blocked with time.

- **Secondary megaureters:** These enlarged ureters appear in association with other conditions such as posterior urethral valves, prune belly syndrome, and neurogenic bladder.

What are the symptoms of megaureter?

In the past, the majority of megaureters were found during the evaluation of a child with a urinary tract infection. These patients usually experience fever, back pain, and vomiting.

But today, because of the widespread use of prenatal fetal sonography, more megaureters are discovered as prenatal hydronephrosis or dilatation of the urinary tract in the fetus.

Because megaureters can cause a severe infection or obstruction that leads to kidney damage, this health issue is potentially serious. Dilatation of the urinary tract may imply a blockage or obstruction, but that is not always the case. In some situations, a dilated ureter may not affect the kidney at all. Also, most patients with prenatally detected megaureters do not experience symptoms related to this wide ureter.

How is a megaureter diagnosed?

If your child develops a urinary tract infection, or other symptoms that could signal this condition, check with your doctor. Further investigation is warranted. You can expect the urologist to conduct a series of tests to clarify the anatomy and function of the urinary tract.

Ultrasound. Also known as sonography, this simple and painless imaging test is usually done to evaluate the appearance of the kidney, ureter, and bladder. The study is highly sensitive in detecting troubled ureters. In fact, while sonography rarely picks up normal ureters because of their narrowed size, this technology produces excellent images of dilated ones.

Voiding cystourethrogram (VCUG). A VCUG is done to determine if vesicoureteral reflux is occurring. A small catheter is inserted through the urethra into the bladder and a contrast dye is injected into the bladder before x-rays are taken. If reflux is present, the image will show the contrast produced by the backflow into the ureter.

Diuretic renal scans. Used to evaluate for a possible obstruction, this test is performed by injecting a radioactive substance into a vein, which is then carried to the kidneys. While the study yields data about a possible blockage, it also gives physicians information about the organ's function.

Intravenous pyelogram (IVP). Also referred to as excretory urogram, IVP is performed by injecting dye into a vein and taking x-ray pictures of the abdomen as the dye is emptied from the kidneys. While renal scans have replaced IVP in evaluating dilated urinary tracts, this test can be extremely helpful in questionable cases.

How is a megaureter treated?

If tests reveal an obstruction or impaired function, your child may need surgery to correct the problem. The typical operation for megaureters is called ureteral reimplantation, the technical term urologists use for trimming the widened ureter. Unless the child has a urinary tract infection or decrease in kidney function, the surgery can be delayed until twelve months of age. Surgery in infants is technically demanding and should be performed by individuals experienced with neonatal surgery. Many babies are kept on antibiotic prophylaxis during this period of observation to minimize the likelihood of infections.

During the procedure, the surgeon makes an incision in the lower abdomen and, depending on the child's anatomy, approaches the ureter either through the bladder (transvesical) or from outside the bladder (extravesical). The ureter is disconnected from the bladder, and if very wide, it may need to be trimmed (tapered) and then replaced in the bladder. If an obstruction exists, it is removed. Your child may have a catheter for a few days to improve healing. Hospitalization is usually between two and four days.

What can be expected after treatment for a megaureter?

Several weeks after surgery, some of the tests that were done before surgery may need to be repeated to determine the success of the surgery. The size of the ureter may not improve immediately after surgery, so evaluation over time will be necessary to ensure a good outcome. Potential complications of surgery are bleeding, obstruction of the ureter, and vesicoureteral reflux. Obstruction may occur soon after the operation or after a long period of time. Fortunately, this complication occurs in only 5 percent of cases and it may require additional surgery. A vesicoureteral reflux complication may occur after surgery in 5 percent of the cases and may improve with time. Most patients are followed for a number of years, using ultrasound, to ensure that the appearance of the kidney and ureter continues to improve.

Is this condition genetic?

At this time scientists do not know if there are genetic links.

Is surgery always necessary to correct a megaureter?

No. Some megaureters may improve over time without the need for surgery. However, it is important to prevent infections during the time of observation so antibiotics are usually prescribed.

Is minimally invasive surgery an option?

It may be possible to place a stent or catheter through the blocked portion of the megaureter as a temporary procedure to improve the drainage of the kidney. Laparoscopic techniques are not presently well developed to correct most megaureters but that may change in the future.

Are there long-term problems if we do not do anything?

Possibly yes. They include ureteral stones, urinary tract infection, deterioration of kidney function, and back pain.

Section 31.7

Ureterocele

Most of us are born with two ureters, one to drain the urine from each kidney into the bladder. Yet what if the portion of the ureter closest to the bladder becomes enlarged because the ureter opening is very tiny and obstructs urine outflow? That is the case for people with a ureterocele. Luckily, medicine has given urologists a range of diagnostic tests and surgical techniques to deal with this abnormality. Read the following to see how your urologist might correct this condition.

What happens under normal conditions?

Within the urinary tract, the kidneys filter and remove waste and water from the blood to produce urine. The urine travels from the kidneys down two narrow tubes called the ureters, where it is then stored in the bladder. Normally, the attachment between the ureters and the bladder is a one-way flap valve that allows unimpeded urinary flow into the bladder but prevents urine from flowing backward (vesicoureteral reflux) into the kidneys. Approximately 1 out of 125 people may have two ureters draining a single kidney. One ureter drains the upper part of the kidney and the second ureter drains the lower portion. This "duplicated collecting system" is not a problem as long as each ureter enters the bladder normally. When the bladder empties, urine flows out of the body through the urethra, a tube at the bottom of the bladder. The opening of the urethra is at the end of the penis in boys and in front of the vagina in girls.

What is a ureterocele?

A ureterocele is a birth defect that affects the kidney, ureter, and bladder. When a person has a ureterocele, the portion of the ureter closest to the bladder swells up like a balloon because the ureter opening is very tiny and obstructs urine outflow. As the urine flow is obstructed, urine backs up in the ureter. Approximately one in two thousand persons are affected by this condition. In 90 percent of girls the ureterocele occurs in the upper half of a duplicated urinary tract. Approximately half of boys have a duplicated urinary tract and half have a single system. Ureteroceles may be "ectopic" when a portion protrudes through the bladder outlet into the urethra, or "orthotopic" when they remain entirely within the bladder. In 5 to 10 percent of cases there is a ureterocele on both sides (bilateral). The majority of ureteroceles are diagnosed in children less than two years of age, although occasionally older children or adults are found to have a ureterocele.

What are some complications of a ureterocele?

This condition often predisposes an individual to a kidney infection. Vesicoureteral reflux is also common, particularly in individuals with a duplication of the urinary tract, because the ureterocele distorts the normal one-way valve attachment between the ureter and bladder. In addition, reflux on the opposite side is common for similar reasons. In rare cases, a ureterocele may prevent the passage of kidney stones. Also, the ureterocele may be so large that it completely obstructs the flow of urine from the bladder into the urethra. Occasionally, in girls, the ureterocele may sink and protrude out from the opening of the urethra.

What are some symptoms of a ureterocele?

Symptoms can include flank or back pain, urinary tract infection, fever, painful urination, foul-smelling urine, abdominal pain, blood in the urine (hematuria), and/or excessive urination.

How is a ureterocele diagnosed?

Although doctors can and often do detect ureteroceles during prenatal ultrasounds, they may not be diagnosed until a patient is being evaluated for another medical condition like a urinary tract infection.

Ultrasonography is the first imaging test used in evaluation. Additional imaging studies may also be necessary to help delineate the anatomy. One such test is a voiding cystourethrogram (VCUG), which is an x-ray examination of the bladder and lower urinary tract. A catheter is inserted through the urethra, the bladder is filled with a water-soluble dye, and then the catheter is withdrawn. Several x-ray images of the bladder and urethra are captured as the patient empties the bladder. These images allow radiologists to diagnose any abnormalities in the flow of urine through the body.

In individuals with a ureterocele, it is also important to evaluate the function of the kidneys, specifically to determine whether the affected portion of the kidney has any function. In most cases, this evaluation is performed with a renal scan.

Abdominal computed tomography (CT) scans, magnetic resonance imaging (MRI) tests, and excretory urograms are additional studies that may also be performed in the evaluation of a patient with a ureterocele. These tests are usually performed in situations where the urinary tract anatomy is extremely ambiguous and will allow the surgeon to better identify anatomical variations.

What are some treatment options?

Timing of therapy and form of treatment are based on the age of the patient, whether the affected portion of the kidney is functioning, and whether vesicoureteral reflux is present. In some cases, more than one procedure is necessary. In rare cases, observation (no treatment) may be recommended.

Because a ureterocele predisposes an individual to a kidney infection, usually an antibiotic is prescribed until the ureterocele and its complicating features have been treated. The following are available treatment options:

- **Transurethral puncture:** A form of minimally invasive therapy is to puncture and decompress the ureterocele using a cystoscope that is inserted through the urethra. The procedure usually takes fifteen to thirty minutes, and often can be done on an outpatient basis. In some cases, this treatment is unsuccessful if the ureterocele wall is thick and difficult to recognize. The advantage of this treatment is that there is no surgical incision. Risks include failure to adequately decompress the ureterocele, possibly causing urine to flow into the ureterocele, which could necessitate an open operation. In addition, there is a slight risk of causing an obstructive flap valve with the ureterocele, which can make it difficult to urinate.

- **Upper pole nephrectomy:** Often, if the upper half of the kidney does not function because of the ureterocele and there is no vesicoureteral reflux, removal of the affected portion of the kidney is recommended. In many cases, this operation is performed through a small incision under the rib cage. In some cases it may be performed laparoscopically.

- **Nephrectomy:** If the entire kidney does not function because of the ureterocele, removal of the kidney is recommended. Usually this can be done laparoscopically, although at some centers it is performed through a very small incision under the rib cage.

- **Removal of the ureterocele and ureteral reimplantation:** If it is deemed necessary to remove the ureterocele, then an operation is performed in which the bladder is opened, the ureterocele is removed, the floor of the bladder and bladder neck are reconstructed, and the ureters are reimplanted in such a way to create a non-refluxing connection between the ureters and the bladder. The operation is performed through a small lower abdominal incision. The success rate with this procedure is 90 to 95 percent and the complications include persistent ureteral obstruction.

- **Ureteropyelostomy or upper-to-lower ureteroureterostomy:** If the upper portion of the ureter shows significant function, one option is to connect the obstructed upper portion to the nonobstructed lower portion of the ureter or pelvis of the kidney. The operation is done through a small lower abdominal incision. The success rate with this procedure is 95 percent.

Is there any way to prevent this condition?

There is no known prevention for this condition; it is present at birth but may not be discovered until later in life.

My baby was diagnosed with a ureterocele on a prenatal ultrasound. She seems very healthy. Is it absolutely necessary for her to undergo treatment?

In the past, most children with a ureterocele had their condition detected following a serious kidney infection, which often required hospitalization for intravenous antibiotics. Consequently, it would be unusual for her not to develop a urinary tract infection unless her ureterocele was treated.

My doctor has recommended that my daughter take antibiotic prophylaxis because she has a ureterocele and urinary reflux. Is it safe to take antibiotics every day?

Many children and adults take a low dose of an antibiotic every day to prevent urinary tract infections. This form of therapy has been used for over thirty-five years and has proven to be relatively safe, as long as the dose is maintained at one-fourth to one-half the full dose. One needs to weigh the risk of taking the antibiotic against the risk of a serious kidney infection if the antibiotic were not taken.

My child was diagnosed with a ureterocele and it was punctured through a small scope. Now there is reflux into the ureterocele and the lower part of the kidney also. Will more surgery be necessary?

In most cases, if there is reflux up the ureter into the lower part of the kidney and/or the ureterocele, the reflux is unlikely to disappear with time, and removal of the ureterocele and ureteral reimplantation is often necessary.

Section 31.8

Vesicoureteral Reflux

Reprinted from the National Kidney and Urologic Diseases Information Clearinghouse, a service of the National Institute of Diabetes and Digestive and Kidney Diseases (NIDDK), National Institutes of Health, NIH Publication No. 03-4555, April 2003.

Urine normally flows in one direction—down from the kidneys, through tubes called ureters, to the bladder. Vesicoureteral reflux (VUR) is the abnormal flow of urine from the bladder back into the ureters.

VUR is most commonly diagnosed in infancy and childhood after the patient has a urinary tract infection (UTI). About one-third of children with UTI are found to have VUR. VUR can lead to infection because urine that remains in the child's urinary tract provides a place for bacteria to grow. But sometimes the infection itself is the cause of VUR.

There are two types of VUR. Primary VUR occurs when a child is born with an impaired valve where the ureter joins the bladder. This happens if the ureter did not grow long enough during the child's development in the womb. The valve does not close properly, so urine backs up (refluxes) from the bladder to the ureters, and eventually to the kidneys. This type of VUR can get better or disappear as the child gets older. The ureter gets longer as the child grows, and the function of the valve improves.

Secondary VUR occurs when there is a blockage anywhere in the urinary system. The blockage may be caused by an infection in the bladder that leads to swelling of the ureter. This also causes a reflux of urine to the kidneys.

Infection is the most common symptom of VUR. As the child gets older, other symptoms, such as bedwetting, high blood pressure, protein in the urine, and kidney failure, may appear.

Common tests to show the presence of urinary tract infection include urine tests and cultures.

Because no single test can tell everything about the urinary tract that might be important to know, more than one of the following imaging tests may be needed:

- **Kidney and bladder ultrasound:** A test that uses sound waves to examine the kidney and bladder. This test shows shadows of the kidney and bladder that may point out certain abnormalities. The test cannot reveal all important urinary abnormalities or measure how well a kidney works.

- **Voiding cystourethrogram (VCUG):** A test that examines the urethra and bladder while the bladder fills and empties. A liquid that can be seen on x-rays is placed in the bladder through a catheter. Pictures are taken when the bladder is filled and when the child urinates. This test can reveal abnormalities of the inside of the urethra and bladder. The test can also determine whether the flow of urine is normal when the bladder empties.

- **Intravenous pyelogram:** A test that examines the whole urinary tract. A liquid that can be seen on x-rays is injected into a vein. The substance travels into the kidneys and bladder, revealing possible obstructions.

- **Nuclear scans:** A number of tests using radioactive materials that are usually injected into a vein to show how well the kidneys work, their shape, and whether urine empties from the kidneys normally. Each kind of nuclear scan gives different information about the kidneys and bladder. Nuclear scans expose a child to about the same amount of radiation as a conventional x-ray. At times, it can be even less.

The goal for treatment of VUR is to prevent any kidney damage from occurring. Infections should be treated at once with antibiotics to prevent the infection from moving into the kidneys. Antibiotic therapy usually corrects reflux caused by infection. Sometimes surgery is needed to correct primary VUR.

Section 31.9

Urachal Anomalies

Before birth, there is a connection between the bellybutton and the bladder. This connection, called the urachus, normally disappears before birth. But what happens if part of the urachus remains after birth? Read on to learn more about what problems can arise.

What happens under normal conditions?

The bladder, located in the lower abdomen, is formed from structures located in the lower half of the developing fetus that are directly connected to the umbilical cord. After the first few weeks of gestation, this thick pathway to and from the placenta contains blood vessels, a merged channel to the future intestine, and a tubular structure called the allantois. The internal part of the allantois is connected to the top of the developing bladder, and in ordinary circumstances, collapses and becomes a cordlike structure called the urachus. The formation and regression of this connection from the top of the bladder to the bellybutton are completed by the middle of the second trimester of pregnancy (approximately twenty weeks).

Although the urachus is easily seen by a surgeon whenever an operation inside the abdomen or around the bladder is performed, it is a remnant of development that serves no further purpose but can be a source of specific health problems. Such problems are rare and usually seen in childhood, but occasionally can be seen for the first time in adults.

What are the symptoms of urachal abnormalities?

Because this remnant of early development is found between the bellybutton and the top of the bladder, diseases of the urachus can appear anywhere in that space. In newborns and infants, persistent drainage or "wetness" of the bellybutton can be a sign of a urachal problem. However, the most common detectable problem at the bellybutton is a granuloma, a reddened area that is present because the base of the umbilical cord stump did not heal properly.

Urachal abnormalities can also be seen without persistent umbilical drainage—35 percent of urachal problems are manifestations of an enclosed urachal cyst or infected urachal cyst (abscess). This type of problem is seen more often in older children and adults. Instead of visible bellybutton drainage, the symptoms of such a cyst consist of lower abdominal pain, fever, a lump that can be felt, pain with urination, urinary tract infection, or hematuria.

How are urachal abnormalities treated?

An umbilical granuloma is usually treated by chemical cauterization in the office of the primary care provider. The condition is a superficial abdominal wall problem that heals after treatment and has no long-term implications; it is not caused by a urachal problem.

In contrast to the simple granuloma, persistent umbilical wetness needs to be further evaluated. Approximately 65 percent of all urachal problems appear as a sinus or drainage opening at the bellybutton. Most of those are not connected all the way to the bladder, but a small percentage represent an open pathway from the bladder to bellybutton, called a patent urachus. The drainage can be analyzed for urea and creatinine levels, which would be high if the fluid was primarily made of urine from a bladder connection instead of inflammatory tissue fluid. There can be associated redness from the drainage itself. Skin infection—indicated by tenderness, fever, or spreading redness of the surrounding skin—can occur and requires prompt antibiotic treatment and possible hospitalization. This is called omphalitis and can be caused by bacteria that have become involved with a urachal sinus or the other embryologic structure in the bellybutton that was once connected to the intestinal system and might also be persistent. Once inflammation is controlled, the nature and extent of an opening at the bellybutton can be determined by a sinogram. This involves placing a small tube into the sinus opening and allowing contrast material to flow in while taking x-rays to determine the direction and extent of the channel. If the channel follows the expected pathway toward the top of the bladder, the diagnosis is urachal sinus. Treatment should be directed toward complete surgical removal of the urachus and all of its connections, including a small amount of the top of the bladder. Leaving any portion of the structure allows for the possible development of a future malignancy. Less than 1 percent of all bladder malignancies occur in the urachus, but once the urachus has become a potential problem, it should be removed.

When there is no draining sinus to investigate, an ultrasound of the lower abdomen will show the typical findings of a fluid-filled, enclosed lump in the location of the urachus. In an adult, where the rare possibility of malignancy could be present, an abdominal and pelvic computed tomography (CT) scan might be helpful. Again, complete removal of the urachus is important. Simple needle or other drainage of the cyst will result in recurrence in at least one-third of patients, since the linings and structures are still present. About 80 percent of infected cysts are populated by *Staphylococcus aureus*, and one-third contain multiple types of bacteria. Almost all the time, such an infected cyst stays confined to its predetermined anatomical location; rarely, an infected cyst can drain into the peritoneal cavity and present with additional signs of peritonitis and febrile illness.

Therefore, most urachal problems can be characterized by the physical examination and a sinogram or ultrasound. Sometimes a combination of these is needed, and occasionally it is useful to obtain a voiding cystourethrogram. This is done when the draining urachus is associated with outlet obstruction of the bladder, which would also need to be treated. This possibility is usually determined by the age, gender, and physical examination of the patient. There are also situations where a direct look inside the bladder (cystoscopy) can add a bit more information to the diagnostic picture, but most urologists recommend that the basic course of action be determined by the previously described approach.

What can be expected after treatment for urachal abnormalities?

After complete surgical removal of a troublesome urachus with no immediate postoperative problems, there should be no further issues and no need for follow-up or evaluation on a regular basis.

Besides the problems that have already been outlined, are there other diseases that appear at the bellybutton?

As you might expect, there have been rare reports of other inflammatory problems involving the structures that are contained in the umbilical cord. These include infections of the remnant blood vessels. In addition, the vitelline duct, which is supposed to regress in its course between the bellybutton and the small intestine, sometimes has its own remnant problems. The sinogram that is useful for identifying urachal problems will also serve to identify a likely vitelline duct problem.

Occasionally, an intra-abdominal process such as appendicitis or ovarian cyst can mimic some of the symptoms of a urachal problem.

Are urachal abnormalities hereditary?

No. There is no evidence that they are inherited.

After my baby's umbilical cord stump came off, his bellybutton was extremely red. Is this normal or does he need immediate evaluation?

Some redness is expected after the stump falls away. Dabbing a small amount of alcohol on the site with a Q-tip twice a day will usually allow complete healing in two to three days. If the redness fails to improve or worsens, contact your primary care provider.

Chapter 32

Defects of the Reproductive Organs

Chapter Contents

Section 32.1—Undescended Testes 510
Section 32.2—Hypospadias 512
Section 32.3—Hydroceles and Inguinal Hernias 514
Section 32.4—Urogenital Sinus 517
Section 32.5—Vaginal Agenesis 519
Section 32.6—Cloacal Exstrophy............................. 523
Section 32.7—Ambiguous Genitalia 525

Section 32.1

Undescended Testes

From *Pediatric Common Questions, Quick Answers,* by Donna D'Alessandro, M.D., Lindsay Huth, B.A., and Susan Kinzer, M.P.H., revised October 2004. Copyright Donna M. D'Alessandro, M.D. All rights reserved. For additional information, visit http://www.virtualpediatrichospital.org.

What is an undescended testicle?

It is when the testicle does not move from the abdominal cavity to the scrotum.

What causes it?

Normally, the testicles move to the scrotum before birth. An undescended testicle does not move to the scrotum.

Who can get it?

This is a condition only in males. It is fairly common in premature infants.

What are the signs and symptoms?

There are usually no symptoms except that the testicle is not found in the scrotum. It can lead to other problems. Undescended testicles are at higher risk of developing cancer, even if they are brought down to the scrotum. It can lead to infertility (testicles are unable to make sperm).

How is it treated?

Often, the testicle descends on its own without treatment before the child is one year old. Testicles that do not descend by one year of age may need treatment. Treatment choices include hormone injections (shots) or surgery. The hormones remind the body that the testicle should move down to the scrotum. Hormone treatment often does not work for children under two years old. Surgery is usually recommended around one year of age. The surgery brings the testicle down and is usually successful. Bringing the testicle down to the scrotum helps it produce sperm and makes it easier to examine the testicle for early signs of cancer. Sometimes, the undescended testicle can be found in the abdominal wall above the scrotum. Whenever there is an undescended testicle, there is also usually a hernia. During the surgery to bring the testicle down, the hernia is usually fixed too. To do the surgery, a small cut is made in the groin and on the scrotum. The child can usually go home on the same day. In very few cases, a second surgery may be needed to bring the testicle down. In a few cases, the testicle can't be found during surgery. This is called a vanished or absent testis. It is a birth defect.

How long does it last?

In many cases, the testicle will descend on its own before the child is nine months old. A testicle that does not descend by one year of age may need surgery.

Can it be prevented?

Doctors do not know how it can be prevented.

When should I call the doctor?

Call your doctor if you think your son has an undescended testicle. Call your doctor if you have questions or concerns about your child's condition or treatment.

Quick Answers

- An undescended testicle does not move from the abdominal cavity to the scrotum.

- Normally, the testicles move to the scrotum before birth.

- It is fairly common in premature infants.

- An undescended testicle can lead to other problems such as infertility.

- A testicle that does not descend on its own may need hormone treatment or surgery.

- In many cases, the testicle will descend on its own before the child is nine months old.

- Doctors do not know how it can be prevented.

- Call your doctor if you think your son has an undescended testicle.

References

MEDLINEplus. *Undescended Testicle*. 2001 May 27 (cited 2002 February 19). URL: http://www.nlm.nih.gov/medlineplus/ency/article/000973.htm

Urology. *Information about Undescended Testicle (Cryptorchidism)*. Virtual Children's Hospital. 2000 May (cited February 19). URL: http://www.vh.org/Patients/IHB/Uro/Peds/UndescendedTesticle.html

Texas Pediatric Surgical Associates. *The Undescended Testicle*. (cited 2002 February 19). URL: http://www.pedisurg.com/PtEduc/Undescended_Testis_or_Testicle.htm.

Section 32.2

Hypospadias

Definition: Hypospadias is a relatively common abnormality in which the opening of the urethra is on the underside, rather than at the end, of the penis.

Causes, Incidence, and Risk Factors: Hypospadias is a congenital defect that affects up to three in one thousand newborn boys. The condition varies in severity. In most cases, the opening of the urethra is located near the tip of the penis on the glans. More severe forms of hypospadias occur when the opening is at the midshaft or the base of the penis. Occasionally, the opening is located in the scrotum or the perineum (behind the scrotum).

This anomaly is often associated with chordee, a downward curvature of the penis during erection. (Erections are common with infant boys.)

Some cases are inherited—others result from unknown causes.

Symptoms:

- The opening of the urethra is not at the tip of the penis but is displaced to the underside.
- The penis has a marked curvature downward.
- The penis looks hooded due to malformation of the foreskin.
- The child must sit down to urinate.

Signs and Tests: Diagnosis is made on physical examination. For hypospadias occurring at the base of the penis, radiologic studies may be necessary to look for other congenital anomalies.

Treatment: Infants with hypospadias should not be circumcised. The foreskin should be preserved for use in later surgical repair.

Surgery is usually completed before the child starts school. Today, most urologists recommend repair before eighteen months of age. During the surgery, the penis is straightened and the hypospadias is corrected using tissue grafts from the foreskin. The repair may need to be performed in stages, requiring multiple surgeries.

Expectations (Prognosis): Results after surgery are typically good, both cosmetically and functionally. Approximately 10 to 20 percent of the operations require revision for fistulas (which result in leaks) and chordee recurrence.

Complications: If hypospadias is untreated, a boy may have difficulty with toilet training and problems with sexual intercourse in adulthood. Urethral strictures and fistulas may form throughout the boy's life, requiring surgical correction.

Calling Your Health Care Provider: Typically a child is diagnosed with hypospadias shortly after birth. If you notice that your son's urethral opening is abnormally located, or if his penis becomes curved during erection, call your health care provider.

Do not have the child circumcised if hypospadias is suspected.

Section 32.3

Hydroceles and Inguinal Hernias

Hydroceles and inguinal (groin) hernias can create problems in males. But do they cause pain and dysfunction? When and how should they be treated? The following information should help you talk to a urologist about these two conditions.

What causes hernias and hydroceles?

Testicles develop near kidneys in the abdomen and descend from that location to their normal position in the scrotum toward the end of pregnancy. In order for the testicles to leave the abdomen, a muscle ring in the groin on each side opens and allows the testicles to drop down to the scrotum. As the testicle descends, the lining of the abdomen also drops to line the scrotum. This channel closes in most boys. If that channel remains open, or reopens, a small amount of fluid can go from the abdomen to the scrotum through this passage. This results in hydrocele. If the channel remains open or reopens widely, then a portion of the intestine can pass down the channel toward the scrotum. This results in an inguinal hernia.

Hydroceles can also develop due to inflammation or injury within the scrotum. These sometimes resolve over a few months but many remain and require medical attention. Hernias can also be the result of increased pressure that forces part of the intestines through a weak spot in the abdominal wall—straining during bowel movements, heavy lifting, coughing, sneezing, or obesity.

What are the symptoms of a hernia?

Only about 25 percent of hernias cause pain or discomfort. However, you may be able to see and feel the bulge that often occurs at the junction of the thigh and groin. About 1 percent of boys develop hernias, with premature infant males having a higher incidence. Sometimes, the protruding intestine enters the scrotum and causes pain and/or swelling in the scrotum.

What are the symptoms of a hydrocele?

About 10 percent of male infants have a hydrocele at birth. Seldom causing symptoms, this swelling of the scrotum does not bother a baby and usually disappears in the first year of life, even though the appearance may worry new parents. In older males, a hydrocele usually remains painless but may cause discomfort due to the increased size of the scrotum.

How are hernias treated?

Surgery to repair the muscle ring that did not close properly is recommended for a hernia in a child. Hernias do not go away on their own and may cause problems with digestion leading to emergency surgery. In infants and children, a small incision is made in the groin through which a urologist sutures or sews the channel shut and repairs the muscle ring. This procedure can be done in an outpatient setting. In teenagers and adults, laparoscopic surgery may be considered.

How are hydroceles treated?

Hydroceles require surgical repair if they cause symptoms, such as growing large or changing size significantly during the day. If the hydrocele is uncomplicated, an incision is made in the scrotum. The hydrocele is cut out, removing the tissues involved in the hydrocele. If there are complications, such as a hernia, an incision is made in the inguinal (groin) area. This approach allows repair of hernias and other complicating factors at the same time.

What can be expected after treatment for hernias and hydroceles?

After surgery, there will be discomfort that will require pain medication. In most cases, pain is reduced during the first week so that pain medication is no longer necessary. It may be necessary to restrict full activity for several weeks, depending on your child's age and whether or not both sides were treated. If your son still plays on straddle toys, such as a rocking horse, he may have to avoid them for a time. The testicle and scrotum may stay swollen for several weeks after surgery before returning to normal. After surgery, less than 1 percent of cases have a hernia or hydrocele return.

Are hernias or hydroceles hereditary?

No. Hernias and hydroceles are common. And while several family members may experience them, there is no evidence that they are inherited.

Is there anything a parent did to cause a hernia or hydrocele in his or her child?

No.

What is the likelihood of a hernia developing on the other side?

This depends on the age of the child. Younger children treated for a hernia are much more likely to develop a hernia on the other side than older children. In younger children, sometimes a laparoscope is used to look at and evaluate the opposite side. If the examination shows that a hernia is present or likely to occur, then surgical repair is done on both sides as a preventive course of action.

What is the likelihood of a hydrocele developing on the other side?

The risk of developing a hydrocele on the other side is about 5 percent. Because of this low risk, many times the laparoscopic evaluation is not performed.

Do girls develop hydroceles and hernias?

Girls do not develop hydroceles. They can develop hernias but because of their anatomy, girls are ten times less likely than boys to develop hernias.

Section 32.4

Urogenital Sinus

The urethra and vagina are separate anatomical entities in normal females. But in rare instances, they are joined in what urologists call a urogenital sinus anomaly. The following information can help you talk to your child's urologist about correcting this rare birth defect.

What are urogenital sinus anomalies?

A urogenital sinus anomaly is a defect present at birth in which the vagina and urethra open into a common channel, rather than separately. There are two general types of urogenital sinus anomalies. In a low confluence urogenital sinus anomaly, the common channel is short, the urethral opening is close to its normal location, and the vagina is almost normal in length. In a high confluence urogenital sinus anomaly, the common channel is long, the urethral opening is internal, and the vagina is quite short. This type is sometimes associated with an anus that is located too far forward.

How are urogenital sinus anomalies diagnosed?

Urogenital sinus malformations are usually diagnosed during infancy by physical examination. If a urogenital sinus defect is suspected in an infant, an examination called a genitogram will be performed. To do a retrograde genitogram, contrast dye will be injected into the common opening. An x-ray will then be taken that will permit the doctors to determine the length of the common channel and the spatial relationship between the urethra and the vagina. This information will allow the urologist to determine the type of urogenital sinus anomaly and implement the appropriate treatment.

If a retrograde genitogram is inadequate, endoscopy may be done. In endoscopy, a fiber-optic camera is inserted into the common channel, which will allow the anatomy to be seen and identified. Other tests used under special situations include an ultrasound and magnetic resonance imaging (MRI).

How are urogenital sinus anomalies treated?

Surgery to separate the vagina and urethra is the only treatment for urogenital sinus anomalies. Since there are many procedures for this operation, you and your child's doctor will decide the best approach, depending on the type of anomaly. If your child is diagnosed with a low confluence urogenital sinus anomaly, the surgeon will perform what is known as a flap vaginoplasty—a procedure to open the sinus so that the vagina and urethra have separate exterior openings. If she has a high confluence urogenital sinus anomaly, the surgeon will perform a pull-through vaginoplasty. In this procedure the vagina is brought to its normal location on the surface of the skin while the urethra continues to drain through what was once the common channel. Sometimes, a piece of skin or a section of bowel may be needed for this procedure.

Will my daughter have control over urination?

If the problem is corrected, urination should be normal.

Will my daughter have a normal sex life?

Yes, once the disorder has been corrected, she will be able to have a normal, enjoyable sex life.

Will she be able to have children?

Yes, once corrected, she should have no problem conceiving or bearing children.

Will she have a normal vaginal delivery?

Yes, she should be able to deliver children normally.

Section 32.5

Vaginal Agenesis

Reprinted from "Congenital Malformations of the Female Reproductive Tract: Vaginal Agenesis/Hypoplasia," prepared by Nada Kawar, M.D., Washington University School of Medicine Class of 2005. Program in Pediatric and Adolescent Gynecology, Washington University School of Medicine, St. Louis, Missouri, Director Diane F. Merritt, M.D., merrittd@wustl.edu. Reprinted with permission.

You may have just learned that you or your child has vaginal agenesis or vaginal hypoplasia, and you probably have many questions and concerns. Vaginal agenesis involves many issues, including concerns about physical abnormality, body image, sexual identity, and sexual/reproductive functioning. It is normal to feel confused, scared, sad, and overwhelmed. The following information is meant to help answer some of the many questions that you may be pondering. This information is by no means comprehensive, but is meant to help address some of the most frequently asked questions, and to help point you in the right direction for additional sources of information.

Introduction

Vaginal agenesis and vaginal hypoplasia are part of a much broader group of congenital malformations of the female reproductive tract. Congenital means "present at birth." Agenesis means "absence of" or "failure to develop." Hypoplasia means "less development than usual."

Vaginal agenesis occurs in approximately one in every five thousand to seven thousand female births. It results from a problem during the very early development of the reproductive system of a fetus while in her mother's uterus.

There are many different conditions that may cause such a developmental problem and lead to vaginal agenesis. By far the most common, representing more than 90 percent of patients with vaginal agenesis, is Rokitansky-Mayer-Küster-Hauser syndrome, named after the doctors who first discovered and reported this medical condition (also referred to as RMKH, Rokitansky-Mayer syndrome, or Rokitansky syndrome).

Rokitansky-Mayer-Küster-Hauser syndrome is a condition that includes abnormal development or absence of the vagina, fallopian tubes, cervix, and/or uterus. Some women have incompletely developed uterine remnants. The ovaries and external genitalia are normal, and the chromosome makeup of individuals is 46XX (normal female). Other symptoms involved to a varying degree are kidney abnormalities, skeletal problems, and hearing loss. The exact cause of these developmental problems is not yet known.

Approximately 7 to 8 percent of the remaining patients with vaginal agenesis have a more unusual genetic abnormality and have a condition known as androgen insensitivity syndrome (AIS). Genetically, these patients are 46XY, and lack a vagina, cervix, uterus, fallopian tubes, and ovaries. External genitalia may have a normal female appearance, or may lie anywhere along the spectrum from male to female. Even fewer patients with vaginal agenesis have other, more rare, conditions and more complex genetic and physical abnormalities.

Regardless of the cause, the concerns surrounding vaginal agenesis are shared by all who have this condition. The remainder of this section will help address some of these issues.

Diagnosis

The diagnosis of vaginal agenesis or hypoplasia is most commonly made between the ages of fifteen and eighteen years. Most young women first present to their physicians with concerns because they have not started menstruating. Women with RMKH syndrome have normal functioning ovaries and have usually gone through puberty and have normal breast and pubic hair by this time. Women with AIS or other conditions may have additional concerns over sexual development. In either case, vaginal agenesis is the most common cause for failing to start menstruating.

Diagnosis of vaginal agenesis is usually made with a physical examination by a qualified physician. Other tests, including hormonal and genetic tests, can help determine what, if any, the exact cause of this condition is. Since there may be associated kidney and uterine abnormalities, imaging studies such as an ultrasound, MRI, or intravenous pyelogram may be useful. Patients are usually referred to a pediatric and adolescent gynecologist for specialized care.

Treatment

After being evaluated by a specialist, questions usually arise about treatment. It is important to know that a variety of treatment options are available for vaginal agenesis. Both nonsurgical and surgical techniques are available to reconstruct the vagina. The nonsurgical approach involves expanding and enlarging the tissue already present at the vaginal entrance by applying pressure (pressure dilation) over an extended period of time. Plastic surgery techniques involve constructing a new vagina out of tissue from various donor sites.

Although there are a variety of treatment approaches, the results of pressure dilation are considered superior to those of surgical construction of a vagina. It is also important to realize that dilation is also required after most surgical methods of creating a vagina, and this postoperative dilation can often be more painful. It is therefore generally recommended that pressure dilation should always be the first intervention tried, with surgery utilized as a last resort.

Pressure Dilation Techniques

As described previously, pressure dilation involves expanding and enlarging the tissue present at the vaginal entrance by applying pressure over a period of time. After dilation, the vagina naturally develops a mucosal lining very similar to that of a normal vagina, and has a more natural sensation. Two approaches to this method are available: the intermittent pressure (Frank method) and the continuous pressure (Vecchietti procedure).

The intermittent pressure method (known as the Frank Method after the doctor who first advocated it) is performed by the girl herself at home. It involves gentle pressure application of rod-shaped appliances at the vaginal opening. This is typically done once or twice per day for twenty to thirty minutes. The dilators are increased in size as dilation of the vagina is achieved. The time necessary to complete treatment varies from less than one month to over a year. A variety of different vaginal dilators are available, and some refinements of the technique have been made. A specialized stool (Ingram Method) is available that allows dilation to be carried out while clothed and in a sitting position.

In the continuous pressure method (Vecchietti Procedure), pressure is applied in the vaginal area by a dilation "olive," a plastic bead through which sutures (or threads) are threaded. A surgical procedure is necessary to set up this method, since the sutures run through the abdomen and a traction device is placed on the outside of the abdomen. Following the surgery, the vagina is stretched over the course of seven to ten days.

Plastic Surgery Techniques

A variety of surgical methods have been developed for constructing a new vagina. All of these procedures should be delayed until after puberty so that dilation can be tried first, and because surgical creation of a vagina in childhood usually has poor results. The most common surgical technique used is the Abbe-McIndoe method. In this surgery, a skin graft is used to create a vagina. The skin is usually taken from the buttocks of the patient, and is then molded to form the vagina. The main problem of this procedure is the tendency of the vagina to contract, necessitating the use of dilators after surgery.

Other surgical techniques are available, such as using a length of colon (gut) or peritoneum (the membrane lining the inside of the abdominal cavity) to create a vagina.

Gender, Sexual Identity and Functioning, and Motherhood

These concerns are common and natural when confronted with the diagnosis of vaginal agenesis. Gender and sexual identity issues may be even more troubling for patients with AIS or other more complicated genetic and physical conditions. These concerns are best addressed with the guidance of a qualified physician and professional counselor. The important thing to remember is that no one can tell that a patient has vaginal agenesis. And, following treatment with dilators or surgery, no one will be able to tell that the patient has had a reconstructive procedure.

Patients also wonder about sexual functioning and sexual pleasure. Much of the sexual pleasure comes from stimulation of the clitoris, and not from the vagina. Therefore, after creation of a vagina and the decision to become sexually active, a patient will have normal sexual sensations and enjoyable sexual relations.

Motherhood is also a very important concern. The question of "Will I be able to have children?" depends on the individual patient. In women with RMKH syndrome that were born with a normal-sized uterus, patients may become pregnant and deliver a baby. In those women that were born without a uterus or if the uterus is small, patients may not be able to carry a pregnancy. However, since these patients have normal functioning ovaries, other options are available. In vitro fertilization can allow an egg to be fertilized by a partner's sperm, and then the pregnancy carried by a surrogate mother. Adoption is another choice for some couples that are not able to have their own children. It is important to realize, however, that not being able to have your own children does not mean that you cannot become a mother.

Assessment and Counseling

An assessment by a qualified physician and professional counseling are both necessary and very useful. Counseling can help patients and parents deal with the complex issues that this diagnosis entails. Feelings of inadequacy and questions about gender/sexual identity and functioning and motherhood are common concerns, and should not be ignored or deferred until a girl is considered old enough to begin her sex life. Counseling should be given near the age of puberty. The girl should be informed truthfully of her anatomical situation and concurrently told what treatment is available. Pediatric and adolescent gynecologists are an excellent resource for this specialized care.

Section 32.6

Cloacal Exstrophy

Sometimes factors can interfere with bladder development, as is the case for children with cloacal exstrophy. If your newborn has been diagnosed with this condition, what can you expect? The following information should help you talk to your child's doctor.

What is cloacal exstrophy?

This is the most severe birth defect in the exstrophy-epispadias complex. A child with this condition will have many lower abdominal organs, like the bladder and intestines, exposed outside the abdomen.

In males the penis is usually flat and short and sometimes split. In females the clitoris is split and there may be two vaginal openings. Also, frequently the intestine is short and the anus is not open. There is a high association with other birth defects, especially spina bifida, which occurs in up to 75 percent of cases. Abnormal development of the kidneys is also common.

How often does it occur?

It is rare, occurring in approximately one in every 250,000 births, and is slightly more common in males than females.

What caused this condition?

There is no known cause but it is also very unlikely that anything could have been done to prevent it.

How is it diagnosed?

Frequently it can be detected before birth during a routine sonogram. Nonetheless, this condition will be obvious at birth.

What is the treatment?

Surgical reconstruction is undertaken when the child is medically stable. The surgery is staged, but the schedule of surgery is very dependent on the individual child. The first surgical consideration is repair of any coexistent spinal abnormality. Once the child has recovered sufficiently from this, the gastrointestinal tract is then treated. Attempts are always made to place the intestines back inside the abdomen but a significant number of cases require diversion to a stoma. Closure of the bladder and reconstruction of the genitalia are similar to that for classic exstrophy. In select cases the abdominal wall and genitourinary system can be repaired at the same time as the bowel. For a successful closure, a pelvic osteotomy is mandatory. Achieving eventual continence almost always involves enlarging the bladder and emptying using a catheter or urinary diversion and a continent stoma.

What can be expected after treatment?

The management of cloacal exstrophy has advanced to provide great improvement in the quality of life of affected children. With advances in pediatric anesthesia the survival rate in the newborn is high and the incidence of life-threatening complications from surgery has reduced significantly. The child born with cloacal exstrophy can usually gain control of urination and bowel movements. The neurological deficit they often have is usually manageable but they will probably continue to depend on medical services.

Will my child be able to have children when he or she reaches adulthood?

In many cases, the answer to this question is yes. However, this will almost certainly require assisted fertility treatment.

Section 32.7

Ambiguous Genitalia

Ambiguous genitalia (also known as atypical genitalia) is a birth defect (or birth variation) of the sex organs that makes it unclear whether an affected newborn is a girl or boy. This condition occurs approximately once in every 4,500 births. The baby seems to have a mixture of both female and male parts—for example, the child may have both a vulva and testicles. Associated intersex conditions for male babies include hypospadias, where the urethral opening is located in an unusual position such as the underside of the penis.

The causes of ambiguous genitalia include genetic variations, hormonal imbalances, and malformations of the fetal tissues that are supposed to evolve into genitals. Tests (including ultrasound, x-rays, and blood tests) are needed before the baby's sex can be identified. Mild forms of ambiguous genitalia may be characterized by a large (penis-like) clitoris in baby girls or undescended testicles in boys.

Sexual Determination during Embryo Development

A baby's sex is decided at conception. The mother's egg provides an X chromosome and the father's sperm determines the baby's sex by contributing either an X or a Y sex chromosome. An XX embryo is female while an XY embryo is male. Both female and male embryos develop in exactly the same way and have identical gonads and genital parts until around the eighth week of gestation. The sexual determination process includes:

- **Girls:** the internal genital parts transform into the uterus, fallopian tubes, and vagina. The gonads turn into ovaries, which start producing female sex hormones. The lack of male hormones is fundamental in allowing the development of female genitalia.

- **Boys:** the internal genital parts transform into the prostate gland and vas deferens. The gonads turn into testes, which start producing male sex hormones. The presence of male hormones allows the penis and scrotum to develop.

Different Types of Ambiguous Genitalia

The different types of ambiguous genitalia are as follows:

- The baby has ovaries and testicles, and the external genitals are neither clearly male nor female.

- The baby has ovaries and a penis-like structure or phallus.

- The baby has undescended testes and external female genitals including a vulva.

A Range of Causes

For typical genital development, the gender "message" must be communicated from the sex chromosomes to the gonads. The gonads must then manufacture appropriate hormones and the genital tissues and structures have to respond to these hormones. Any deviations along the way can cause ambiguous genitalia. Some specific causes include:

- **Androgen insensitivity syndrome (AIS):** a genetic condition characterized by the fetal tissue's insensitivity to male hormones. This affects genital development. For example, a newborn may have some of the female reproductive organs but also have testicles.

- **Congenital adrenal hyperplasia (CAH):** an inherited condition that affects hormone production. A child with CAH lacks particular enzymes, and this deficiency triggers the excessive manufacture of male hormones. For example, female genitals are masculinized.

- **Sex chromosome disorders:** instead of having either XX or XY sex chromosomes, a baby may have a mixture of both ("mosaic" chromosomes); or specific genes on the Y chromosome may be inactive; or one of the X chromosomes may have a tiny Y segment attached to it. Research at the University of California at Los Angeles (UCLA) indicates that ambiguous genitalia can be caused by the doubling up of a particular gene (named WNT-4) on the sex chromosome. This variation will interfere with male sexual development so that a genetically male baby will appear female.

- **Maternal factors:** the pregnant mother may have had an androgen-secreting tumor while pregnant, and the excess of this male hormone affected her baby's genital development. In other cases, the placenta may have lacked a particular enzyme which failed to deactivate male hormones from the baby; as a result, both the mother and the female baby were masculinized by the excess of these hormones.

Diagnosis Methods

There are currently no prenatal tests that can detect ambiguous genitalia. Research into the WNT-4 gene suggests that a prenatal test could one day be developed. Tests performed at birth to determine the baby's gender can take about one week and may include:

- Physical examination;
- Hormone tests using blood, urine, or both;
- Genetic tests using blood, urine, or both;
- Ultrasound scan;
- X-rays.

Treatment Options

Treatment options to help assign the baby a definite gender may include the following:

- **Parental counseling:** successful sex assignment and identity for the child depends largely on the attitude of the parents. It is important that both the mother and father are fully informed about their child's condition. Support groups may provide help in this area.

- **Surgery:** for example, an overly large clitoris may be trimmed, or a fused vulva separated, or undescended testicles relocated into the scrotum. However, surgical gender assignment depends heavily on what genital structures the surgeons have to work with. The majority of babies with ambiguous genitalia have been brought up as girls. A few operations may be needed, usually begun in the child's first year. Further surgery might be required during adolescence. Some intersex support groups feel that surgery is not always the answer, particularly when the gender of the child is not clear. Others suggest that surgery should wait until the child is old enough to decide for him- or herself. However, most medical professionals advocate early surgical and hormonal intervention for the sake of clearly establishing the child's gender and sense of belonging in society.

- **Counseling for the child:** the child needs to be informed and talked to about his or her diagnosis in a very careful way.

- **Hormone therapy:** during his or her teenage years, the child may need hormone supplementation therapy to help bring on puberty. A child with CAH will need to have daily hormone therapy.

Possible Long-Term Problems

Some of the possible problems faced by a person born with ambiguous genitalia may include:

- Infertility;
- Problems with sexual functioning;
- Feelings of insecurity and uncertainty about gender identity, such as feeling like the opposite gender to the sex that was determined earlier in life.

Where to Get Help

- Your doctor
- Endocrinologist

- Genetic counselor
- Endocrinology clinic counselor
- Congenital adrenal hyperplasia support group

Things to Remember

- "Ambiguous genitalia" is a birth defect of the sex organs that makes it unclear whether an affected newborn is a girl or a boy.
- Causes include genetic variations, hormonal imbalances, and malformations of the fetal tissues that would have otherwise evolved into genitals.
- Treatment aims at assigning the baby a specific gender.
- Treatment options include corrective surgery, hormone therapy, peer support, and counseling.

Chapter 33

Musculoskeletal Defects

Chapter Contents

Section 33.1—Arthrogryposis 532
Section 33.2—Clubfoot 534
Section 33.3—Congenital Amputation 542
Section 33.4—Congenital Torticollis 544
Section 33.5—Fibrous Dysplasia 546

Section 33.1

Arthrogryposis

What is arthrogryposis?

Arthrogryposis (arthrogryposis multiplex congenita) is a term describing the presence of a muscle disorder that causes multiple joint contractures at birth. A contracture is a limitation in the range of motion of a joint.

In some cases, few joints may be affected and the range of motion may be nearly normal. In the "classic" case of arthrogryposis, hands, wrists, elbows, shoulders, hips, feet, and knees are affected. In the most severe cases, nearly every body joint may be involved, including the jaw and back. Frequently, the contractures are accompanied by muscle weakness, which further limits movement. Arthrogryposis is relatively rare, occurring in approximately one in three thousand births.

Can arthrogryposis occur again in the same family?

In most cases, arthrogryposis is not a genetic condition and does not occur more than once in a family. In about 30 percent of the cases, a genetic cause can be identified. The risk of recurrence for these cases varies with the type of genetic disorder.

What causes arthrogryposis?

Research has shown that anything that prevents normal joint movement before birth can result in joint contractures. The joint itself may be normal. However, when a joint is not moved for a period of time, extra connective tissue tends to grow around it, fixing it in position. Lack of joint movement also means that tendons connecting to the joint are not stretched to their normal length; short tendons, in turn, make normal joint movement difficult. (This same kind of problem can develop after birth in joints that are immobilized for long periods of time in casts.)

In general, there are four causes for limitation of joint movement before birth:

1. Muscles do not develop properly (atrophy). In most cases, the specific cause for muscular atrophy cannot be identified. Suspected causes include muscle diseases (for example, congenital muscular dystrophies), maternal fever during pregnancy, and viruses, which may damage cells that transmit nerve impulses to the muscles.

2. There is not sufficient room in the uterus for normal movement. For example, the mother may lack a normal amount of amniotic fluid, or have an abnormally shaped uterus.

3. The central nervous system and spinal cord are malformed. In these cases, a wide range of other conditions usually accompanies arthrogryposis.

4. Tendons, bones, joints, or joint linings may develop abnormally. For example, tendons may not be connected to the proper place in a joint.

What is the treatment?

For most types of arthrogryposis, physical therapy has proven very beneficial in improving the range of motion of affected joints. Parents are encouraged to become active participants in a therapy program and to continue therapy at home on a daily basis.

Splints can be made to augment the stretching exercises to increase range of motion. Casting is often used to improve foot position. However, emphasis should be placed on achieving as much joint mobility as possible. Some type of removable splint (perhaps a bi-valve cast) may be used on knees and feet so that the joints can be moved periodically. In some cases, merely wearing a splint at night may be sufficient.

Surgery may be used to treat the congenital deformities that frequently occur in conjunction with arthrogryposis or should be viewed as a supportive measure once physical therapy has achieved maximum results but more range of motion is needed. Surgeries are commonly performed on feet, knees, hips, elbows, and wrists to achieve better position or greater range of motion. In some cases, tendon transfers have been done to improve muscle function. Congenital deformities of the feet, hips, and spine may require surgical correction at or about one year of age.

What is the outlook?

There is a wide variation in the degree to which muscles and joints are affected in those with arthrogryposis. In some cases, arthrogryposis may be accompanied by other conditions, such as central nervous system disorders, which complicate the picture. However, in most cases, the outlook for those with arthrogryposis is a positive one. Unlike many other conditions, arthrogryposis is nonprogressive; it does not worsen with age. Furthermore, with physical therapy and other available treatments, substantial improvement in function is usually possible. Most people with arthrogryposis are of normal intelligence and are able to lead productive, independent lives as adults.

Section 33.2

Clubfoot

Reprinted with permission from "Help for Patients with Clubfoot," © 2005 Shriners Hospitals for Children. All rights reserved. Reviewed by Dr. Norman Otsuka in July 2006.

Talipes equinovarus, or clubfoot, is a relatively common foot deformity, affecting one in one thousand children each year. Clubfoot is readily identifiable at birth, making it easy to diagnose. Yet how to best treat clubfoot generates more controversy among physicians than almost any other orthopedic condition. Nonsurgical approaches are usually attempted first, but when surgery is indicated there is no clear consensus on which type of surgery is better, when surgery should be performed, or how to evaluate the results of treatment. Following, you will read about the latest techniques, research, and recommendations related to the treatment of this condition.

In referring a child for treatment of clubfoot, please remember these two basic rules:

- Treatment must begin immediately at birth. There is consensus that casting and manipulation is best started in the newborn infant.

- A child with clubfoot should be referred to a pediatric orthopedic physician specializing in the treatment of clubfoot both by casting and manipulation and by surgical means. Many highly qualified orthopedists specialize in hand, knee, or hip problems, to name a few. The child with clubfoot, however, needs a pediatric orthopedic physician specializing in clubfoot.

With proper treatment, a child with clubfoot should develop normally and be able to participate in whatever activities he or she desires.

A Case Study

Like most fourteen-year-old boys, Brandon Santee enjoys video games, action movies, and most of all, sports. His bedroom bookshelves are adorned with gold, silver, and bronze medals awarded for excellence in basketball, track, and football. Brandon dreams someday of playing college and professional football, and counts Dallas Cowboys starting quarterback Troy Aikman among his heroes.

But Brandon and Aikman share something else besides a love of sports. Both were born with talipes equinovarus, or clubfoot.

One in one thousand children in the United States are born with clubfoot each year. Boys are twice as likely as girls to be born with the condition, but clubfoot is usually more severe in girls. Half of all patients have only one foot affected; the other half have a left and right clubfoot.

Brandon was born with a right clubfoot and a normal left foot. Although he endured casts, corrective shoes, and surgery as a toddler, he never slowed down.

"He was very active and even wore out two casts before the age of three," said Brandon's mom Leatrice.

What Is Clubfoot?

Readily apparent at birth, clubfoot is a birth deformity in which the foot turns inward and points down, causing walking on the toes and outer sole of the foot, explained Dr. Douglas Barnes, assistant chief of staff at Shriners Hospital for Children in Houston.

535

"Clubfoot may cause various deformities in the foot," Barnes said, "but to qualify as true clubfoot, the following components must be present."

- A tightened Achilles tendon, or heel cord, causes the heel to be drawn up toward the leg, making it impossible to place the foot flat on the floor. This position is referred to as an "equinus" or "plantar flexed" position.

- The foot turns on its side, coming to rest on the outer border of the sole, a condition known as "varus" or "supinated."

- The front half of the foot is adducted or turned inward, giving the foot a kidney bean shape.

In some but not all cases, the arch is abnormally high at the mid-foot, a condition called "cavus."

"A true clubfoot is usually stiff and will lack normal motion, be smaller than a normal foot, and the muscles in the adjoining calf will be noticeably smaller," explained Barnes.

Some of the bones in clubfoot are abnormal not only in their relationship to each other, he said, but also in shape and size. Shortened tendons on the inside of the lower leg together with abnormally shaped bones that restrict movement outward cause the foot to turn inward. A tightened Achilles tendon (the tendon that joins calf muscles to the heel of the foot) causes the heel to be drawn up and the foot to point downward.

The diagnosis of clubfoot is not difficult and is seldom confused with other foot deformities, Barnes said.

"Occasionally, another foot deformity known as metatarsus varus is confused with clubfoot. However, the 'equinus' or raised heel and heel varus (heel turned to the outside) seen in clubfoot are not present in metatarsus varus," he explained.

The presence of clubfoot should prompt a careful search for other musculoskeletal problems, including examination of the back, hip, and knees, Barnes said. "A malformed foot sometimes relates to problems elsewhere," he explained.

Why Clubfoot Occurs

The majority of clubfoot cases result from abnormal development of the muscles, tendons, and bones while the fetus is forming in the uterus. The disturbance in normal growth of the foot probably occurs at about the eighth week of pregnancy.

In pinpointing the specific causes of clubfoot, researchers classify the condition, based on reasons for occurrence, into four major groups: congenital, teratologic, syndrome complex, or positional.

Congenital clubfoot is by far the most common form of clubfoot and is also referred to as "idiopathic" clubfoot, meaning that the condition arises spontaneously from an unknown cause. A child with congenital clubfoot has no other abnormalities, and the clubfoot is an isolated incident. The condition occurs more frequently within certain families, prompting scientists to believe that genetics play an important role in causing congenital clubfoot. Shriners Hospital researcher Jacqueline Hecht, Ph.D., currently is conducting a study to locate the gene or genes connected with congenital clubfoot.

Teratologic clubfoot occurs as a part of an underlying neuromuscular disorder, such as spina bifida or arthrogryposis multiplex congenita. Clubfoot may or may not be present in children with these disorders. Teratologic clubfoot often is severe and nearly always requires early, radical surgery to achieve correction.

Syndrome complex clubfoot occurs when a child is born with one of a number of genetic disorders, and clubfoot is part of the bigger disorder. Children with chromosomal abnormalities such as Down syndrome may also have syndrome complex clubfoot.

Positional clubfoot occurs when an otherwise normal foot is held in a deformed position in utero, and thus is "molded" incorrectly. A small uterus, the presence of twins, and abnormal fetal position have all been associated with positional clubfoot, although many such pregnancies result in babies without clubfoot. Positional clubfoot responds readily to nonsurgical treatments, such as splinting and casting. Because positional clubfoot is not an inherent defect, but instead a "packaging" problem, some physicians do not consider it a true clubfoot.

"In many cases, clubfoot may be neither purely genetic nor purely environmental," Barnes said. "Abnormal intrauterine pressures at a critical time in fetal development may produce clubfoot in a genetically predisposed patient," he explained.

Like his brother Brandon, six-year-old Brett Santee also was born with congenital clubfoot. While Brandon's right foot only was involved, both Brett's feet were affected. After surgery at Shriners Hospital, Brett is following in his big brother's footsteps. He proudly displays two gold medals earned for "best tug of war team member" at his elementary school's field day, and faithfully attends all his brother's football games. Brett has become so popular in the stands that the cheerleaders occasionally invite him on the field. In addition, Brett is picking up his brother's love of music. Brandon plays tuba in the school band and won first place in solo and ensemble competitions this year, while Brett is learning to play the piano.

Both boys have completed treatment for clubfoot and are considered "success stories" at Shriners Hospital. They return now and again for checkups, and receive excellent medical reports every time.

"Be patient, keep your appointments regularly, and do what the doctors tell you to do," advised mom Leatrice. "Clubfoot can be corrected if health professionals, parents, and children work together . . . it's a team effort all the way."

Methods of Treatment

Clubfoot is one of the most common, yet challenging pediatric foot deformities, said Shriners Hospital pediatric orthopedic surgeon Dr. Allison Scott. How to best treat clubfoot continues to be a controversial subject among orthopedic surgeons, Scott said.

"Over the past several decades, considerable advances have been made toward understanding the cause and treatment of clubfoot. However, there is still no universally accepted method for classifying the severity of the deformity; no consensus on which type of operation is better; and no standardized method for evaluating the results of treatment," Scott stated.

The goal in treating clubfoot is to achieve and maintain as normal a foot as possible. The extent of treatment varies, depending on the severity of each child's condition. Congenital clubfoot is usually mild to moderate, while clubfoot that accompanies other conditions is more severe.

To Begin, Be Conservative

Most physicians agree that all infants should be given an initial trial of treatments that do not involve surgery, no matter how rigid the deformity. Nonoperative treatments include physical therapy, taping and splinting, and serial manipulation and casting. The earlier these conservative treatments are begun, the more likely they are to be successful, Scott said.

"With the passage of time, untreated clubfoot only becomes more resistant to conservative treatments, so treatment should begin immediately in the newborn," she advised.

To begin, doctors or physical therapists slowly "manipulate," or stretch out the tightened muscles and hold the foot in an improved position with a plaster cast. (Plastic splints and tape may be substituted if the child is premature and too small for casting). Casts extend from the toes to either just above or just below the knee. They are changed frequently, each time repositioning the foot a little closer to normal. For the first two to three weeks, the casts are changed every week. Cast changes are then decreased to once every two weeks.

This treatment, known as "serial casting," continues until the child is three to six months old and involves between five and ten applications of plaster casts. Manipulation and casting may be distressing to the infant for a short period only, Scott said, but the baby soon settles once rewrapped and cuddled. Complete correction, if it happens, will occur by the time the child is three to six months of age.

Doctors differ widely in their opinions regarding the success rate of serial casting. Some say the procedure works only a small percentage of the time, while some believe almost all cases of clubfoot, when treated early and correctly, can be corrected with conservative therapy. Recent research (studies completed between 2002 and 2006) indicates that the Ponseti method of nonoperative clubfoot treatment, which employs manipulation and casting, is successful in more than 90 percent of the cases.

"Physicians with limited experience should not attempt to correct clubfoot with manipulation and casting. They may succeed in correcting mild clubfoot," Barnes said, "but the severe cases require experienced hands." A well-intentioned doctor with inadequate training in serial casting can actually compound the deformity, he said, making further treatment difficult.

"Clubfoot patients should be referred to a center with expertise in the management of clubfoot. An orthopedic hospital such as Shriners Hospital for Children, or a university medical school with a pediatric orthopedic practice have such experts on staff," Barnes explained.

If All Else Fails

If the foot is too resistant to allow for adequate correction, then surgery is performed to lengthen or release the tight or shortened tendons and ligaments, allowing them to be positioned in normal alignment. Although at this point manipulation and serial casting have failed to correct the clubfoot, months of stretching and casting have prepared the skin well for surgery by stretching and making it more supple, Barnes said.

Some surgeons prefer to operate when a child is six months old, while others opt to delay until nine to twelve months of age. Those who prefer early surgery feel that the rapid growth of the foot during the first year of life should occur when the foot has already been corrected, resulting in better alignment. Those desiring to delay surgery say anesthesia is safer when a child is older, a larger-sized foot is easier to operate on, and weight bearing on a recently corrected foot helps maintain the correction.

Still other physicians believe the size of the foot is more important than the child's age and recommend surgery when the foot is eight centimeters or longer in length.

At four months of age, Mitch Beito had surgery at Shriners Hospital to correct a left and right clubfoot. Now six months old, Mitch is well on his way to recovery. Not surprising, since the expert care Mitch received at Shriners Hospital was supplemented with personalized medical care from his dad Steve, a podiatrist specializing in medical care of the human foot. Mitch, Steve, mom Colleen, and sister Allie regularly make the three-hour trip to Houston from their home in New Braunfels, Texas, to monitor Mitch's progress. So far, the prognosis is excellent, said Steve.

"We brought Mitch to Shriners Hospital in Houston because as a doctor, I knew that's where he would receive the ultimate care from specialists who see clubfoot cases every day," he said.

Surgical treatment can be divided into three major categories:

- Soft tissue releases that release the tight tissues around the joints and result in lengthening of tendons.

- Bony procedures such as osteotomies that divide or remove bone to correct deformities, or arthrodeses, which surgically stabilize joints to enable the bones to grow solidly together.

- Tendon transfers to place the tendons, or ligaments, in an improved position.

Occasionally, a combination of these procedures may be necessary.

Surgery usually means a day or two in the hospital, and ten to twelve weeks in plaster "holding" casts that are applied under anesthesia immediately after the surgery.

Whether correction is achieved through manipulation and casting or surgery, Barnes said, the corrected foot will need to be maintained with a splint until the child learns to walk. The ankle-foot orthosis (AFO) is the splint most commonly used for this purpose. The device is made of lightweight plastic and held on by Velcro. AFOs can be worn twenty-four hours a day, or at night only. From the time a child begins walking to age two or three years, splints are typically worn at night only.

What to Expect

Children with clubfoot do well with treatment, develop normally, and participate in most athletic or recreational activities they choose. But it is important for families to understand that a clubfoot will never be a normal foot, Barnes cautioned. There will always be some degree of deformity, although the corrected foot may appear nearly normal, and a child with one affected foot may require two different shoe sizes. Usually the calf muscle will be slightly smaller on the affected side. No two cases of clubfoot are identical, Barnes said.

"Each clubfoot behaves differently and each case has its own personality," he said, stressing that a careful and detailed plan of care must be custom made for each child.

Patients should be regularly monitored through maturity, he advised, because the growing foot may begin to revert to its uncorrected state. Recurrence is most common within the first two to three years of life, but may happen up to age seven. Relapses are not uncommon in severe clubfoot, and may be corrected by manipulation and two to three plaster casts. However, if the recurrence remains untreated, surgical correction is often required with repeat casting. Subsequent surgeries are much more difficult than the first procedure, Barnes said.

"Having a clubfoot means many months of treatment and years of observation," he said. "It can be tedious and frustrating at times, but the reward is a foot that allows children to participate in all activities without restrictions."

Section 33.3

Congenital Amputation

Reprinted from *The Gale Encyclopedia of Medicine*, by Jeffrey P. Larson, RPT, 2, Gale Group, © 2002, Gale Group. Reprinted by permission of The Gale Group.

Definition

Congenital amputation is the absence of a fetal limb or fetal part at birth. This condition may be the result of the constriction of fibrous bands within the membrane that surrounds the developing fetus (amniotic band syndrome) or the exposure to substances known to cause birth defects (teratogenic agents). Other factors, including genetics, may also play a role.

Description

An estimated one in two thousand babies are born with all or part of a limb missing, ranging from a missing part of a finger to the absence of both arms and both legs. Congenital amputation is the least common reason for amputation. However, there are occasional periods in history where the number of congenital amputations increased. For example, the thalidomide tragedy of the early 1960s occurred after pregnant mothers in Western Europe were given a tranquilizer containing the drug. The result was a drastic increase in the number of babies born with deformed limbs. In this example, the birth defect usually presented itself as very small, deformed versions of normal limbs. More recently, birth defects as a result of radiation exposure near the site of the Chernobyl disaster in Russia have left numerous children with malformed or absent limbs.

Causes and Symptoms

The exact cause of congenital amputations is unknown. However, according to the March of Dimes, most birth defects have one or more genetic factors and one or more environmental factors. It is also known that most birth defects occur in the first three months of pregnancy, when the organs of the fetus are forming. Within these crucial first weeks, frequently prior to when a woman is aware of the pregnancy, the developing fetus is most susceptible to substances that can cause birth defects (teratogens). Exposure to teratogens can cause congenital amputation. In other cases, tight amniotic bands may constrict the developing fetus, preventing a limb from forming properly, if at all. It is estimated that this amniotic band syndrome occurs in between one in twelve thousand and one in fifteen thousand live births.

An infant with congenital amputation may be missing an entire limb or just a portion of a limb. Congenital amputation resulting in the complete absence of a limb beyond a certain point (and leaving a stump) is called transverse deficiency or amelia. Longitudinal deficiencies occur when a specific part of a limb is missing; for example, when the fibula bone in the lower leg is missing, but the rest of the leg is intact. Phocomelia is the condition in which only a mid-portion of a limb is missing, as when the hands or feet are attached directly to the trunk.

Diagnosis

Many cases of congenital amputation are not diagnosed until the baby is born. Ultrasound examinations may reveal the absence of a limb in some developing fetuses, but routine ultrasounds may not pick up signs of more subtle defects. However, if a doctor suspects that the fetus is at risk for developing a limb deficiency (for example, if the mother has been exposed to radiation), a more detailed ultrasound examination may be performed.

Treatment

Successful treatment of a child with congenital amputation involves an entire medical team, including a pediatrician, an orthopedist, a psychiatrist or psychologist, a prosthetist (an expert in making prosthetics, or artificial limbs), a social worker, and occupational and physical therapists. The accepted method of treatment is to fit the child early with a functional prosthesis because this leads to normal development and less wasting away (atrophy) of the muscles of the limbs present. However, some parents and physicians believe that the child should be allowed to learn to play and perform tasks without a prosthesis, if possible. When the child is older, he or she can be involved in the decision of whether or not to be fitted for a prosthesis.

Recently, there have been cases in which physicians have detected amniotic band constriction interfering with limb development fairly early in its course. In 1997, doctors at the Florida Institute for Fetal Diagnosis and Therapy reported two cases in which minimally invasive surgery freed constricting amniotic bands and preserved the affected limbs.

Alternative Treatment

Prevention of birth defects begins with building the well-being of the mother before pregnancy. Prenatal care should be strong and educational so that the mother understands both her genetic risks and her environmental risks. Several disciplines in alternative therapy also recommend various supplements and vitamins that may reduce the chances of birth defects. If a surgical procedure is planned, naturopathic and homeopathic pre- and post-surgical therapies can speed recovery.

Section 33.4

Congenital Torticollis

Reproduced with permission from Congenital Torticollis, in Johnson TR, (ed): *Your Orthopaedic Connections*. Rosemont, Illinois, American Academy of Orthopaedic Surgeons, 2004. Available at http://orthoinfo.aaos.org.

Description

Parents of a newborn are often fascinated by their child's every move. When a child doesn't move in a normal way, the parents are rightly concerned.

An infant who keeps his or her head tilted to one side may have a condition called congenital muscular torticollis. Congenital means that the condition is present at birth. Torticollis means twisted or bent neck. It is caused by a tight muscle on one side of the head that pulls the head (ear) down toward one shoulder as the chin tilts to the opposite side.

Within the first month after birth, a lump or pseudotumor may be felt on the tight muscle, but this gradually disappears. As many as one in five babies born with congenital muscular torticollis also has developmental dysplasia of the hip. Early diagnosis and treatment is required to avoid permanent deformities.

If you notice that your child consistently holds the head tilted to one side, consult your physician. Conditions other than congenital muscular torticollis may result in this head position, and the physician must eliminate them as possible causes. The physician will also want to check the child's hips to ensure that no dysplasia is present. He or she may request x-rays or an ultrasound of the hips.

Congenital muscular torticollis generally is painless and can be treated with a consistent program of exercises and stretching.

Risk Factors / Prevention

No one knows exactly what causes this condition, which is more common in firstborn children. One theory is that the muscle was stretched or torn during the delivery. Bleeding and swelling create pressure on the muscle. Eventually, scar tissue forms and replaces some of the muscle. Another theory suggests that the condition develops while the infant is still in the womb.

Symptoms

- Head tilts to one side, and chin points to the opposite shoulder. Usually, the head tilts right and the chin points left, meaning the muscle on the right side is affected.

- There is a lump or swelling in the muscle that gradually disappears.

- There is a limited range of motion in neck muscles.

- One side of face may flatten and the skull may appear oblong instead of round.

Treatment Options

The initial treatment consists of a series of exercises that must be done several times a day. The physician may refer you to a physical therapist, but most of the time, the parents will be doing the exercises with the child, turning and bending the child's head to stretch the muscle.

Placing toys and other objects in positions where the infant has to turn the head to see them encourages the infant to stretch the muscle. So does carrying the infant in a side-lying position, with the face away from you. Support the infant by putting one arm under the head on the side of the tight muscle, which will stretch the muscle. Place the other arm between the child's legs to hold the body.

Treatment Options: Surgical

Most of the time, this condition resolves by the time the child is a year old. If not, the physician may recommend surgical treatment to release and lengthen the tight muscle.

Section 33.5

Fibrous Dysplasia

What is fibrous dysplasia?

Fibrous dysplasia is a condition of the skeleton (bones). It is a birth defect that is a noncancerous disease. It is not hereditary so your child did not get it from you nor will he or she pass it along to his or her children.

How do I recognize this condition in my child?

Fibrous dysplasia is usually detected in early childhood as a result of swelling of the jaw. Also, in some cases it may cause the teeth to separate.

How does the disease progress?

Fibrous dysplasia gets progressively worse from birth until the bones finish growing. As it progresses, normal bone is replaced by various amounts of structurally weak fibrous and osseous (bone-like) tissue. In normal bone formation, woven bone appears first and later matures into lamellar bone. In fibrous dysplasia, bone does not mature and development stops in the woven bone stage.

Fibrous dysplasia causes misshapen bones. It can occur in the bones in the front of the head and/or sphenoid bones that are situated at the base of the skull. If this happens, it can eventually lead to deformation of facial features and affect the shape of the skull.

How many types of fibrous dysplasia are there?

There are three types of fibrous dysplasia.

Monostotic disease is the most common type of fibrous dysplasia, occurring in 70 percent of cases. Monostotic simply means involving one bone. It most often occurs on the long bones such as the femur (thigh bone), ribs, and skull.

Polyostotic disease affects 30 percent of patients. Polyostotic means occurring in more than one bone. The head and neck are involved in half of these patients.

The third type is **McCune-Albright syndrome**. It occurs in only 3 percent of cases. It is characterized by polyostotic fibrous dysplasia (fibrous dysplasia occurring in more than one bone); skin pigmentation; and, in females, early puberty.

How often does fibrous dysplasia affect the face and head?

Skull involvement occurs in 27 percent of monostotic and up to 50 percent of polyostotic patients. Fibrous dysplasia involving the face and skull is called "leontiasis ossea." Without treatment, one or more bones progressively increase in size, and move into the cavities of the eye, mouth, and/or the nose and its sinuses. Also, abnormal protrusion of the eyeball (exophthalmos) may develop and eventually cause complete loss of sight because it presses on the optic nerve. In addition, there may be interference of the nasal passage and with eating.

What are the effects of fibrous dysplasia of the skull base?

When fibrous dysplasia of the frontal (forehead bone) and/or sphenoid (bone at the base of the skull) bones progresses, these bones become thick and dense. This increase in size eventually causes the facial features and skull to become misshapen. In these cases more than one bone is usually involved. It can also result in cranial nerve problems. If the temporal bone is affected, the patient may suffer as much as

80 percent hearing loss when the inner ear canal narrows. It may also cause facial nerve paralysis or dizziness. However, any of our twelve cranial nerves can be involved with fibrous dysplasia. The more common results could include cranial nerve problems, and sight and hearing loss.

Are there any other effects of fibrous dysplasia?

It is estimated that patients with fibrous dysplasia are four hundred times more likely than the general population to develop a malignant bone tumor.

What is the treatment for fibrous dysplasia?

Physicians decide on treatment options after assessing a patient's symptoms. First the doctor observes the patient. Then he will consider conservative treatment such as surgically shaving or removing the fibrous tissue. In more severe cases the doctor may recommend complete removal of the bone.

Surgery is used to return the face to its normal structure and/or to relieve effects when a cranial nerve is being pinched. In these cases the abnormal bone must be completely removed. It is best to wait until adolescence for surgery. However, if the progression of the disease affects nerve function, a decompressive procedure should be considered early in childhood to keep normal function.

If surgery is recommended, how many will be necessary?

Sometimes the fibrous tissue can be completely removed successfully by a single procedure. However, most fibrous tissue can be managed through staged procedures with overall very favorable results and good long-term prognosis.

Chapter 34

Fetal Tumors

Chapter Contents

Section 34.1—Cervical Teratoma 550
Section 34.2—Sacrococcygeal Teratoma 553
Section 34.3—Fetal Surgery for Sacrococcygeal Teratoma 556

Section 34.1

Cervical Teratoma

What is a cervical teratoma?

A cervical teratoma is a very rare congenital tumor in the neck. These tumors tend to be large, disfiguring masses, partly solid and partly fluid, that encircle essential structures, such as the esophagus, thyroid, and trachea, making it impossible for a newborn to breathe upon birth.

Advances in medical technology, early detection, and careful monitoring during pregnancy now make it possible for these babies to be saved, usually by a procedure that enables surgeons to create an airway for the baby as it's being delivered and is still attached to and sustained by the mother's placenta.

What causes a cervical teratoma?

The cause of a cervical teratoma is unknown. It has never been linked to maternal lifestyle, so it is likely that there is nothing an expecting mother can do to prevent it.

How is it diagnosed?

An abnormality leading to a diagnosis is usually first discovered during a routine prenatal ultrasound, sometime around the eighteenth week of pregnancy. The first sign of a problem in the fetus could be an empty stomach indicating a blockage in the esophagus, polyhydramnios (excess amniotic fluid), or even discovery of the mass itself. The fetus's neck may also appear hyperextended.

If your obstetrician suspects a problem, you will be referred to an obstetrician who specializes in high-risk cases or a pediatric surgeon specializing in fetal and neonatal care for further ultrasound and possibly magnetic resonance imaging (MRI.)

How is it treated?

The initial stages of treatment for a cervical teratoma involve careful monitoring of the mother and fetus along with the development of a surgical plan. Your treatment will likely be handled by a multidisciplinary team of medical professionals including a perinatologist; general pediatric surgeon; radiologist; ears, nose and throat surgeon; and a nurse practitioner.

Repeated ultrasounds will be used to monitor amniotic fluid volume, tumor size, and the overall well-being of the fetus. The multidisciplinary team will be paying close attention to the tumor, which may not grow, but can grow rapidly, becoming large and bulky, sometimes extending out of the fetus's mouth, displacing the fetus's ear, and disfiguring the jaw.

The medical team will be monitoring the lungs for hyperinflation, a sign that the airway is completely blocked by the tumor. They will also be closely watching the heart, looking for signs of impending heart failure (hydrops) which is a complication that can occur if the heart is overextending itself to supply blood to the tumor.

In most cases involving cervical teratoma, surgery is done as the baby is delivered via cesarean section and still attached to mother's placenta. This method, known as an EXIT (ex utero intrapartum treatment) procedure, gives surgeons time to perform multiple procedures to secure the baby's airway while the blood flow and exchange of gases that normally occurs in the womb between the fetus and the placenta is preserved.

During an EXIT procedure, the fetus is only partially exposed during surgery, so that the volume of the uterus is maintained. Doctors may use inhalation agents to ensure relaxation of the mother's uterus. As with all prenatal surgeries there are risks to the mother, including excessive bleeding and infection. Be sure to discuss these risks fully with your doctor.

At this stage, the main goal for surgeons is to secure the airway by inserting a breathing tube (endotracheal tube) into it, bypassing the obstruction. Some combination of the following procedures will be used to facilitate this:

- **Laryngoscopy:** examination of the interior of the larynx (voice box) using an instrument called a laryngoscope;

- **Bronchoscopy:** examination of the bronchi (the two primary divisions of the trachea that lead to the lungs) using a tubular illuminated instrument (bronchoscope);

- **Tracheostomy:** the surgical formation of an opening into the trachea through the neck to allow the passage of air. This is done if surgeons cannot establish an airway with a breathing tube.

Once an airway is established, the umbilical cord is cut, and while the mother's cesarean section is completed and she is moved into recovery, doctors will surgically remove the tumor. This can be a long process since doctors must be extremely careful to avoid affecting any of the surrounding structures in the neck, including nerves, the larynx (voice box), the trachea (windpipe), and the esophagus. Subsequent surgeries may be needed either for complete removal of the tumor or for reconstruction of the trachea or other neck structures that were distorted by the tumor.

What happens after surgery?

Infants who undergo successful surgery have a high survival rate and grow up to live healthy, normal lives with perhaps one complication. These babies may develop transient or permanent hypothyroidism, both of which can be treated with medication. These conditions develop when the cervical teratoma either completely or partially replaces the thyroid gland. In this case, a pediatric endocrinologist should be consulted.

After surgery, doctors will want to monitor the baby routinely to ensure that the cervical teratoma doesn't recur. Most cervical teratomas are benign; however there is the possibility that a recurring tumor could be malignant.

Section 34.2

Sacrococcygeal Teratoma

What is sacrococcygeal teratoma?

Sacrococcygeal teratoma (SCT) is an unusual tumor that, in the newborn, is located at the base of the tailbone (coccyx). This birth defect is more common in female than in male babies. Although the tumors can grow very large, they are usually not malignant (that is, cancerous). They can usually be cured by surgery after birth, but occasionally cause trouble before birth.

SCT is usually discovered either because a blood test done at sixteen weeks shows a high alpha-fetoprotein amount, or because a sonogram is done because the uterus is larger than it should be. The increased size of the uterus is caused by extra amniotic fluid, called polyhydramnios. The diagnosis of SCT can be made by an ultrasound examination.

What is the outcome for a fetus with SCT?

Most fetuses with sacrococcygeal teratoma do well with surgical treatment after birth. These tumors are generally not malignant. Babies with small tumors that can be removed along with the coccyx bone after birth can be expected to live normal lives, although they should be followed for development of tumors later in life, using a simple blood test for alpha-fetoprotein. Fetuses with larger tumors or tumors that go up inside the baby's abdomen will require more complex surgery after birth, but in general do well. Again, they will have to be followed with blood tests for several years. Fetuses with very large tumors, which can reach the size of the fetus itself, pose a difficult problem both before and after birth.

We have found that those SCTs that are largely cystic (fluid-filled) generally do not cause a problem for the fetus. However, when the SCT is made up of mostly solid tissue and has a lot of blood flow in it, the fetus can suffer adverse effects. This is because the fetus's heart has to pump not only to circulate blood to its body, but also to all the blood vessels of the tumor, which can be as big as the fetus. In essence, the heart is performing twice its normal amount of work. The amount of work the heart is doing can be measured by fetal echocardiography. This sensitive test can determine when the fetus is approaching heart failure.

Fetuses with large tumors and a great deal of blood flow to the tumor have to be followed closely for the development of hydrops or fetal heart failure which can forecast fetal death. If hydrops does not develop, these babies will require cesarean-section delivery and extensive operation after birth. Most babies will do well once the tumor is completely removed. There can be long-term consequences which include the need to monitor (with blood tests) the development of a malignant tumor or difficulty with urination as a consequence of the surgical procedure. If hydrops does develop, usually in solid, rapidly growing tumors, the fetus usually will not survive without immediate intervention before birth.

How serious is my fetus's diaphragmatic hernia?

For you to make the best decision, you must have accurate and complete information about your fetus's condition. This includes:

- The type of defect—distinguishing it from other similar-appearing problems;

- The severity of the defect—determining whether your fetus's defect is mild or severe;

- Associated defects—determining if there is another problem or a cluster of problems (syndrome).

Amniocentesis may be necessary for chromosome testing. Sonography is the best imaging tool, but is dependent on the experience and expertise of the operator. Magnetic resonance imaging may be necessary in some cases. Many problems are first detected during routine screening procedures performed in your doctor's office (amniocentesis, maternal serum screening, routine sonography), but assessment of complex problems usually requires a tertiary perinatal/neonatal center with experience managing complex and rare fetal problems.

Fortunately, we can now predict before birth how good or bad your fetus's congenital diaphragmatic hernia (CDH) is. Careful and accurate prenatal assessment (level II sonogram, echocardiogram, sometimes magnetic resonance imaging [MRI]) is critical for your decision making and planning. One of the most important issues is to make sure there are no other birth defects (like heart problems) that will affect outcome. When CDH is the only problem, we have learned that severity and, thus, outcome is determined by two factors: 1) liver position, and 2) lung-to-head ratio or LHR. Liver position refers to whether or not any portion of the liver has herniated, or gone up into the chest of the fetus. Fetuses with the liver up in the chest have a more severe form of CDH and a low survival rate. About 75 percent of all CDH patients have some portion of the liver herniated into the chest. The lung-to-head ratio, or LHR, is a numeric estimate of the size of the fetal lungs, based on measurement of the amount of visible lung. High LHR values are associated with a good outcome.

The severity of sacrococcygeal teratoma is directly related to the size of the tumor and the amount of blood flow to the tumor. Both the size and the blood flow can now be accurately assessed by sonography and echocardiography. Small or medium-sized tumors without excessive blood flow will not cause a problem in the fetus. These babies should be followed with serial ultrasounds to make sure the tumor does not enlarge or the blood flow does not increase. They can be then delivered vaginally near term, and the tumor successfully taken care of after birth. However, very large tumors are prone to develop excessive blood flow, which causes heart failure in the fetus. Fortunately, this is easy to detect by sonography. These babies need to be closely followed for the development of excess fluid in the abdomen (ascites), in the chest (pleural effusion), in the pericardium (pericardial effusion), or under the skin (skin edema). It is the extra blood flowing to the tumor that strains the fetal heart enough to cause heart failure (hydrops).

Section 34.3

Fetal Surgery for Sacrococcygeal Teratoma

Most newborns with Sacrococcygeal Teratoma survive and do well. Malignant tumors are unusual. Fetuses with large cystic SCTs rarely develop hydrops and therefore are rarely candidates for fetal intervention. These cases are best handled with surgical removal of the tumor after delivery. A cesarean-section delivery of the baby may be necessary if the tumor is larger than 10 cm.

Because all sacrococcygeal teratomas require complete surgical resection after birth, babies with this condition should be born at a tertiary center with pediatric surgery expertise. Fetuses with large, mostly solid tumors need to be monitored frequently between eighteen and twenty-eight weeks of gestation for rapid growth of the tumor and the development of excessive blood flow and heart failure (hydrops). A small number of these fetuses with large solid tumors develop hydrops, due to extremely high blood flow through the tumor. These fetuses may be candidates for fetal intervention. Fetal intervention is only offered to women in whom there is evidence of heart failure in the fetus. Heart Failure is usually diagnosed by ultrasound. The fetus may have abdominal ascites (fluid in the abdomen), pleural or pericardial effusions (excess fluid around the heart or lungs), and skin or scalp edema (excess fluid under the skin or scalp). The mother may have polyhydramnios (too much amniotic fluid), or a slightly thickened placenta (placentomegaly). Women who have fetuses with advanced hydrops-placentomegaly or maternal preeclampsia (high blood pressure, protein in the urine) are not candidates for fetal intervention, as we have found that these symptoms (the so-called mirror syndrome) indicate an irreversible situation.

Fetuses who develop evidence of heart failure (hydrops) require fetal intervention. If late enough in gestation, past thirty-two weeks, the fetus may be delivered for intensive management after birth.

Before that, fetal intervention may be necessary to reverse the otherwise fatal heart failure. Open fetal surgery is performed in which the SCT is removed. This procedure was developed at the University of California, San Francisco (UCSF) Fetal Treatment Center, and has proven successful in a number of cases. As with all fetal interventions, we have tried to develop minimally invasive methods to treat this condition without opening the uterus, in this case, by stopping the high blood flow to the tumor. Instead of surgically opening the uterus and removing the tumor, a needle is inserted through the mother's abdomen and the uterine wall and into the blood vessels that feed the tumor. Radiofrequency waves are used to destroy the blood vessels and, without blood flow, the tumor does not grow and the heart failure (hydrops) is reversed. However, damage caused by the probe itself. may be difficult to control. Another method of cutting off blood flow to the tumor is injection of drugs (for example, alcohol) that cause blood to clot. None of these methods has so far proven effective in all cases.

What will happen after birth?

All babies with sacrococcygeal teratoma should be delivered at a tertiary center with pediatric surgery expertise. Tumors larger than 10 cm in diameter will require C-section delivery. The neonatologist will provide support in the intensive care nursery until the baby is stable enough for surgery. Surgical removal of small tumors is straightforward, but removal of large tumors can be very difficult and dangerous. The baby may require a blood transfusion(s) and intensive support for days or weeks after surgery. Most will get through this difficult period and enjoy a normal life. All babies should have yearly blood tests for elevated alpha-fetoprotein, which can signal development of a malignant tumor. A few babies may have difficulty with voiding urine because of nerve damage.

Chapter 35

Birthmarks

There are two main categories of birthmarks—red birthmarks and pigmented birthmarks. Red birthmarks are a vascular type of birthmark. Pigmented birthmarks are areas in which the color of the birthmark is different from the color of the rest of the skin.

What are red birthmarks?

Red birthmarks are colored, vascular (blood vessel) skin markings that develop before or shortly after birth.

What are the types of red birthmarks?

One common kind of vascular birthmark is the hemangioma. It usually is painless and harmless and its cause is not known. Color from the birthmark comes from the extensive development of blood vessels at the site.

Strawberry hemangiomas (strawberry mark, nevus vascularis, capillary hemangioma, hemangioma simplex) may appear anywhere on the body, but are most common on the face, scalp, back, or chest. They consist of small, closely packed blood vessels. They may be absent at birth, and develop at several weeks. They usually grow rapidly,

"Birthmarks," © 2005 The Cleveland Clinic Foundation, 9500 Euclid Avenue, Cleveland, Ohio 44195, www.clevelandclinic.org. Additional information is available from the Cleveland Clinic Health Information Center, 216-444-3771, toll-free 800-223-2273 extension 43771, or at http://www.clevelandclinic.org/health.

remain a fixed size, and then subside. In most cases, strawberry hemangiomas disappear by the time a child is nine years old. Some slight discoloration or puckering of the skin may remain at the site of the hemangioma.

Cavernous hemangiomas (angioma cavernosum, cavernoma) are similar to strawberry hemangiomas but are more deeply situated. They may appear as a red-blue spongy mass of tissue filled with blood. Some of these lesions disappear on their own, usually as a child approaches school age.

Port-wine stains are flat purple-to-red birthmarks made of dilated blood capillaries. These birthmarks occur most often on the face and may vary in size. Port-wine stains often are permanent (unless treated) and may result in emotional distress.

Salmon patches (also called stork bites) appear on 30 to 50 percent of newborn babies. These marks are small blood vessels (capillaries) that are visible through the skin. They are most common on the forehead, eyelids, upper lip, between the eyebrows, and the back of the neck. Often, these marks fade as the infant grows.

What are the symptoms of red birthmarks?

Symptoms of red birthmarks include:

- Skin markings that develop before or shortly after birth;
- Red skin rashes or lesions;
- Skin markings that resemble blood vessels;
- Possible bleeding;
- Skin that may break open.

How are red birthmarks diagnosed?

In most cases, a health professional can diagnose a red birthmark based on the appearance of the skin. Deeper birthmarks can be confirmed with tests such as magnetic resonance imaging (MRI), ultrasound, computed tomography (CT) scans, or biopsies.

What is the treatment for red birthmarks?

Many capillary birthmarks such as salmon patches and strawberry hemangiomas are temporary and require no treatment. For permanent lesions, concealing cosmetics such as Covermark may be helpful. Cortisone (oral or injected) can reduce the size of a hemangioma that is growing rapidly and obstructing vision or vital structures.

Port-wine stains on the face can be treated at a young age with a yellow pulsed dye laser for best results. Treatment of the birthmarks may help prevent psychosocial problems that can result in individuals who have a port-wine stain.

Permanent red birthmarks may be treated with methods including:

- Cryotherapy (freezing);
- Laser surgery;
- Surgical removal.

In some cases, birthmarks are not treated until a child reaches school age. However, birthmarks are treated earlier if they result in unwanted symptoms or if they compromise vital functions like vision or breathing.

Can red birthmarks be prevented?

Currently, there is no known way to prevent red birthmarks.

What are pigmented birthmarks?

Pigmented birthmarks are skin markings that are present at birth. The marks may range from brown or black to bluish or blue-gray in color.

What are the types of pigmented birthmarks?

Mongolian spots usually are bluish and appear as bruises. They often appear on the buttocks and/or lower back, but they sometimes also appear on the trunk or arms. The spots are seen most often in people who have darker skin.

Pigmented nevi (moles) are growths on the skin that usually are flesh-colored, brown, or black. Moles can appear anywhere on the skin, alone or in groups.

Congenital nevi are moles that are present at birth. These birthmarks have a slightly increased risk of becoming skin cancer depending on their size. Larger congenital nevi have a greater risk of developing skin cancer than do smaller congenital nevi. All congenital nevi should be examined by a healthcare provider and any change in the birthmark should be reported.

Café-au-lait spots are light tan or light brown spots that are usually oval in shape. They usually appear at birth but may develop in the first few years of a child's life.

What causes pigmented birthmarks?

The cause of pigmented birthmarks is not known. However, the amount and location of melanin (a substance that determines skin color) determines the color of pigmented birthmarks. Café-au-lait spots may be a normal type of birthmark, but the presence of several café-au-lait spots larger than a quarter may occur in neurofibromatosis (a genetic disorder that causes abnormal cell growth of nerve tissues). Moles occur when cells in the skin grow in a cluster instead of being spread throughout the skin. These cells are called melanocytes, and they make the pigment that gives skin its natural color. Moles may darken after exposure to the sun, during the teen years and during pregnancy.

What are the symptoms of pigmented birthmarks?

Symptoms of pigmented birthmarks include skin that is abnormally dark or light, or bluish, brown, black, or blue-gray in color. Discolorations of the skin may vary in size and be smooth, flat, raised, or wrinkled. Pigmented birthmarks may increase in size, change colors, become itchy, and occasionally bleed.

How are pigmented birthmarks diagnosed?

In most cases, health care professionals can diagnose birthmarks based on the appearance of the skin. If a mole exhibits potentially cancerous changes, a biopsy may be performed.

How are pigmented birthmarks treated?

In most cases, no treatment is needed for the birthmarks themselves. When birthmarks do require treatment, however, that treatment varies based on the kind of birthmark and its related conditions.

Large or prominent nevi that affect the appearance and self-esteem may be covered with special cosmetics.

Moles may be removed surgically if they affect the appearance or if they have an increased cancer risk.

What are the complications of pigmented birthmarks?

Some complications of pigmented birthmarks can include psychological effects in cases in which the birthmark is prominent. Pigmented birthmarks also can pose an increased skin cancer risk.

A doctor should check any changes that occur in the color, size, or texture of a nevus or other skin lesion. See a doctor right away if there is any pain, bleeding, itching, inflammation, or ulceration of a congenital nevus or other skin lesion.

Can pigmented birthmarks be prevented?

There is no known way to prevent birthmarks. People with birthmarks should use a good quality sunscreen when outdoors in order to prevent complications.

Part Four

Additional Help and Information

Chapter 36

Glossary of Terms Related to Congenital Disorders

abdomen: the area between the chest and the hips in the front of the body.[2]

acquired cerebral palsy: cerebral palsy that occurs as a result of injury to the brain after birth or during early childhood.[2]

agenesis corpus callosum: congenital absence of the part of the brain which connects the two cerebral hemispheres.[1]

agenesis, aplasia: congenital absence of a body part or organ, implying that the structure never formed. Result of an error in development, as opposed to an external process.[1]

amniotic band sequence: highly variable group of defects (or single defect) due to encirclement (strangulation) of a body part by strands of a fragmented amniotic sac. Includes terminal transverse limb defects, clefts, and body wall defects.[1]

anemia: not enough red blood cells in the blood.[2]

The terms in this glossary are from "Glossary of Selected Birth Defects Terms," © 2002 The Massachusetts Department of Public Health. Reprinted with permission [these terms are marked 1]. Other terms are from documents produced by the National Institute of Diabetes and Digestive and Kidney Diseases and the National Institute of Neurological Disorders and Stroke [marked 2], including "What I Need to Know about Hirschsprung's Disease," NIH Publication No. 05-4384 (2004) and "Cerebral Palsy: Hope through Research," NIH Publication No. 93-159 (2006).

anencephaly: congenital absence of the skull and brain.[1]

aniridia: congenital complete absence of the iris of the eye.[1]

anophthalmia: congenital complete (or essentially complete) absence of the eye globe.[1]

anotia: congenital absence of the ear.[1]

anticholinergic drugs: a family of drugs that inhibit parasympathetic neural activity by blocking the neurotransmitter acetylcholine.[2]

anus: the opening at the end of the large intestine. Stool leaves the body through this opening.[2]

aortic valve stenosis: congenital heart defect characterized by aortic valve narrowing reducing the flow of blood.[1]

Apgar score: a numbered scoring system doctors use to assess a baby's physical state at the time of birth.[2]

arthrogryposis: multiple congenital contractures of various joints.[1]

asphyxia: a lack of oxygen due to trouble with breathing or poor oxygen supply in the air.[2]

ataxia (ataxic): the loss of muscle control.[2]

athetoid: making slow, sinuous, involuntary, writhing movements, especially with the hands.[2]

atresia/imperforation: congenital absence or closure of a normal opening (valve or lumen).[1]

atresia or stenosis of large intestine, rectum, and anus: congenital absence, closure, or constriction of the large intestine, rectum, or anus (commonly known as imperforate anus).[1]

atresia or stenosis of small intestine: congenital absence, closure, or constriction of the small intestine (duodenal, jejunal, ileal atresia/stenosis).[1]

atrial septal defect (ASD): congenital heart defect characterized by one or more openings in the atrial septum (wall between the right and left atria). Most common type is called ASD, secundum.[1]

biliary atresia: congenital absence of the ducts in the biliary tract.[1]

bilirubin: a bile pigment produced by the liver of the human body as a byproduct of digestion.[2]

birth defect: congenital abnormalities of structure, function, or metabolism present before birth.[1]

bisphosphonates: a family of drugs that strengthen bones and reduce the risk of bone fracture in elderly adults.[2]

bladder exstrophy: congenital exposure of the bladder mucosa caused by incomplete closure of the anterior bladder wall and the abdominal cavity.[1]

botulinum toxin: a drug commonly used to relax spastic muscles; it blocks the release of acetylcholine, a neurotransmitter that energizes muscle tissue.[2]

branchial cleft, fistula, tag, cyst: congenital abnormality of the neck or area just below the collarbone (clavicle). Includes skin pits (cleft), tissue tags, or cysts.[1]

cataract: congenital opacity (clouding) of the lens of the eye.[1]

cerebral: relating to the two hemispheres of the human brain.[2]

cerebral dysgenesis: defective brain development.[2]

chemodenervation: a treatment that relaxes spastic muscles by interrupting nerve impulse pathways via a drug, such as botulinum toxin, which prevents communication between neurons and muscle tissue.[2]

choanal atresia, choanal stenosis: congenital absence (or narrowing) of the passageway between the nose and pharynx due to a thick bone or thin "membranous" bone.[1]

choreoathetoid: a condition characterized by aimless muscle movements and involuntary motions.[2]

cleft lip: congenital defect of the upper lip in which there is incomplete closure.[1]

cleft palate: congenital defect in the closure of the palate; the structure which separates the nasal cavities and the back of the mouth. May involve the soft palate, hard palate, or alveolus (gum).[1]

coarctation of the aorta: congenital heart defect characterized by narrowing of the descending aorta. Usually occurs as an indentation at a specific location, less commonly diffuse narrowing.[1]

colostomy: surgery to connect the colon to a hole in the abdomen.[2]

computed tomography (CT) scan: an imaging technique that uses x-rays and a computer to create a picture of the brain's tissues and structures.[2]

congenital cerebral palsy: cerebral palsy that is present at birth from causes that have occurred during fetal development.[2]

congenital heart defect (CHD), cardiovascular malformation (CVM): abnormal heart structure present at birth. Includes defects detected prenatally and those recognized after the newborn period.[1]

congenital: abnormality or problem present at birth. Includes defects detected prenatally and those not recognized until after the newborn period.[1]

contracture: a condition in which muscles become fixed in a rigid, abnormal position, which causes distortion or deformity.[2]

craniosynostosis: congenital abnormality of skull shape due to premature fusion of the sutures between the skull bones. Head may be elongated, foreshortened, tower-like, or asymmetrically flattened.[1]

cytokines: messenger cells that play a role in the inflammatory response to infection.[2]

Dandy-Walker malformation: congenital defect of the cerebellum involving a small cerebellar vermis and cystic dilation of the fourth ventricle.[1]

developmental delay: behind schedule in reaching the milestones of early childhood development.[2]

diaphragmatic hernia: congenital defect of the muscular diaphragm resulting in herniation of the abdominal contents into the chest. Incomplete, asymptomatic variation is called eventration.[1]

diarrhea: loose, watery stool.[2]

disuse atrophy: muscle wasting caused by the inability to flex and exercise muscles.[2]

Down syndrome (trisomy 21): distinctive and common chromosome abnormality syndrome caused by an extra copy of chromosome 21. Can be complete (Trisomy 21), attached to another chromosome (translocation), or mixed with cells containing normal chromosomes (mosaic).[1]

dyskinetic: the impairment of the ability to perform voluntary movements, which results in awkward or incomplete movements.[2]

dysplasia: abnormal cell organization of an organ. Usually congenital, may be acquired.[1]

dystonia (dystonic): a condition of abnormal muscle tone.[2]

Ebstein anomaly: congenital heart defect characterized by downward displacement of the tricuspid valve into the right ventricle, associated with tricuspid valve regurgitation.[1]

electroencephalogram (EEG): a technique for recording the pattern of electrical currents inside the brain.[2]

electromyography: a special recording technique that detects muscle activity.[2]

encephalocele: congenital defect of the skull resulting in herniation (protrusion) of the brain.[1]

endocardial cushion defect (ECD), atrioventricular canal (AVC) defect, atrioventricular septal defect (AVSD): congenital heart defect characterized by a combined atrial and ventricular septal defect, and common atrioventricular valve (instead of distinct tricuspid and mitral valves). In contrast to complete AVC, the partial AVC includes an atrial septal defect, primum type, plus a cleft mitral valve.[1]

enterocolitis: infection of the small and large intestines.[2]

esophageal atresia: congenital discontinuity of the lumen of the esophagus. Usually associated with a tracheoesophageal fistula (TEF) which is an abnormal connection between the esophagus and trachea.[1]

failure to thrive: a condition characterized by a lag in physical growth and development.[2]

fistula: abnormal connection between an internal organ and the body surface, or between two internal organs or structures. Can be congenital or acquired.[1]

focal (partial) seizure: a brief and temporary alteration in movement, sensation, or autonomic nerve function caused by abnormal electrical activity in a localized area of the brain.[2]

gait analysis: a technique that uses cameras, force plates, electromyography, and computer analysis to objectively measure an individual's pattern of walking.[2]

ganglion cells: a type of nerve cell involved in moving stool through the large intestine. A person with Hirschsprung disease is missing these cells from part of the large intestine.[2]

gastroesophageal reflux disease (GERD): also known as heartburn, which happens when stomach acids back up into the esophagus.[2]

gastroschisis: congenital opening of the abdominal wall with protrusion of the abdominal contents. Can be distinguished from omphalocele by location usually to the right of the umbilicus.[1]

gastrostomy: a surgical procedure that creates an artificial opening in the stomach for the insertion of a feeding tube.[2]

gestation: the period of fetal development from the time of conception until birth.[2]

hemianopia: defective vision or blindness that impairs half of the normal field of vision.[2]

hemiparesis: paralysis affecting only one side of the body.[2]

heterotaxy (situs anomalies): congenital malposition of the abdominal organs often associated with a congenital heart defect.[1]

Hirschsprung disease: congenital aganglionic megacolon (enlarged colon) due to absent nerves in the wall of the colon.[1]

holoprosencephaly: spectrum of congenital defects of the forebrain due to failure of the brain to develop into two equal halves. Includes alobar (single ventricle), semilobar, and lobar types.[1]

hydrocephalus: accumulation of fluid within the spaces of the brain. Can be congenital or acquired.[1]

hydronephrosis: enlargement of the urine-filled chambers (pelves, calyces) of the kidney.[1]

hyperplasia: overgrowth due to an increase in the number of cells of tissue.[1]

hypertonia: increased muscle tone.[2]

hypertrophy: overgrowth due to enlargement of existing cells.[1]

hypoplasia: small size of organ or part due to arrested development.[1]

hypoplastic left heart syndrome (HLHS): congenital heart defect characterized by extreme smallness of left-sided structures. Classically, aortic valve/mitral valve atresia or marked hypoplasia, ascending aorta, and left ventricle hypoplasia.[1]

hypospadias: congenital defect of the penis in which the urethral meatus (urinary outlet) is not on the glans (tip). Severity based on location from shaft to scrotum and perineum.[1]

hypotonia: decreased muscle tone.[2]

hypoxic-ischemic encephalopathy: brain damage caused by poor blood flow or insufficient oxygen supply to the brain.[2]

ileostomy: surgery to connect the bottom of the small intestine (ileum) to a hole in the abdomen.[2]

intracranial hemorrhage: bleeding in the brain.[2]

intrapartum asphyxia: the reduction or total stoppage of oxygen circulating in a baby's brain during labor and delivery.[2]

intrathecal baclofen: baclofen that is injected into the cerebrospinal fluid of the spinal cord to reduce spasticity.[2]

intrauterine infection: infection of the uterus, ovaries, or fallopian tubes (see pelvic inflammatory disease for a more detailed explanation).[2]

jaundice: a blood disorder caused by the abnormal buildup of bilirubin in the bloodstream.[2]

kernicterus: a neurological syndrome caused by deposition of bilirubin into brain tissues. Kernicterus develops in extremely jaundiced infants, especially those with severe Rh incompatibility.[2]

kyphosis: a humpback-like outward curvature of the upper spine.[2]

large intestine: a long tube that makes stool and carries it out of the body.[2]

limb deficiency, upper (arms) / lower (legs): congenital absence of a portion or entire limb. Types include transverse (resembling an amputation), longitudinal (missing ray), and intercalary (missing bone in-between).[1]

lordosis: an increased inward curvature of the lower spine.[2]

macrocephaly: large head due to extra fluid or extra volume.[1]

magnetic resonance imaging (MRI): an imaging technique that uses radio waves, magnetic fields, and computer analysis to create a picture of body tissues and structures.[2]

meninges: membranes that cover the brain and spinal cord.[1]

microcephaly: small head, with corresponding smallness of the brain.[1]

microphthalmia: congenital smallness of the eye globe.[1]

microtia: congenital smallness or maldevelopment of the external ear, with or without absence or narrowing of the external auditory canal.[1]

mosaic: in genetics, two or more different chromosome types in cell lines. Proportion of normal to abnormal cells usually correlated to severity.[1]

nerve cells: nerves are long fibers that carry messages from the body to the brain, and back again, like telephone lines. The messages often tell a body part what to do. Nerve cells are part of nerves. In the intestine, the nerve cells tell muscles how to push the stool along.[2]

nerve entrapment: repeated or prolonged pressure on a nerve root or peripheral nerve.[2]

neural tube defect (NTD): congenital opening from head to the base of the spine resulting from failure of the neural tube to close in the first month of pregnancy. Includes anencephaly, spina bifida, and encephalocele.[1]

neuronal migration: the process in the developing brain in which neurons migrate from where they are born to where they settle into neural circuits. Neuronal migration, which occurs as early as the second month of gestation, is controlled in the brain by chemical guides and signals.[2]

neuroprotective: describes substances that protect nervous system cells from damage or death.[2]

neurotrophins: a family of molecules that encourage survival of nervous system cells.[2]

obstructive genitourinary defect: congenital narrowing or absence of the urinary tract structure at any level. Severity often depends upon the level of the obstruction. Often accompanied by hydronephrosis.[1]

off-label drugs: drugs prescribed to treat conditions other than those that have been approved by the Food and Drug Administration.[2]

omphalocele: congenital opening of the abdominal wall with protrusion of the abdominal contents. Can be distinguished from gastroschisis by location within umbilical ring.[1]

orthotic devices: special devices, such as splints or braces, used to treat posture problems involving the muscles, ligaments, or bones.[2]

osteopenia: reduced density and mass of the bones.[2]

ostomy: surgery to connect part of the intestine to a hole in the abdomen.[2]

palsy: paralysis, or the lack of control over voluntary movement.[2]

paresis or plegia: weakness or paralysis. In cerebral palsy, these terms are typically combined with other phrases that describe the distribution of paralysis and weakness; for example, quadriplegia means paralysis of all four limbs.[2]

patent ductus arteriosus (PDA): congenital heart defect characterized by persistence of the fetal blood vessel connecting the pulmonary artery and the aorta.[1]

pelvic inflammatory disease (PID, also sometimes called pelvic infection or intrauterine infection): an infection of the upper genital tract (the uterus, ovaries, and fallopian tubes) caused by sexually transmitted infectious microorganisms. Symptoms of PID include fever, foul-smelling vaginal discharge, abdominal pain and pain during intercourse, and vaginal bleeding. Many different organisms can cause PID, but most cases are associated with gonorrhea and chlamydia.[2]

periventricular leukomalacia (PVL): "peri" means near; "ventricular" refers to the ventricles or fluid spaces of the brain; and "leukomalacia" refers to softening of the white matter of the brain. PVL is a condition in which the cells that make up white matter die near the ventricles. Under a microscope, the tissue looks soft and sponge-like.[2]

placenta: an organ that joins a mother with her unborn baby and provides nourishment and sustenance.[2]

polydactyly: extra fingers or toes which may be medial (pre-axial) or lateral (postaxial).[1]

post-impairment syndrome: a combination of pain, fatigue, and weakness due to muscle abnormalities, bone deformities, overuse syndromes, or arthritis.[2]

pulmonary atresia: congenital heart defect characterized by absence of the pulmonary valve or pulmonary artery itself. May occur with an intact ventricular septum (PA/IVS) or with a ventricular septal defect, in which it is more properly called tetralogy of Fallot with pulmonary atresia (TOF/PA).[1]

pulmonary stenosis (PS): congenital heart defect characterized by narrowing of the pulmonary valve.[1]

quadriplegia: paralysis of both the arms and legs.[2]

rectum: the last section of the large intestine.[2]

renal agenesis: congenital absence of the kidney.[1]

Rh incompatibility: a blood condition in which antibodies in a pregnant woman's blood attack fetal blood cells and impair an unborn baby's supply of oxygen and nutrients.[2]

rubella (also known as German measles): a viral infection that can damage the nervous system of an unborn baby if a mother contracts the disease during pregnancy.[2]

scoliosis: a disease of the spine in which the spinal column tilts or curves to one side of the body.[2]

selective dorsal rhizotomy: a surgical procedure in which selected nerves are severed to reduce spasticity in the legs.[2]

spastic (or spasticity): describes stiff muscles and awkward movements.[2]

spastic diplegia (or diparesis): a form of cerebral palsy in which spasticity affects both legs, but the arms are relatively or completely spared.[2]

spastic hemiplegia (or hemiparesis): a form of cerebral palsy in which spasticity affects an arm and leg on one side of the body.[2]

spastic quadriplegia (or quadriparesis): a form of cerebral palsy in which all four limbs are paralyzed or weakened equally.[2]

spina bifida: neural tube defect with protrusion of the spinal cord and/or meninges. Includes myelomeningocele (involving both spinal cord and meninges) and meningocele (involving just the meninges).[1]

stenosis: narrowing or constriction of the diameter of a bodily passage or orifice.[1]

stereognosia: difficulty perceiving and identifying objects using the sense of touch.[2]

stoma: a hole on the outside of the body, made by surgery. Stool leaves the body through the hole, instead of through the anus.[2]

stool: solid waste from the body. The material that gets passed in a bowel movement.[2]

strabismus: misalignment of the eyes, also known as cross eyes.[2]

tetralogy of Fallot (TOF): congenital heart defect composed of ventricular septal defect, pulmonary stenosis or atresia, displacement of the aorta to the right, and hypertrophy of right ventricle.[1]

tonic-clonic seizure: a type of seizure that results in loss of consciousness, generalized convulsions, loss of bladder control, and tongue biting followed by confusion and lethargy when the convulsions end.[2]

tracheoesophageal fistula (TEF): see esophageal atresia.[1]

translocation: chromosome rearrangement in which a piece of genetic material is transferred from one segment to another. May be balanced (no chromosome material gained or lost), or unbalanced (material has been gained or lost).[1]

transposition of the great vessels (arteries) (dTGA): congenital heart defect in which the aorta arises from the right ventricle, and the pulmonary artery arises from the left ventricle (opposite of normal).[1]

tremor: an involuntary trembling or quivering.[2]

tricuspid atresia: congenital heart defect characterized by the absence of the tricuspid valve.[1]

trisomy: chromosome abnormality characterized by a third copy of a chromosome. Includes complete and partial formation of an extra chromosome.[1]

trisomy 13: chromosome abnormality caused by an extra chromosome 13.[1]

trisomy 18: chromosomal abnormality caused by an extra chromosome 18.[1]

trisomy 21: see Down syndrome.[1]

truncus arteriosus: congenital heart defect characterized by a single great arterial trunk, instead of a separate aorta and pulmonary artery.[1]

ultrasound: a technique that bounces sound waves off tissue and bone and uses the pattern of echoes to form an image, called a sonogram.[2]

ventricular septal defect (VSD): congenital heart defect characterized by one or several openings in the ventricular septum. Includes subtypes based on location of the "hole" in the septum, i.e., membranous, muscular, conoventricular, subtricuspid/canal.[1]

Chapter 37

Congenital Disorders: Resources for Information and Support

General Information

American Pregnancy Association
1425 Greenway Drive
Suite 440
Irving, TX 75038
Toll-Free: 800-672-2296
Fax: 972-550-0800
Website: http://
www.americanpregnancy.org
E-mail: questions@
americanpregnancy.org

Resources in this chapter were compiled from many sources deemed accurate. This list is intended as a starting point for further research and is not considered all-inclusive; inclusion does not constitute endorsement. All contact information was updated and verified in July 2006.

Birth Defect Research for Children, Inc.
930 Woodcock Road, Suite 225
Orlando, FL 32803
Phone: 407-895-0802
Fax: 407-895-0824
Website: http://
www.birthdefects.org
E-mail: staff@birthdefects.org

International Birth Defects Information Systems
Website: http://www.ibis-birthdefects.org

March of Dimes Birth Defects Foundation
1275 Mamaroneck Avenue
White Plains, NY 10605
Toll-Free: 888-663-4637
Phone: 914-997-4488
Fax: 914-428-8203
Website: http://
www.marchofdimes.com

**National Birth Defects
Prevention Network**
Website: http://www.nbdpn.org

**National Center on Birth
Defects and Developmental
Disabilities**
Centers for Disease Control
and Prevention
1600 Clifton Rd
Atlanta, GA 30333
Toll-Free: 800-232-4636
Phone: 404-639-3534
Website: http://www.cdc.gov/
ncbddd

**National Dissemination
Center for Children with
Disabilities (NICHCY)**
P.O. Box 1492
Washington, DC 20013
Toll-Free: 800-695-0285
Fax: 202-884-8441
Website: www.nichcy.org
E-mail: nichcy@aed.org

**National Institute of Child
Health and Human
Development (NICHD)**
P.O. Box 3006
Rockville, MD 20847
Toll-Free: 800-370-2943
Fax: 301-984-1473
TTY: 1-888-320-6942
Website: http://
www.nichd.nih.gov
E-mail:
NICHDInformationResourceCenter
@mail.nih.gov

**National Organization for
Rare Disorders (NORD)**
P.O. Box 1968
Danbury, CT 06813-1968
Toll-Free: 800-999-6673
Phone: 203-744-0100
Fax: 203-798-2291
Website: http://
www.rarediseases.org
E-mail:
orphan@rarediseases.org

Nemours Foundation
Website: http://kidshealth.org

Anencephaly

**Anencephaly Support
Foundation**
Website: http://www.asfhelp.com
E-mail: info@asfhelp.com

Cerebral Palsy

**American Academy for
Cerebral Palsy and
Developmental Medicine**
555 E. Wells Street, Suite 1100
Milwaukee, WI 53202
Phone: 414-918-3014
Fax: 414-276-3349
Website: http://www.aacpdm.org

Children's Neurobiological Solutions (CNS) Foundation
610 Annacapa Street
Santa Barbara, CA 93103
Phone: 866-267-5580
or 805-965-8838
Website: http://
www.cnsfoundation.org
E-mail: info@cnsfoundation.org

United Cerebral Palsy Association, Inc.
1660 L Street NW, Suite 700
Washington, DC 20036
Toll-Free: 800-USA-5-UCP
Phone: 202-776-0406
Fax: 202-776-0414
Website: http://www.ucp.org
E-mail: national@ucp.org

Cleft Palate

American Cleft Palate-Craniofacial Association/ Cleft Palate Foundation
1504 East Franklin Street
Suite 102
Chapel Hill, NC 27514-2820
Phone: 919-933-9044
Website: http://www.cleftline.org
E-mail: info@cleftline.org

Congenital Diaphragmatic Hernia

Association of Congenital Diaphragmatic Hernia Research, Advocacy, and Support (CHERUBS)
270 Coley Road
Henderson, NC 27537
Phone: 252-492-6003
or 252-492-9066
Fax: 815-425-9155
Website:
http://www.cherubs-cdh.org
E-mail: info@cherubs-cdh.org

Craniofacial Disorders

American Cleft Palate-Craniofacial Association/ Cleft Palate Foundation
1504 East Franklin Street
Suite 102
Chapel Hill, NC 27514-2820
Phone: 919-933-9044
Website: http://www.cleftline.org
E-mail: info@cleftline.org

Children's Craniofacial Association
13140 Coit Road, Suite 307
Dallas, TX 75240
Toll-Free: 800-535-3643
Phone: 214-570-9099
Fax: 214-570-8811
Website: http://www.ccakids.com
E-mail:
contactCCA@ccakids.com

Cleft Lip and Palate Association
First Floor Green Man Tower
332B Goswell Road
London EC1V 7LQ
United Kingdom
Website: http://www.clapa.com

National Craniofacial Association
P.O. Box 11082
Chattanooga, TN 37401
Toll-Free: 800-332-2373
Website:
http://www.faces-cranio.org

Pierre Robin Network
3604 Biscayne
Quincy, IL 62305
Website:
http://www.pierrerobin.org
E-mail: info@pierrerobin.org

Drug/Environmental Exposure

Collaborative on Health and the Environment
c/o Commonweal
P.O. Box 316
Bolinas, CA 94924
Website: http://
www.healthandenvironment.org
E-mail:
info@healthandenvironment.org

Organization of Teratology Information Services (OTIS)
OTIS Information/Pregnancy
Riskline
University of Arizona
501 N Campbell, Room 1156
Tucson AZ 85724
Toll-Free: 866-626-6847
Website:
http://www.otispregnancy.org

Fetal Alcohol Syndrome

Fetal Alcohol Syndrome Prevention Section
Division of Birth Defects and
Developmental Disabilities
National Center for
Environmental Health, MS F-15
Centers for Disease Control and
Prevention
4770 Buford Highway NE
Atlanta, GA 30341-3724
Phone: 770-488-7370
Fax: 770-488-7361
E-mail: ncehinfo@cdc.gov

National Institute on Alcohol Abuse and Alcoholism (NIAAA)
5635 Fishers Lane, MSC 9304
Bethesda, MD 20892-9304
Website:
http://www.niaaa.nih.gov

National Organization on Fetal Alcohol Syndrome

900 17th Street NW, Suite 910
Washington, DC 20006
Toll-Free: 800-66NOFAS
Phone: 202-785-4585
Fax: 202-466-6456
Website: http://www.nofas.org
E-mail: information@nofas.org

Substance Abuse and Mental Health Services Administration (SAMHSA) Fetal Alcohol Spectrum Disorders Center for Excellence

2101 Gaither Road, Suite 600
Rockville, MD 20850
Phone: 866-STOPFAS(786-7327)
Website:
http://fascenter.samhsa.gov
E-mail: fasdcenter@samhsa.gov

Fetal Surgery

Center for Fetal Diagnosis and Treatment

Children's Hospital of
Philadelphia
Toll-Free: 800-468-8376

Fetal Care Center of Cincinnati

3333 Burnet Ave., MLC 2023
Cincinnati, Ohio 45229-3039
Toll-Free: 888-338-2559
Phone: 513-636-9608
Fax: 513-636-5959
Website:
http://www.fetalcarecenter.org
E-mail: info@fetalcarecenter.org

Fetal Treatment Center

University of California San
Francisco
513 Parnassus Avenue
HSW 1601
San Francisco, CA 94143-0570
Toll-Free: 800-RX-FETUS
Fax: 415-502-0660
Website: http://
fetalsurgery.ucsf.edu
E-mail: fetus@surgery.ucsf.edu

Texas Center for Fetal Surgery

8th Floor, Clinical Care Center
Texas Children's Hospital
6621 Fannin Street
Houston, TX 77030
Toll-Free: 800-364-5437
Phone: 832-824-1000
Fax: 832-825-3141
Website: http://
www.texaschildrenshospital.org/
carecenters/FetalSurgery

University of California, San Diego Fetal Surgery Program

200 West Arbor Drive
MC 8825
San Diego, CA 92103-8825
Phone: 866-638-0601
Website: http://health.ucsd.edu/
specialties/fetalsurgery

583

Gastrointestinal Disorders

*International Foundation
for Functional
Gastrointestinal Disorders,
Inc. (IFFGD)*
P.O. Box 170864
Milwaukee, WI 53217-8076
Toll-Free: 888-964-2001
Phone: 414-964-1799
Fax: 414-964-7176
Website: http://www.iffgd.org
E-mail: iffgd@iffgd.org

Mothers of Omphaloceles
Website:
http://www.omphalocele.com

Pull-thru Network
2312 Savoy Street
Hoover, AL 35226
Phone: 205-978-2930
Website: http://
www.pullthrough.org
E-mail: info@pullthrough.org

Goldenhar Syndrome

*Goldenhar Syndrome
Support Network*
9325 163rd Street
Edmonton, Alberta,
T5P 2P4
Canada
Phone: 403-465-9534
Website: http://
www.goldenharsyndrome.org
E-mail:
support@goldenharsyndrome.org

Heart Defects

*Adult Congenital Heart
Association (ACHA)*
6757 Greene Street
Philadelphia, PA, 19119
Phone: 215-849-1260
Fax: 215-849-1261
Website: http://
www.achaheart.org
E-mail: info@achaheart.org

American Heart Association
National Center
7272 Greenville Avenue
Dallas, TX 75231
Toll-Free: 800-242-8721
Website: http://
www.americanheart.org

*Canadian Adult Congenital
Heart Network*
Phone: 416-417-6523
Website: http://www.cachnet.org

*Congenital Heart
Information Network
(C.H.I.N.)*
600 North Third Street
First floor
Philadelphia, PA 19123-2902
Phone: 215-627-4034
Fax: 215-627-4036
Website: http://tchin.org
E-mail: mb@tchin.org

Little Hearts, Inc.
P.O. Box 171
Cromwell, CT 06416
Toll-Free: 866-435-HOPE
Phone/Fax: 860-635-0000
Website: http://
www.littlehearts.org

Holoprosencephaly

Carter Centers for Research in Holoprosencephaly
c/o Texas Scottish Rite Hospital
2222 Welborn Street
P.O. Box 190567
Dallas, TX 75219-9982
Phone: 214-559-8411
Fax: 214-559-8383
Website: http://
www.stanford.edu/group/hpe
E-mail: hpe@tsrh.org

Hydrocephalus

Guardians of Hydrocephalus Research Foundation
2618 Avenue Z
Brooklyn, NY 11235-2023
Phone: 718-743-4473
Fax: 718-743-1171
Website: http://
ghrf.Homestead.com/ghrf.html
E-mail: GHRF2618@aol.com

Hydrocephalus Association
870 Market Street, Suite 705
San Francisco, CA 94102
Toll-Free: 888-598-3789
Phone: 415-732-7040
Fax: 415-732-7044
Website: http://
www.hydroassoc.org
E-mail: info@hydroassoc.org

Hydrocephalus Support Group, Inc.
P.O. Box 4236
Chesterfield, MO 63006-4236
Phone: 636-532-8228
Fax: 314-251-5871
E-mail: hydrodb@earthlink.net

National Hydrocephalus Foundation
12413 Centralia Road
Lakewood, CA 90715-1623
Toll-Free: 888-857-3434
Phone/Fax: 562-924-6666
Website: http://nhfonline.org
E-mail: hydrobrat@earthlink.net

Kidney Disorders

American Kidney Fund
6110 Executive Blvd.
Suite 1010
Rockville, MD 20852
Toll-free: 800-638-8299
Phone: 301-881-3052
Website: http://www.akfinc.org
E-mail: helpline@akfinc.org

Herman B. Wells Research Center
702 Barnhill Drive, 2600A
Indianapolis, IN 46202
Phone: 317-274-8900
Website: http://www.wellscenter
.iupui.edu/home.html

National Kidney Foundation
30 East 33rd Street
New York, NY 10016
Toll-Free: 800-622-9010
Phone: 212-889-2210
Website: http://www.kidney.org
E-mail: info@kidney.org

Liver Disorders

American Liver Foundation
75 Maiden Lane, Suite 603
New York, NY 10038
Toll-Free: 800-GO-Liver (465-4837)
or 888-4HEP-USA (443-7872)
Phone: 212-668-1000
Fax: 212-483-8179
Website:
http://www.liverfoundation.org
E-mail: info@liverfoundation.org

Multiple Births

Center for Study of Multiple Birth (CSMB)
333 E Superior St., Suite 464
Chicago, IL 60611
Phone: 312-695-1677
Fax: 312-908-8777
Website: http://
www.multiplebirth.com

Conjoined Twins International (CTI)
P.O. Box 10895
Prescott, AZ 86304
Phone: 928-445-2777
Website: http://
www.conjoinedtwinsint.com/
home.htm

RESOLVE: The National Infertility Association
Toll-Free Helpline:
888-623-0744
Website: http://www.resolve.org

Triplet Connection
P.O. Box 429
Spring City, UT 84662
Phone: 435-851-1105

Respiratory Disorders

American Lung Association
61 Broadway, 6th Floor
New York, NY 10006
Toll-Free: 800-548-8252
Phone: 212-315-8700
Website: http://www.lungusa.org

Retinopathy of Prematurity

American Association for Pediatric Ophthalmology and Strabismus
P.O. Box 193832
San Francisco, CA 94119-3832
Phone: 415-561-8505
Website: http://www.aapos.org
E-mail: aapos@aao.org

Association for Retinopathy of Prematurity and Related Diseases (ROPARD)

P.O. Box 250425
Franklin, MI 48025
Toll-Free: 800-788-2020
Website: http://www.ropard.org

National Eye Institute (NEI)

31 Center Drive MSC 2510,
Building 31, Room 6A32
Bethesda, MD 20892-2510
Phone: 301-496-5248
Website: http://www.nei.nih.gov

Spina Bifida

Management of Meningocele Study (MOMS)

GWU Biostatistics Center
6110 Executive Blvd., Suite 750
Rockville, MD 20852
Toll-Free: 866-ASK-MOMS
(275-6667)
Fax: 866-458-4621
Website: http://
spinabifidamoms.com
E-mail:
MOMS@biostat.bsc.gwu.edu

Spina Bifida Association of America

4590 MacArthur Blvd. NW
Suite 250
Washington, DC 20007-4266
Toll-Free: 800-621-3141
Phone: 202-944-3285
Fax: 202-944-3295
Website: http://www.sbaa.org
E-mail: sbaa@sbaa.org

Umbilical Cord Abnormalities

International Vasa Previa Foundation, Inc.

P.O. Box 272293
Boca Raton, FL 33427-2293
Phone: 309-797-1995
Fax: 267-790-6693
Website: http://
www.vasaprevia.com

Urological Disorders

American Urological Association

Website: http://
www.urologyhealth.org

National Kidney and Urologic Diseases Information Clearinghouse

3 Information Way
Bethesda, MD 20892-3580
Toll-Free: 800-891-5390
Fax: 703-738-4929
Website: http://
kidney.niddk.nih.gov
E-mail:
nkudic@info.niddk.nih.gov

Index

Index

Page numbers followed by 'n' indicate a footnote. Page numbers in *italics* indicate a table or illustration.

A

abdomen, defined 567
"Abdominal Wall Defects: Gastroschisis" (University of California) 437n
"Abdominal Wall Defects: Omphalocele" (University of California) 441n
About Cesarean Childbirth (American College of Surgeons) 246n
abruption *see* placental abruption
abruptio placentae *see* placental abruption
"Acardiac Twin (TRAP Sequence)" (University of California) 228n
acardiac twin (TRAP sequence), described 231
ACC *see* agenesis corpus callosum
Accutane (isotretinoin)
  birth defects 4, 72–76
  pregnancy safety concerns 70
"Accutane (Isotretinoin) and Pregnancy" (OTIS) 72n

ACE inhibitors *see* angiotensin converting enzyme inhibitors
acephaly, described 330
acetaminophen, pregnancy safety concerns 69
acetylcholine
  cerebral palsy 376
  described 568, 569
acetylsalicylate, pregnancy safety concerns 70
ACHA *see* Adult Congenital Heart Association
achondroplasia, prenatal testing 19
acitretin, pregnancy safety concerns 70
acquired cerebral palsy, defined 567
acquired hydrocephalus, described 317
acrosyndactyly, amniotic band syndrome 170
adactyly, maternal tobacco use 50
A.D.A.M., Inc., publications
  Apgar score 254n
  congenital rubella 134n
addiction, maternal drug abuse 63
Adult Congenital Heart Association (ACHA), contact information 584
Advil (ibuprofen), pregnancy safety concerns 69

591

AFI *see* amniotic fluid index
AFP *see* alpha-fetoprotein
age factor
  amniocentesis 28
  Down syndrome 20
  fetal alcohol spectrum
    disorders 56–59
  fifth disease 130
  maternal blood screening 27
  placenta previa 174
  preeclampsia 117
  pregnancy 16
Agency for Healthcare Research and
  Quality (AHRQ), hyperbaric oxygen
  therapy publication 386n
agenesis
  defined 567
  described 519
agenesis corpus callosum (ACC)
  defined 567
  described 333–34
"Agenesis of the Corpus Callosum
  Information Page" (NINDS) 333n
AHRQ *see* Agency for Healthcare
  Research and Quality
AIS *see* androgen insensitivity
  syndrome
albuterol, maternal asthma 99
alcohol-related birth defects (ARBD),
  described 53
alcohol-related neurodevelopmental
  disorders (ARND), described 53
alcohol use
  fetal alcohol syndrome 4
  preconception counseling 7
  pregnancy 36, 52–56
  pregnancy safety concerns 69
  prenatal care 13, 14
  see also fetal alcohol syndrome
Alexander, Duane 54
allantois, described 504
allergic reactions, thalidomide 81
alobar holoprosencephaly 324
alpha-fetoprotein (AFP)
  sacrococcygeal teratoma 553
  spina bifida 399
Alving, Barbara 98
ambiguous genitalia, described
  525–29

American Academy for Cerebral
  Palsy and Developmental Medicine,
  contact information 580
American Association for Pediatric
  Ophthalmology and Strabismus,
  contact information 586
American Cleft Palate-Craniofacial
  Association/Cleft Palate
  Foundation, contact information
  581
American College of Surgeons 246n
American Heart Association
  contact information 584
  publications
    congenital cardiovascular
      defects 276n
    fetal echocardiography 276n
American Kidney Fund, contact
  information 585
American Liver Foundation,
  contact information 586
American Lung Association
  contact information 586
  smoking cessation publication 45n
American Pregnancy Association
  contact information 579
  publications
    drug abuse, pregnancy 61n
    fetal growth restriction 160n
    premature baby care 200n
American Society of Clinical
  Oncology, maternal cancer
  publication 101n
American Urological Association,
  Web site address 587
American Urological Association
  Foundation, vaginal anomalies
  publication 517n
ammonia, pregnancy 95
Amnesteem (isotretinoin), birth
  defects 4, 72
amniocentesis
  birth defect diagnosis 7
  versus chorionic villus
    sampling 26
  congenital diaphragmatic hernia
    433–34
  prenatal testing 28–29
  spina bifida 399

amnioreduction, twin to twin
   transfusion 229, 232–33
amniotic band constriction,
   congenital amputation 544
amniotic band sequence, defined 567
"Amniotic Band Syndrome"
   (University of Missouri Children's
   Hospital) 163n
amniotic band syndrome,
   described 169–70
amniotic fluid
   color 163, 168
   described 163
   urinary tract obstruction 478
"Amniotic Fluid Abnormalities
   (March of Dimes Birth Defects
   Foundation) 3n
amniotic fluid abnormalities,
   overview 163–70
amniotic fluid index (AFI),
   described 164
amniotic septostomy, twin to twin
   transfusion syndrome 236
amphetamines, maternal drug use 64
androgen insensitivity syndrome
   (AIS), described 526
anemia
   defined 567
   percutaneous umbilical blood
      sampling (PUBS) 30
   premature birth 198–99
   prenatal testing 22
anencephaly
   amniocentesis 28
   defined 568
   described 41, 323
   prenatal testing 20
Anencephaly Support Foundation,
   Web site address 580
angiography, patent foramen ovale
   293
angiotensin converting enzyme
   inhibitors (ACE inhibitors), birth
   defect risks 77–78
animals
   fifth disease 132–33
   toxoplasmosis 150–51
aniridia, defined 568
annular pancreas, described 422–23

anophthalmia, defined 568
anotia, defined 568
antenatal hydronephrosis 468–69
"Antenatal Hydronephrosis" (Texas
   Pediatric Surgical Associates) 468n
antibiotic medications
   group B streptococcus 261–63, 265
   listeriosis 148–49
   pregnancy safety concerns 69
   toxoplasmosis 153
   urinary tract obstruction 483
anticholinergic medications
   cerebral palsy 376
   defined 568
antidepressant medications,
   pregnancy safety concerns 69, 78–79
antihypertensive medications,
   pregnancy 77–78
anus, defined 568
AOP *see* apnea of prematurity
aortic valve stenosis
   defined 568
   described 281
"APGAR" (A.D.A.M., Inc.) 254n
Apgar, Virginia 254
Apgar score
   cerebral palsy 367–68
   defined 568
   overview 254–56
aplasia, defined 567
apnea of prematurity (AOP)
   described 197–98
   overview 206–9
aqueductal stenosis 317
ARBD *see* alcohol-related birth
   defects
Arizona, prenatal substance abuse
   legislation 64
ARND *see* alcohol-related
   neurodevelopmental disorders
Arnold-Chiari malformation,
   described 334–35
arrhinencephaly *see*
   holoprosencephaly
arsenic, pregnancy 92
ART *see* assisted reproductive
   techniques
arteriovenous malformation (AVM),
   described 294–305

"Arteriovenous Malformation and Other Vascular Lesions of the Central Nervous System Fact Sheet" (NINDS) 294n
arthrogryposis
    defined 568
    described 532–34
ASD *see* atrial septal defect
aspartame, pregnancy safety concerns 69
asphyxia, defined 568
aspirin, pregnancy safety concerns 70
assisted reproductive techniques (ART)
    high order multiple gestations 238
    multiple births 222
    see also in vitro fertilization
Association for Retinopathy of Prematurity and Related Diseases (ROPARD), contact information 587
Association of Congenital Diaphragmatic Hernia Research, Advocacy, and Support (CHERUBS), contact information 581
asthma, pregnancy 71, 98–100
asymmetric growth restriction, described 160
ataxia, defined 568
ataxic cerebral palsy, described 363
athetoid, defined 568
athetoid cerebral palsy
    described 363
    treatment 376
atresia
    defined 568
    described 430, 448
atresia of large intestine, defined 568
atresia of small intestine, defined 568
atrial septal defect (ASD)
    defined 568
    described 283
atrioventricular canal defect (AVC defect)
    defined 571
    described 284–85
atrioventricular septal defect (AVSD), defined 571
atypical genitalia *see* ambiguous genitalia

AVC defect *see* atrioventricular canal defect
AVM *see* arteriovenous malformation
AVSD *see* atrioventricular septal defect
AZT (zidovudine), pregnancy 70

B

baclofen, described 573
bacterial vaginosis (BV), pregnancy 139
Barnes, Douglas 535–36, 537, 539, 541
behavioral disorders, maternal drug use 62
benztropine 376
beta agonists, maternal asthma 100
beta thalassemia, prenatal testing 19
bicuspid aortic valve, described 282
biliary atresia
    defined 568
    described 425–27
bili light, described 202
bilirubin
    defined 569
    jaundice 573
    kernicterus 573
biopsy
    Hirschsprung disease 457
    maternal cancer 102
biotin dependence, prenatal diagnosis 7
Birth Defect Research for Children, Inc., contact information 579
birth defects
    amniotic band syndrome 169–70
    Cesarean section 248
    coping strategies 270–71
    defined 569
    maternal diabetes mellitus 108–9
    maternal drug abuse 61–65
    maternal obesity 119–20
    maternal phenylketonuria 121–23
    oligohydramnios 165
    overview 3–9, 269–72
    polyhydramnios 166–67
    prevention 6–7, 32
    sexually transmitted diseases 137
    statistics 72

"Birth Defects" (March of Dimes
Birth Defects Foundation) 3n
"Birthmarks" (Cleveland Clinic)
559n
birthmarks, overview 559–63
bisphosphonates, defined 569
bladder exstrophy
defined 569
described 484–86
blindness
diabetes mellitus 105
retinopathy of prematurity 215
blood pressure, described 113
see also hypertension
blood sugar *see* glucose levels
blood tests
birth defect diagnosis 7
prenatal screening 27–28
prenatal testing 21–22
see also tests
blood types, Rh factor 155
blue babies, tetralogy of Fallot 285
BMI *see* body mass index
"BMI-Body Mass Index: BMI for
Adults" (CDC) 119n
body chemistry birth defects,
described 5
body mass index (BMI)
high order multiple gestations 238
pregnancy 120
botulinum toxin (Botox)
cerebral palsy 384–85
defined 569
bowel obstruction, described 448–49
BPD *see* bronchopulmonary
dysplasia
brachycephaly, described 331
bradycardia
described 206
premature birth 197–98
brain damage
fetal alcohol syndrome 53
isotretinoin 73
branchial cleft, defined 569
breast cancer, pregnancy 101
breastfeeding
isotretinoin 75
maternal cancer 103
phenylketonuria 123

breastfeeding, continued
premature birth 203
thalidomide 81
vaccinations 84
breech presentation
cerebral palsy 367
umbilical cord prolapse 178
bronchogenic cysts, described 415
bronchopulmonary dysplasia (BPD)
described 197
overview 210–14
bronchopulmonary sequestrations,
described 415, 416
bronchoscopy, cervical teratoma 551
bruit, arteriovenous malformation
295
budesonide, maternal asthma 100
bump (slang) 62
Busse, William W. 98–99
BV *see* bacterial vaginosis

C

C (slang) 62
cadmium, pregnancy 92
café-au-lait spots 562
caffeine, pregnancy 14, 36–37, 68
CAH *see* congenital adrenal
hyperplasia
calcium
food sources 35
pregnancy 34–36
Canadian Adult Congenital Heart
Network, contact information 584
cancer, diethylstilbestrol 71–72
candy (slang) 62
capillary telangiectases,
described 300
carbohydrates, food sources 35
carbon dioxide, maternal drug use 61
carbon monoxide
maternal drug use 61
maternal tobacco use 46
cardiac catheterization, patent
foramen ovale 293
"Care for the Premature Baby"
(American Pregnancy Association)
200n

Carter Centers for Research in Holoprosencephaly contact information 585
casts, clubfoot 539–40
cataracts, defined 569
cat feces, toxoplasmosis 14, 37, 70
CAT scan *see* computed tomography
cavernous hemangiomas 560
cavernous malformations, described 300
CCAM *see* cystic adenomatoid malformations
CDC *see* Centers for Disease Control and Prevention
CDH *see* congenital diaphragmatic hernia
cebocephaly 325
Center for Fetal Diagnosis and Treatment, contact information 583
Center for Study of Multiple Birth (CSMB), contact information 586
Centers for Disease Control and Prevention (CDC), publications
  diabetes, pregnancy 104n
  folic acid 39n
  group B streptococcal disease 260n
  maternal obesity 119n
central line, premature birth 202
cephalic disorders, overview 322–32
"Cephalic Disorders Fact Sheet" (NINDS) 322n
cereals, folic acid 42
cerebral, defined 569
cerebral dysgenesis, defined 569
cerebral palsy
  acquired, defined 567
  botulinum toxin 384–85
  congenital, defined 570
  hyperbaric oxygen therapy 386–91
  hypothermia 391–93
  overview 360–83
  see also spastic diplegia; spastic hemiplegia; spastic quadriplegia
"Cerebral Palsy: Hope Through Research" (NINDS) 360n, 567n
cerebrospinal fluid (CSF), hydrocephalus 316–21

cervical cancer
  pregnancy 102
  prenatal testing 22
  prenatal tests 18
cervical teratoma, described 550–52
cervical tests, prenatal testing 22
Cesarean section
  group B streptococcus 264
  multiple gestations 226
  overview 246–48
Chang, Benjamin 49–50
CHD *see* congenital heart disease
chemicals, pregnancy 89–96
chemodenervation, defined 569
chemotherapy
  maternal cancer 102–3
  pregnancy safety concerns 69
CHERUBS *see* Association of Congenital Diaphragmatic Hernia Research, Advocacy, and Support
Chiari malformation
  described 334–35
  spina bifida 398
"Chiari Malformation Information Page" (NINDS) 334n
chickenpox *see* varicella
childbirth education classes, pregnancy 14
Children's Craniofacial Association
  contact information 581
  publications
    facial palsy 347n
    fibrous dysplasia 546n
Children's Hospital of Philadelphia, publications
  spina bifida surgery 407n
  tobacco use during pregnancy 45n
Children's Memorial Hospital of Chicago, multicystic dysplastic kidney publication 470n
Children's Neurobiological Solutions Foundation (CNS Foundation), contact information 581
C.H.I.N. *see* Congenital Heart Information Network
chlamydia, pregnancy 137–38
chlorinated drinking water, pregnancy 94
choanal atresia, defined 569

choanal stenosis, defined 569
choreoathetoid, defined 569
chorionic villus sampling (CVS)
    birth defect diagnosis 7
    prenatal testing 26–27
chromosomal birth defects,
    described 3–4
chromosomal disorders
    described 527
    prenatal testing 20
chromosomes
    birth defects 3–4
    Down syndrome 570
    mosaic, defined 574
    trisomy, defined 577
chronic cerebellar stimulation,
    cerebral palsy 377
chronic hypertension, described 113,
    114
cigarette smoking *see* tobacco use
Cipro (ciprofloxacin), pregnancy
    safety concerns 69
ciprofloxacin, pregnancy safety
    concerns 69
Claravis (isotretinoin), birth defects
    4, 72
cleaning products, pregnancy 94–95
cleft lip
    defined 569
    overview 340–47
"Cleft Lip and Palate" (Nemours
    Foundation) 340n
Cleft Lip and Palate Association,
    contact information 582
cleft palate
    defined 569
    overview 340–47
clefts
    amniotic band syndrome 170
    described 5
    holoprosencephaly 325
    isotretinoin 73
cleft spine *see* spina bifida
Cleveland Clinic, publications
    birthmarks 559n
    patent foramen ovale 290n
cloacal exstrophy
    described 523–25
    omphalocele 442

Clomiphene 238
closed neural tube defects,
    described 396–97
clubfoot, described 534–41
CMV *see* cytomegalovirus
CNS Foundation *see* Children's
    Neurobiological Solutions
    Foundation
coarctation of aorta
    defined 569
    described 281–82
cocaine, maternal drug use 62–63
coke (slang) 62
Collaborative on Health and the
    Environment, contact information
    582
colon, described 448
    see also large intestine; rectum
colostomy
    defined 570
    Hirschsprung disease 457–59
colpocephaly, described 324
communicating hydrocephalus,
    described 317
Compazine (prochlorperazine),
    pregnancy safety concerns 69
computed tomography (CAT scan;
    CT scan)
    cerebral palsy 371
    defined 570
    ectopic ureter 491
    hydrocephalus 319
    lissencephaly 327
    porencephaly 329
    urachal anomalies 506
    ureterocele 500
congenital, described 430, 519
congenital adrenal hyperplasia
    (CAH)
    described 527
    newborn screening 258
congenital amputation, described
    542–44
"Congenital Cardiovascular Defects"
    (American Heart Association) 276n
congenital cardiovascular defects,
    overview 279–90
congenital cerebral palsy,
    defined 570

congenital diaphragmatic hernia
(CDH)
    fetal surgery 435–37
    overview 432–35
    sacrococcygeal teratoma 554–55
"Congenital Diaphragmatic Hernia:
    Learn More" (University of
    California) 432n
"Congenital Diaphragmatic Hernia:
    Treatments" (University of
    California) 435n
congenital heart disease (CHD),
    described 276–78
Congenital Heart Information
    Network (C.H.I.N.), contact
    information 584
congenital hydrocephalus,
    described 317
congenital lung lesions,
    overview 415–20
"Congenital Malformations of the
    Female Reproductive Tract: Vaginal
    Agenesis/Hypoplasia" (Kawar) 519n
congenital nevi 561–62
"Congenital Rubella"
    (A.D.A.M., Inc.) 134n
congenital rubella, described 134–36
"Congenital Torticollis" (Johnson) 544n
congenital torticollis, described
    544–46
Conjoined Twins International
    (CTI), contact information 586
continuous positive airway pressure
    (CPAP)
    apnea of prematurity 207–8
    premature birth 201
contractions, premature labor 194–95
contraction stress test, described 30
contracture
    defined 570
    described 532
cord accident, described 180
corticosteroids
    maternal asthma 99–100
    placental previa 174
    premature labor 195
cortisone
    birthmarks 561
    pregnancy safety concerns 69

counseling
    ambiguous genitalia 528
    congenital heart disease 278
    substance abuse 65
    vaginal agenesis 523
CPAP *see* continuous positive
    airway pressure
crack (slang) 62
craniosynostosis
    defined 570
    described 336–37
"Craniosynostosis" (NINDS) 336n
cromolyn, maternal asthma 100
crossed renal ectopia 467
cryotherapy, retinopathy of
    prematurity 217
CSF *see* cerebrospinal fluid
CSMB *see* Center for Study of
    Multiple Birth
CTI *see* Conjoined Twins
    International
CT scan *see* computed tomography
CVS *see* chorionic villus sampling
cyanotic defects, described 285–89
cyclopia, described 325
cystic adenomatoid malformations
    (CCAM), described 415, 416
cystic fibrosis, prenatal testing 19, 22
cystoscopy, urachal anomalies 506
cysts, umbilical cord 180–81
cytokines, defined 570
cytomegalovirus (CMV)
    birth defects 4
    pregnancy 143–46

D

D'Alessandro, Donna 510n
Dandy-Walker malformation
    defined 570
    described 337–38
"Dandy-Walker Syndrome
    Information Page" (NINDS) 337n
dental care, clefts 343–44
DES *see* diethylstilbestrol
developmental delays
    defined 570
    maternal drug use 62

"Diabetes and Pregnancy: Frequently
    Asked Questions" (CDC) 104n
diabetes mellitus
    neural tube defects 41
    pregnancy 71, 104–13
    see also gestational diabetes
diabetic coma, described 105–6
diaphragm, described 432
diaphragmatic hernia, defined 570
diarrhea, defined 570
diastolic pressure, described 113
diet and nutrition
    folic acid 42
    Hirschsprung disease 459–60
    listeriosis 149–50
    maternal phenylketonuria 121–23
    mercury 91
    pregnancy 33–39
    prenatal care 13, 14
dietary guidelines, pregnancy 34–36
diethylstilbestrol (DES), pregnancy
    safety concerns 70, 71–72
Diflucan (fluconazole), pregnancy
    safety concerns 69
digestive system
    pregnancy 38
    premature birth 198
digit anomalies
    amniotic band syndrome 169–70
    maternal tobacco use 49–50
Dilantin (phenytoin), pregnancy
    safety concerns 69
disuse atrophy, defined 570
"Does a Parent's Age Increase Risk of
    Conceiving Child with Oral Clefts?"
    (NIDCR) 340n
Dombrowski, Mitchell 99
dominant gene disorders, prenatal
    testing 19
"Do Multivitamin Supplements
    Reduce the Risk for Diabetes-
    Associated Birth Defects?"
    (CDC) 104n
Doppler ultrasound *see* ultrasound
Down syndrome
    amniocentesis 28
    blood tests 27–28
    chorionic villus sampling 27
    defined 570

drug abuse
    placenta previa 174
    preconception counseling 7
    pregnancy 4, 61–65
    prenatal care 13, 14
dTGA *see* transposition of great
    arteries
duodenum, described 448
dyskinetic, defined 571
dyskinetic cerebral palsy,
    described 363
dysphagia, vascular rings 313
dysplasia
    defined 571
    described 210
dystonia, defined 571

E

"Eating During Pregnancy"
    (Nemours Foundation) 33n
Ebstein anomaly
    defined 571
    described 282–83
ECD *see* endocardial cushion defect
ECG *see* electrocardiogram
Echinacea 71
echocardiogram
    congenital heart disease 276–78
    patent foramen ovale 292
echogram *see* ultrasound
eclampsia, described 115
ECMO *see* extracorporeal membrane
    oxygenation
ectopic kidneys, described 466–67
ectopic pregnancy, sexually
    transmitted diseases 137
ectopic ureter, described 489–93
Edwards syndrome 325
EEG *see* electroencephalogram
Eisenmenger complex,
    described 284
EKG *see* electrocardiogram
electrocardiogram (ECG; EKG),
    patent foramen ovale 292
electroencephalogram (EEG)
    cerebral palsy 371
    defined 571

electromyography, defined 571
encephalocele, defined 571
endocardial cushion defect (ECD),
    defined 571
endocarditis, cardiovascular defects
    281–90
endoscopy
    fetal surgery 184–85
    twin to twin transfusion s
        yndrome 233
enterocolitis, defined 571
environmental factors
    birth defects 4
    digit anomalies 50
    pregnancy 89–96
"Environmental Risks and
    Pregnancy" (March of
    Dimes Birth Defects
    Foundation) 89n
environmental tobacco smoke,
    pregnancy 47
epilepsy, cerebral palsy 364
epispadias, described 487–88
erythema infectiosum *see* fifth
    disease
esophageal atresia
    defined 571
    described 430–31
esophagus, described 430
estriol, maternal blood screening 27
ethmocephaly, described 325
ethnic factors
    digit anomalies 50
    neural tube defects 41
etretinate, pregnancy safety
    concerns 70, 75
exchange transfusions, Rh
    incompatibility 157
exencephaly, described 330
exomphalos *see* omphalocele
extracorporeal membrane
    oxygenation (ECMO)
    congenital diaphragmatic
        hernia 433
    persistent pulmonary
        hypertension of newborn
        309–10
extra-large babies, diabetes
    mellitus 109–10

F

facial features, fetal alcohol
    syndrome 53
facial palsy, described 347–51
FAE *see* fetal alcohol effects
failure to thrive
    cerebral palsy 364
    defined 571
famotidine, pregnancy safety
    concerns 69
FAS *see* fetal alcohol syndrome
FASD *see* fetal alcohol spectrum
    disorders
FDA *see* US Food and Drug
    Administration
"FDA Advising of Risk of Birth
    Defects with Paxil" (FDA) 78n
feeding methods, premature birth
    201–2
feeding tubes, bronchopulmonary
    dysplasia 212
fertility
    age factor 16
    ambiguous genitalia 528
    maternal cancer 104
    phenylketonuria 123
    see also in vitro fertilization
fetal alcohol effects (FAE),
    described 53
    see also alcohol-related birth
        defects; alcohol-related
        neurodevelopmental disorders
fetal alcohol spectrum disorders
    (FASD), lifespan implications 56–59
fetal alcohol syndrome (FAS),
    overview 52–59
"Fetal Alcohol Syndrome" (NWHIC)
    52n
Fetal Alcohol Syndrome Prevention
    Section, contact information 582
Fetal Care Center of Cincinnati,
    contact information 583
fetal distress, Cesarean section 247
"Fetal Echocardiography" (American
    Heart Association) 276n
fetal echocardiography, congenital
    heart defects 276–78

fetal growth restriction, described 160–62

"Fetal Growth Restriction: Intrauterine Growth Restriction (IUGR); Small for Gestational Age" (American Pregnancy Association) 160n

fetal image-guided surgery (FIGS-IT), described 185–86, *187*

fetal intervention, described 183–87

"Fetal Multicystic Dysplastic Kidney (Children's Memorial Hospital of Chicago) 470n

fetal nerve damage, alcohol use 54–55

fetal surgery
  congenital diaphragmatic hernia 435–37
  overview 183–87
  sacrococcygeal teratoma 556–57
  spina bifida 407–9
  twin to twin transfusion syndrome 232–36
  urinary tract obstruction 480–83

"Fetal Surgery for Spina Bifida Shows Early Benefits in Leg Function, Fewer Shunts" (Children's Hospital of Philadelphia) 407n

Fetal Treatment Center, contact information 583

Fetal Treatment Program *see* University of California

fetal tumors, birth defects 550–57

Fetendo fetal surgery
  depicted *185*
  described 184–85

fiber consumption, pregnancy 38

fibrous dysplasia, described 546–48

fifth disease, pregnancy 130–33

"Fifth Disease (Parvovirus B19) and Pregnancy" (OTIS) 130n

FIGS-IT *see* fetal image-guided surgery

financial considerations
  multivitamins 43
  neural tube defects 41–42
  prenatal care 16–17

fingers, maternal tobacco use 49–50

fish, pregnancy 37–38

fistula
  defined 571
  described 430

flake (slang) 62

Florida, prenatal substance abuse legislation 65

flu *see* influenza

fluconazole, pregnancy safety concerns 69

FluMist 83

focal seizure, defined 571

folic acid
  food sources *35*
  neural tube defects prevention 20
  overview 39–44
  preconception counseling 6–7
  pregnancy safety concerns 69
  prenatal care 13
  recommendations 14–15, 34, 42
  spina bifida 401

follicle-stimulating medications 240

Fontan procedure
  hypoplastic left heart syndrome 289
  pulmonary atresia 288

Food and Drug Administration (FDA) *see* US Food and Drug Administration

food cravings, pregnancy 36

food labels, pregnancy 34–36

food safety, pregnancy 147

foscarnet 145

"Frequently Asked Questions Concerning Thalidomide" (FDA) 80n

Freud, Sigmund 360

G

gait analysis, defined 572

galactosemia, newborn screening 257

Gale Encyclopedia of Medicine 425n, 542n

ganciclovir 145–46

ganglion cells, defined 572

gastroesophageal reflux disease (GERD), defined 572

gastrointestinal system
   birth defects 430–63
   premature birth 198
gastroschisis
   defined 572
   overview 437–41
gastrostomy, defined 572
GBS *see* group B streptococcus
genes
   birth defects 3, 272
   phenylketonuria 123
genetic counseling
   hereditary birth defects 21
   prenatal birth defects diagnosis 8
   prenatal testing 31
genital herpes, pregnancy 140
genital warts, pregnancy 140–41
GERD *see* gastroesophageal reflux
   disease
German measles *see* rubella
gestation, defined 572
gestational diabetes
   described 105, 106–7
   glucose screening 25
   prenatal testing 22
   prenatal tests 18
gestational hypertension, described
   113, 114–18
   see also hypertension; preeclampsia
gingko biloba 71
"Glossary of Selected Birth Defects
   Terms" (Massachusetts Department
   of Public Health) 567n
glucose levels
   diabetes mellitus 105–13
   prenatal testing 25–26
glycol ethers, pregnancy 94
"Goldenhar Syndrome" (Mayfield) 351n
Goldenhar syndrome, described 351–
   52
Goldenhar Syndrome Support
   Network, contact information 584
gonorrhea, pregnancy 138
grass (slang) 61
"Group B Strep Disease: Frequently
   Asked Questions" (CDC) 260n
group B streptococcus (GBS)
   overview 260–65
   prenatal testing 22

growth problems, cerebral palsy
   364–65
growth retardation, fetal alcohol
   syndrome 53
Guardians of Hydrocephalus
   Research Foundation, contact
   information 585
"A Guide to Understanding Facial
   Palsy" (Children's Craniofacial
   Association) 347n
"A Guide to Understanding Fibrous
   Dysplasia" (Children's Craniofacial
   Association) 546n

H

hallucinogens, maternal drug
   abuse 63–64
HBOT *see* hyperbaric oxygen
   therapy
health care team
   birth defects 271–72
   cerebral palsy 372–73
   clefts 342–43
   premature birth 202–3
   prenatal testing 31–32
hearing impairment
   cerebral palsy 365
   newborn screening 258
heartburn *see* gastroesophageal
   reflux disease
heart defects
   isotretinoin 73
   omphalocele 441
   overview 276–89
   Paxil 79
heart disorders
   diabetes mellitus 105
   prenatal diagnosis 8
   statistics 5
heavy drinking, described 55
Hecht, Jacqueline 537
HELLP (hemolysis, elevated liver
   enzymes, low platelet count)
   syndrome 116–17
"Help for Patients with Clubfoot"
   (Shriners Hospitals for Children)
   534n

hemianopia
  cerebral palsy 365
  defined 572
"Hemifacial Microsomia"
  (Mayfield) 353n
hemifacial microsomia, described
  353–54
hemiparesis, defined 572
hepatitis B virus
  newborn infections 266–68
  prenatal testing 22
Hepatitis C Support Project,
  hepatitis B prevention
  publication 260n
herbal remedies
  preconception counseling 7
  pregnancy 68, 71
  prenatal care 13
heredity
  amniocentesis 28
  birth defects 4–5
  bronchopulmonary dysplasia 211
  diabetes mellitus 106, 107
  Hirschsprung disease 455–56
  phenylketonuria 123
  preeclampsia 117
  Rh factor 155
heroin, maternal drug use 63
heterotaxy, defined 572
high blood pressure *see* hypertension
"High Blood Pressure During
  Pregnancy" (March of Dimes
  Birth Defects Foundation) 113n
Hirschsprung disease
  defined 572
  overview 454–61
HIV *see* human immunodeficiency
  virus
HLHS *see* hypoplastic left heart
  syndrome
holoprosencephaly
  defined 572
  described 324–25
horse (slang) 63
horseshoe kidney *see* renal fusion
hot tubs
  neural tube defects 41
  pregnancy 14
H-stuff (slang) 63

human chorionic gonadotropin
  (HCG), maternal blood screening 27
human immunodeficiency virus (HIV)
  pregnancy 70–71, 141
  prenatal testing 22
  thalidomide 81
Huntington disease, prenatal
  testing 19
Huth, Lindsay 510n
hyaline membrane disease,
  bronchopulmonary dysplasia 211
hydranencephaly, described 325–26
hydroceles, described 514–16
hydrocephalus
  defined 572
  described 41
  labor and delivery 251
  overview 316–21
Hydrocephalus Association, contact
  information 585
"Hydrocephalus Fact Sheet" (NINDS)
  316n
Hydrocephalus Support Group, Inc.,
  contact information 585
hydronephrosis
  defined 572
  described 468–69
  ectopic ureter 490
hyperbaric oxygen therapy (HBOT),
  cerebral palsy 386–91
"Hyperbaric Oxygen Therapy for
  Brain Injury, Cerebral Palsy, and
  Stroke" (AHRQ) 386n
hyperplasia, defined 572
hypertension (high blood pressure)
  diabetes mellitus 105, 108
  maternal asthma 99
  pregnancy 71, 113–19
  see also persistent pulmonary
    hypertension of newborn
hypertonia, defined 572
hypertrophy, defined 572
hypoglycemia
  described 105–6
  maternal drug abuse 63
hypoplasia
  defined 573
  described 519
  urinary tract obstruction 478

hypoplastic left heart syndrome
(HLHS)
defined 573
described 289–90
hypospadias
defined 573
described 512–13
hypothermia, cerebral palsy
prevention 391–93
"Hypothermia in Newborn Infants"
(United Cerebral Palsy Research
and Education Foundation) 391n
hypothyroidism, newborn
screening 257
hypotonia, defined 573
hypoxic-ischemic encephalopathy
defined 573
described 366

I

ibuprofen, pregnancy safety
concerns 69
IFFGD *see* International Foundation
for Functional Gastrointestinal
Disorders, Inc.
ileostomy
defined 573
Hirschsprung disease 457–59
ileum, described 448
illicit drugs *see* drug abuse
Illinois, prenatal substance abuse
legislation 64, 65
immunity
fifth disease 131
prenatal testing 18, 22
rubella 134, 136
varicella 128–30
imperforate anus, described
462–63, 568
imperforation, defined 568
inactivated vaccine, described 81
incubators, described 202
Indiana, prenatal substance
abuse legislation 65
infections
amniocentesis 29
birth defects 4

infections, continued
bronchopulmonary dysplasia 213
cerebral palsy 366
hepatitis B 266–68
Hirschsprung disease 460
premature birth 198
prenatal testing 22
streptococcal disease 260–65
see also sexually transmitted
diseases
"Infertility Treatment and
Multiple-Gestation Pregnancy"
(RESOLVE: The National
Infertility Association) 236n
influenza, vaccines 83
inguinal hernias, described 514–16
iniencephaly, described 326
insulin
diabetes mellitus 105, 110
pregnancy safety concerns 69
intercalary limb deficiency, defined
573
International Birth Defects
Information Systems, Web site
address 579
International Foundation for
Functional Gastrointestinal
Disorders, Inc. (IUFFGD), contact
information 584
International Vasa Previa
Foundation, Inc., contact
information 587
intestinal malrotation, overview
450–54
intestines *see* colon; large intestine;
small intestine
intracranial hemorrhage, defined
573
intrapartum asphyxia, defined 573
intrathecal baclofen, defined 573
intrauterine growth restriction
(IUGR) *see* fetal growth
restriction
intrauterine infection, described
575
intravenous pyelogram (IVP)
ectopic ureter 490–91
megaureter 496
vesicoureteral reflux 503

intraventricular hemorrhage (IVH),
premature birth 198
in vitro fertilization (IVF)
high order multiple gestations
238, 240–41
multiple births 222–23
see also assisted reproductive
techniques
Iowa, prenatal substance abuse
legislation 64
iPLEDGE program 74
iron, food sources 35
isotretinoin, birth defects 4, 72–76
IUGR (intrauterine growth
restriction) see fetal growth
restriction
IVF see in vitro fertilization
IVH see intraventricular
hemorrhage
IVP see intravenous pyelogram

J

jaundice
biliary atresia 426
bili light 202
cerebral palsy 366, 369
defined 573
kernicterus 573
premature birth 198, 250
jejunum, described 448
Johnson, Mark 407–8
Johnson, T. R. 544n
junk (slang) 63

K

kangaroo care, described 203
Kawar, Nada 519n
kernicterus, defined 573
kidney disorders
birth defects 466–75
diabetes mellitus 105
tests 473–75
kidneys, described 466
Kinzer, Susan 510n
kyphosis, defined 573

L

labor and delivery
asphyxia 366–67
fetal health problems 249–52
preeclampsia 115–17
sexually transmitted diseases 137,
140–41
umbilical cord abnormalities 177
umbilical cord knots 180
see also premature labor
lactose intolerance, calcium
supplements 36
Ladd bands 451
laparoschisis see gastroschisis
large intestine
defined 573
depicted 455
described 448
see also colon; rectum
Larsen, Jeffrey P. 542n
laryngoscopy, cervical teratoma 551
laser therapy
retinopathy of prematurity 217
twin to twin transfusion syndrome
233–36
latex allergy, spina bifida 41, 405–7
"Latex (Natural Rubber) Allergy in
Spina Bifida" (Spina Bifida
Association) 405n
lead exposure, pregnancy 89–91
learning disabilities
maternal drug abuse 62
maternal drug use 62
spina bifida 41
leukomalacia, described 575
leukotriene receptor antagonists,
maternal asthma 100
limb deficiency, defined 573
lissencephaly, described 326–27
Listeria monocytogenes 147–50
listeriosis, pregnancy 37, 147–50
lithium, pregnancy safety
concerns 69
Little, William 360, 362
Little Hearts, Inc., contact
information 585
liver disorders, biliary atresia 425–27

live vaccine, described 81
lobar holoprosencephaly 324
longitudinal limb deficiency,
  defined 573
long-segment Hirschsprung
  disease 460–61
lordosis, defined 574
low birth weight
  bronchopulmonary dysplasia 211
  cerebral palsy 368, 381
  maternal asthma 99
  maternal diabetes mellitus 110
  maternal drug abuse 63, 64
  maternal drug use 62
  maternal tobacco use 46
lower limb deficiency, defined 573
LSD, maternal drug use 63–64
lumbar puncture, persistent
  pulmonary hypertension of
  newborn 309
lung disorders
  congenital lung lesions 415–20
  maternal tobacco use 48
  premature birth 196–97, 201,
    206–14, 251–52

M

macrocephaly
  defined 574
  described 330
magnesium sulfate, premature labor 195
magnetic resonance imaging (MRI)
  cerebral palsy 371
  cervical teratoma 550
  defined 574
  hydrocephalus 319
  lissencephaly 327
  maternal cancer 102
  patent foramen ovale 293
  porencephaly 329
  twin to twin transfusion
    syndrome 234
  ureterocele 500
"Major Congenital Malformations
  after First-Trimester Exposure to
  ACE Inhibitors" (Massachusetts
  Medical Society) 77n

malrotation, described 450–51
Man, Li-Xing 49
Management of Meningocele
  Study (MOMS), contact
  information 587
manometry, Hirschsprung
  disease 457
March of Dimes Birth Defects
  Foundation
  contact information 579
  publications
    amniotic fluid abnormalities 3n
    birth defects overview 3n
    environmental risks, pregnancy
      89n
    high blood pressure, pregnancy
      113n
    multiple births 222n
marijuana, maternal drug use
  61–62
Maryland, prenatal substance
  abuse legislation 65
Massachusetts, prenatal substance
  abuse legislation 64
Massachusetts Department of
  Public Health, glossary of terms
  publication 567n
Massachusetts Medical Society, ACE
  inhibitors publication 77n
Material Safety Data Sheets 94
maternal asthma, overview 98–100
maternal diabetes mellitus,
  overview 104–13
maternal obesity, birth defects
  119–20
"Maternal Obesity and Risk for
  Birth Defects" (CDC) 119n
maternal PKU effects, described 121
maternal serum alpha fetoprotein
  (MSAFP) 398–99
Mayfield, Lynn 351n, 353n, 355n,
  357n
McCune-Albright syndrome,
  described 547
MCDK *see* multicystic dysplastic
  kidney
mechanical aids, cerebral palsy 378
meconium aspiration, described 249,
  251

medications
  apnea of prematurity 208
  birth defects 4
  bronchopulmonary dysplasia 213
  cerebral palsy 376
  HELLP syndrome 116
  maternal asthma 98–100
  multiple gestations 240–41
  neural tube defects 41
  pregnancy 68–81, 69–70
  premature labor 195
  prenatal care 14
megalencephaly, described 327–28
megaureter, described 494–97
men, vaccinations 84
meninges, defined 574
meningitis, group B streptococcus
  260–61
meningocele, described 397, 577
mental retardation, isotretinoin 73
mercury, pregnancy 37–38, 91–92
Merritt, Diane F. 519n
metabolic disorders
  amniocentesis 28
  described 5
methylmalonic academia, prenatal
  diagnosis 7
Michigan, prenatal substance
  abuse legislation 64
micrencephaly, described 330
microcephaly
  cerebral palsy 368
  defined 574
  described 328
microphthalmia, defined 574
microtia
  defined 574
  described 355–56
"Microtia" (Mayfield) 353n
Mills, James L. 55
Minnesota, prenatal substance
  abuse legislation 64, 65
miscarriage
  amniocentesis 29
  diabetes mellitus 71
  maternal cancer 102
  maternal drug abuse 62, 64
  multiple gestations 242
  sexually transmitted diseases 137

moles 561–63
MOMS *see* Management of
  Meningocele Study
Mongolian spots 561
monitors, apnea of prematurity
  208–9
monostotic disease, described 547
mosaic, defined 574
Mothers of Omphaloceles, Web site
  address 584
Motrin (ibuprofen), pregnancy safety
  concerns 69
MRI *see* magnetic resonance imaging
MSAFP *see* maternal serum alpha
  fetoprotein
multicystic dysplastic kidney
  (MCDK), described 470–71
multifactorial birth defects,
  described 4–5
multifactorial disorders, prenatal
  testing 20
multifetal reduction, multiple
  gestations 242–43
multiple births
  cerebral palsy 368
  Cesarean section 247
  overview 222–44
multiple gestation, described 222
"Multiples: Twins, Triplets and
  Beyond" (March of Dimes Birth
  Defects Foundation) 222n
multivitamins
  diabetes-associated birth defects
    112–13
  folic acid 42, 43
  preconception counseling 6
  prenatal care 12, 13
myelomeningocele, described 397, 577

N

National Birth Defects Prevention
  Network, Web site address 580
National Center on Birth Defects and
  Developmental Disabilities, contact
  information 580
National Craniofacial Association,
  contact information 582

National Dissemination Center for
Children with Disabilities
(NICHCY), contact information 580
National Eye Institute (NEI), contact
information 587
National Heart, Lung, and Blood
Institute (NHLBI), maternal
asthma publication 98n
National Hydrocephalus Foundation,
contact information 585
National Institute of Child Health
and Human Development (NICHD),
contact information 580
National Institute of Dental and
Craniofacial Research (NIDCR),
clefts publication 340n
National Institute of Diabetes and
Digestive and Kidney Diseases
(NIDDK)
contact information 587
Hirschsprung disease publication
454n
National Institute of Environmental
Health Sciences (NIEHS),
toxoplasmosis, pregnancy
publication 150n
National Institute of Neurological
Disorders and Stroke (NINDS),
publications
agenesis of corpus callosum 333n
arteriovenous malformations 294n
cephalic disorders 322n
cerebral palsy 360n, 567n
Chiari malformation 334n
craniosynostosis 336n
Dandy-Walker syndrome 337n
hydrocephalus 316n
spina bifida 396n
National Institute on Alcohol Abuse
and Alcoholism (NIAAA), contact
information 582
National Institutes of Health
(NIH), publications
cerebral palsy 567n
fetal damage with maternal
alcohol use 54n
Hirschsprung disease 567n
National Kidney Foundation, contact
information 586

National Organization for Rare
Disorders (NORD), contact
information 580
National Organization on Fetal
Alcohol Syndrome
contact information 583
fetal alcohol syndrome
publication 56n
National Women's Health
Information Center (NWHIC),
publications
fetal alcohol syndrome 52n
medications, pregnancy 68n
prenatal care 12n
nausea, pregnancy 38
NEI *see* National Eye Institute
Nemours Foundation
publications
birth defects 269n
cleft lip and palate 340n
diet and nutrition during
pregnancy 33n
newborn health problems 249n
prenatal tests 17n
Rh incompatibility 155n
Web site address 580
neonatal intensive care unit (NICU)
overview 200–204
persistent pulmonary hypertension
of newborn 309
nephrectomy
ectopic ureter 491–92
ureterocele 501
nerve cells, defined 574
nerve damage
diabetes mellitus 105, 110
thalidomide 81
nerve entrapment, defined 574
neural tube defects (NTD)
defined 574
described 40–42
folic acid 34
prenatal testing 20
neuronal migration, defined 574
neuroprotective, defined 574
neurotrophins, defined 574
Nevada, prenatal substance abuse
legislation 65
newborn scoring *see* Apgar score

"New Study Finds Babies Born to Mothers Who Drink Alcohol Heavily May Suffer Permanent Nerve Damage" (NIH) 54n
"New Treatment Guidelines for Pregnant Women with Asthma: Monitoring and Managing Asthma Important for Healthy Mother and Baby" (NHLBI) 98n
NHLBI *see* National Heart, Lung, and Blood Institute
NIAAA *see* National Institute on Alcohol Abuse and Alcoholism
NICHCY *see* National Dissemination Center for Children with Disabilities
NICHD *see* National Institute of Child Health and Human Development
nicotine, maternal tobacco use 46
see also smoking cessation; tobacco use
NICU *see* neonatal intensive care unit
NIDCR *see* National Institute of Dental and Craniofacial Research
NIDDK *see* National Institute of Diabetes and Digestive and Kidney Diseases
NIEHS *see* National Institute of Environmental Health Sciences
NINDS *see* National Institute of Neurological Disorders and Stroke
nitrous oxide
congenital diaphragmatic hernia 433
persistent pulmonary hypertension of newborn 309
noncommunicating hydrocephalus, described 317
nonstress test (NST), prenatal screening 29–30
NORD *see* National Organization for Rare Disorders
North Dakota, prenatal substance abuse legislation 64
Novarel 240
NST *see* nonstress test
NTD *see* neural tube defect

nuchal loops, described 179–80
nuclear scans, vesicoureteral reflux 503
nutrients
food sources 35
pregnancy 34–36
see also diet and nutrition
NWHIC *see* National Women's Health Information Center

O

obesity
diabetes mellitus 106
neural tube defects 41
pregnancy 119–20
obstructive genitourinary defect, defined 575
occupational therapy, cerebral palsy 373
off-label drugs, defined 575
Ohio, prenatal substance abuse legislation 65
oligohydramnios
described 163–66, 180
multiple gestations 228
omphalocele
defined 575
overview 441–45
open fetal surgery, described 184
oral clefting *see* clefts
organic solvents, pregnancy 93–94
Organization of Teratology Information Services (OTIS)
contact information 582
publications
Accutane 72n
fifth disease, pregnancy 130n
maternal phenylketonuria 121n
vaccines, pregnancy 82n
orthotic devices, defined 575
osteopenia, defined 575
ostomy
defined 575
Hirschsprung disease 457–59
OTIS *see* Organization of Teratology Information Services
otocephaly, described 331

Otsuka, Norman 534n
ovarian cancer, pregnancy 102
"Overview of Bowel Obstruction"
    (University of California) 448n
overweight, preeclampsia 117
Ovidrel 240
oxycephaly, described 331
oxygen hood, premature birth 201
oxygen shortage, cerebral palsy
    366–67
oxytocin 30

P

pain medications, pregnancy
    safety concerns 70
palsy, defined 575
pancreas
    annular pancreas 422–23
    diabetes mellitus 105
pancreas divisum, described 424–25
Pap tests
    maternal cancer 102
    prenatal testing 22
paresis, defined 575
paroxetine, birth defect risks 78–79
partial seizure, defined 571
parvovirus B19 see fifth disease
Patau syndrome 325
patent ductus arteriosus (PDA)
    defined 575
    described 199, 280
patent foramen ovale (PFO)
    depicted *291*
    described 290–94
"Patent Foramen Ovale (PFO)"
    (Cleveland Clinic) 290n
Paxil (paroxetine), birth defect risks
    78–79
PCOS see polycystic ovarian
    syndrome
PCP, maternal drug use 63–64
PDA see patent ductus arteriosus
*Pediatric Common Questions, Quick
    Answers* (D'Alessandro, et al.) 510n
peel, described 443
pelvic infection, described 575
pentalogy of Cantrell 441–42

Pepcid (famotidine), pregnancy
    safety concerns 69
percutaneous umbilical blood
    sampling (PUBS), prenatal
    screening 30–31
peri, described 575
peripheral nervous system, alcohol
    use 54
peripheral neuropathy, alcohol use 55
periventricular leukomalacia (PVL),
    defined 575
persistent pulmonary hypertension of
    newborn (PPHN), overview 305–10
pesticides, pregnancy 93
pets
    fifth disease 132–33
    toxoplasmosis 14, 37, 70, 150–51
    see also animals
PFO see patent foramen ovale
Phe see phenylalanine
phenylalanine (Phe) 121
phenylketonuria (PKU)
    newborn screening 257
    pregnancy 121–25
phenytoin, pregnancy safety
    concerns 69
physical therapy
    arthrogryposis 533
    cerebral palsy 372, 373–76
pica, described 36
PICC line see central line
Pierre Robin Network, contact
    information 582
"Pierre Robin Sequence" (Mayfield)
    357n
Pierre Robin sequence, described
    357–58
pigmented birthmarks, described
    561–62
Pitocin (oxytocin) 30
PKU see phenylketonuria
placenta
    defined 576
    described 171
    maternal cancer 102–3
    maternal drug abuse 62, 63
    maternal tobacco use 46
    twin to twin transfusion 228–30
placenta accreta, described 174–75

placental abruption
Cesarean section 247
described 171–73, 180
hypertension 115
maternal drug abuse 62, 64
placental disorders, overview 171–76
placenta previa
Cesarean section 247
described 173–74
plagiocephaly, described 331
plegia, defined 575
pneumonia
bronchopulmonary dysplasia 211
premature birth 197
Polsdorfer, J. Ricker 425n
polycystic ovarian syndrome (PCOS),
multiple gestations 238
polydactyly
defined 576
maternal tobacco use 50
polyhydramnios
birth defects 166–67
multiple gestations 228
sacrococcygeal teratoma 553
twin to twin transfusion syndrome
233–34
polyostotic disease, described 547
porencephaly, described 328–29
port-wine stains 560
positional clubfoot, described 537
postconceptual age, apnea of
prematurity 209
post-impairment syndrome,
defined 576
pot (slang) 61
PPHN *see* persistent pulmonary
hypertension of newborn
PPROM *see* preterm premature
rupture of membranes
preconception counseling,
described 6
prednisone, pregnancy safety
concerns 69
preeclampsia
described 114–18
maternal asthma 99
multiple gestations 224
prenatal testing 22
preemie *see* premature birth

pregnancy
angiotensin converting enzyme
inhibitors 77–78
chemicals 89–96
chickenpox 128–30
constipation 38
cytomegalovirus 143–46
diabetes 104–13
fifth disease 130–33
folic acid recommendations 14–15,
39–44
food avoidance 37
hot tubs 14, 41
hypertension 113–18
isotretinoin 4, 70, 72–76
listeriosis 147–50
maternal hypertension 113–19
medication use 68–81
nausea 38
normal length 192
obesity 119–20
phenylketonuria 121–25
rubella 134–36
saunas 41
sexually transmitted diseases
137–42
tobacco use 45–50
toxoplasmosis 150–53
vaccines 81–84
weight gain 33–34, 39
x-rays 14, 85–87
"Pregnancy and Cancer" (American
Society of Clinical Oncology) 101n
"Pregnancy and Medications"
(NWHIC) 68n
pregnancy registries, described 70
Pregnyl 240
premature birth
cerebral palsy 368
complications 196–99
maternal asthma 99
multiple gestations 239–40
see also neonatal intensive care
unit
premature labor, overview 192–96
premaxillary agenesis 325
prenatal care
eclampsia 115
hypertension 113

prenatal care, continued
  maternal diabetes mellitus 104
  overview 12–17
  umbilical cord abnormalities 178
"Prenatal Care" (NWHIC) 12n
prenatal surgical procedures,
  described 7–8
"Prenatal Tests" (Nemours
  Foundation) 17n
prenatal tests, overview 17–32
  see also tests
pressure dilation, vaginal agenesis
  521
preterm delivery
  multiple gestations 226
  sexually transmitted diseases 137
preterm premature rupture of
  membranes (PPROM), twin to twin
  transfusion syndrome 232, 234
primary growth restriction,
  described 160
prochlorperazine, pregnancy safety
  concerns 69
procyclidine hydrochloride 376
prolapsed cord, Cesarean section 247
proteins, food sources 35
PS *see* pulmonary stenosis
psychologists, cerebral palsy 373
PUBS *see* percutaneous umbilical
  blood sampling
Pull-thru Network, contact
  information 584
pulmonary atresia
  defined 576
  described 287–88
pulmonary edema,
  bronchopulmonary dysplasia 213
pulmonary hypertension,
  bronchopulmonary dysplasia 213
pulmonary stenosis (PS)
  defined 576
  described 280–81
PVL *see* periventricular leukomalacia

Q

quadriplegia, defined 576
quadruple screen, described 27–28

R

rabies, vaccine 83
racial factor, preeclampsia 117
radiation, pregnancy 85–86
radiation therapy, maternal cancer 103
radio-frequency ablation device (RFA
  device), acardiac twin 231
radiologists, described 25
RDA *see* recommended daily
  allowance
RDS *see* respiratory distress
  syndrome
recessive gene disorders, prenatal
  testing 19
recommended daily allowance (RDA),
  nutrients 34–36, 42
rectum, defined 576
  see also colon; large intestine
red birthmarks, described 559–61
reefer (slang) 61
renal agenesis, defined 576
renal ectopia, described 466–67
renal flow scan
  ectopic ureter 491
  megaureter 496
renal fusion, described 471–72
reproductive organs, birth defects
  510–29
RESOLVE: The National Infertility
  Association
  contact information 586
  multiple gestation pregnancy
    publication 236n
respiratory distress syndrome (RDS)
  bronchopulmonary dysplasia 211
  described 197
retinopathy of prematurity (ROP)
  described 199
  overview 215–19
RFA device *see* radio-frequency
  ablation device
Rh factor, prenatal testing 21, 155
Rh incompatibility
  cerebral palsy 366, 369
  defined 576
  kernicterus 573
  pregnancy 155–57

Rhode Island, prenatal substance
abuse legislation 64, 65
Rokitansky-Mayer-Küster-Hauser
syndrome 519–20
ROP *see* retinopathy of
prematurity
ROPARD *see* Association for
Retinopathy of Prematurity
and Related Diseases
rubella (German measles)
cerebral palsy 369
defined 576
preconception counseling 6
pregnancy 134–36
prenatal care 13
prenatal testing 22

S

sacrococcygeal teratoma (SCT)
described 553–55
fetal surgery 556–57
"Sacrococcygeal Teratoma: Learn
More" (University of California)
553n
"Sacrococcygeal Teratoma:
Treatments" (University of
California) 556n
St. John's wort 71
salicylate, pregnancy safety
concerns 70
salmon patches 560
SAMHSA *see* Substance Abuse
and Mental Health Services
Administration
saunas
neural tube defects 14, 41
pregnancy 14
scaphocephaly, described 331
Schatz, Michael 100
schizencephaly, described 329–30
scleral bucket, retinopathy of
prematurity 217–18
scoliosis, defined 576
Scott, Allison 538
SCT *see* sacrococcygeal teratoma
secondary growth restriction,
described 160

secondhand smoke
see environmental tobacco smoke
seizures
cerebral palsy 364, 368
focal, defined 571
maternal asthma 99
partial, defined 571
selective dorsal rhizotomy,
defined 576
semilobar holoprosencephaly 324
sepsis, premature birth 199
septal defects, described 283–85
sequestrations *see* bronchopulmonary
sequestrations
sexually transmitted diseases (STD)
birth defects 4
pregnancy 137–42, 143–46
prenatal testing 22
prenatal tests 18
SGA (small for gestational age)
see fetal growth restriction
Shriners Hospitals for Children,
publications
arthrogryposis 532n
clubfoot 534n
sickle cell anemia, newborn screening
257
sickle cell disease, prenatal testing
19, 22–23
side effects
thalidomide 81
x-rays 86
simple renal ectopia 466–67
single gene birth defects, described 3
single umbilical artery, described
177–78
sinogram, urachal anomalies 506
situs anomalies, defined 572
smack (slang) 63
small for gestational age (SGA) *see*
fetal growth restriction
small intestine, described 448
smoking *see* tobacco use
smoking cessation, pregnancy 47–49
"Smoking during Pregnancy May
Affect Baby's Fingers and Toes"
(Children's Hospital of
Philadelphia) 45n
snow (slang) 62

social workers, cerebral palsy 373
solvents, pregnancy 94
sonography
  described 578
  fetal surgery 184
  see also ultrasound
Soriatane (acitretin), pregnancy
  safety concerns 70
Sotret (isotretinoin), birth defects
  4, 72
South Carolina, prenatal substance
  abuse legislation 65
South Dakota, prenatal substance
  abuse legislation 65
spastic, defined 576
spastic cerebral palsy, described
  362–63
spastic diparesis, defined 576
spastic diplegia, defined 576
spastic hemiparesis, defined 576
spastic hemiplegia, defined 576
spasticity, defined 576
spastic quadriparesis, defined 577
spastic quadriplegia, defined 577
speech therapy
  cerebral palsy 373
  clefts 345
speed (slang) 64
spina bifida
  amniocentesis 28
  defined 577
  described 40–41
  fetal surgery 407–9
  labor and delivery 251
  latex allergy 405–7
  overview 396–402
  prenatal diagnosis 7
  prenatal testing 20, 28
  spinal cord tethering 409–14
  statistics 5
  urinary tract disorders 403–4
Spina Bifida Association, latex
  allergy publication 405n
Spina Bifida Association of
  America, contact information
  587
"Spina Bifida Fact Sheet"
  (NINDS) 396n
spina bifida occulta, described 396

"Spina Bifida: Urinary Tract
  Concerns" (Texas Pediatric
  Surgical Associates) 403n
spinal cord tethering, described
  409–14
spinal tap *see* lumbar puncture
spiramycin 153
Staphylococcus aureus 506
statistics
  acardiac twin 231
  ambiguous genitalia 525
  arteriovenous malformation 295
  bacterial vaginosis 139
  birth defects 3, 72, 269
  bronchopulmonary dysplasia 210
  cerebral palsy 362, 365
  chlamydia 137
  clefts 5
  cloacal exstrophy 524
  congenital amputation 542
  congenital birth defects 18
  congenital syphilis 4
  cytomegalovirus 144
  Down syndrome 20
  fetal alcohol syndrome 4
  gastroschisis 437–38
  genital herpes 140
  genital warts 140
  gestational diabetes 25
  gonorrhea 138
  group B streptococcus 260
  HIV infection 141
  listeriosis 147
  maternal asthma 99
  maternal drug abuse 62
  multicystic dysplastic kidney 470
  multiple births 222
  oligohydramnios 164
  omphalocele 441
  placental abruption 172
  polyhydramnios 166
  preterm multiple births 224
  renal fusion 472
  retinopathy of prematurity 215
  Rh factor 155
  sexually transmitted diseases 4
  spina bifida 5, 396
  syphilis 139
  tobacco use 45

statistics, continued
toxoplasmosis 150, 152
vaginal agenesis 519
STD *see* sexually transmitted
diseases
stenosis
defined 577
described 280
stenosis of large intestine, defined 568
stenosis of small intestine, defined
568
stereognosia
cerebral palsy 365
defined 577
stereotaxic thalamotomy, cerebral
palsy 377–78
stillbirth
diabetes mellitus 71, 109
sexually transmitted diseases 137
umbilical cord prolapse 178
stoma, defined 577
stool, defined 577
strabismus
cerebral palsy 365
defined 577
Strategies for Daily Living: FAS/
FASD through the Lifespan"
(National Organization on Fetal
Alcohol Syndrome) 56n
strep throat, group B streptococcus
265
stress management, pregnancy 47–48
stridor, vascular rings 313–14
stroke
arteriovenous malformation 297
cerebral palsy 367, 381
subaortic stenosis, described 282
Substance Abuse and Mental Health
Services Administration
(SAMHSA), contact information 583
Sudafed, pregnancy safety concerns 69
sugar *see* diabetes mellitus
supplements
calcium 36
diabetes-associated birth defects
112–13
folic acid 401
preconception counseling 6
pregnancy 68

surgical procedures
arthrogryposis 533–34
bladder exstrophy 485–86
cerebral palsy 377–78
cervical teratoma 551–52
clefts 343
clubfoot 539–40
ectopic ureter 491–92
epispadias 488
facial palsy 349–50
Goldenhar syndrome 352
hemifacial microsomia 353–54
Hirschsprung disease 457–59
hydroceles 515
hypoplastic left heart syndrome
289
imperforate anus 463
intestinal malrotation 453
maternal cancer 102
megaureter 496–97
microtia 356
persistent pulmonary hypertension
of newborn 309
Pierre Robin sequence 358
retinopathy of prematurity 217–18
spina bifida 400–401
spinal cord tethering 409–14
tetralogy of Fallot 286
urogenital sinus 518
vaginal agenesis 522
vascular rings 313
ventricular septal defect 283
see also fetal surgery; prenatal
surgical procedures
symmetric growth restriction,
described 160
syndrome complex clubfoot,
described 537
syphilis
pregnancy 4, 138–39
prenatal testing 22
systolic pressure, described 113

T

talipes equinovarus *see* clubfoot
Tay-Sachs disease, prenatal testing
19

"Techniques of Fetal Intervention"
(University of California) 183n
TEF *see* tracheoesophageal fistula
Tegison (etretinate), pregnancy safety
concerns 70, 75
teratogens, described 4
tests
ambiguous genitalia 527
birth defect diagnosis 7
cerebral palsy 370–72
congenital diaphragmatic hernia
433–34
cytomegalovirus 143–44
diethylstilbestrol 72
ectopic ureter 490–91
fifth disease 131, 132
Hirschsprung disease 456–57
hydrocephalus 318–19
maternal cancer 102
newborns 256–58
patent foramen ovale 292–93
persistent pulmonary hypertension
of newborn 308–9
phenylketonuria 122
preeclampsia 117
pregnancy 16
Rh factor 21, 155
sexually transmitted diseases 137
spina bifida 398–99
urachal anomalies 505–6
ureterocele 499–500
urinary tract abnormalities 473–75
urinary tract obstruction 483
vascular rings 312–13
see also blood tests; prenatal tests
tetanus, vaccine 83
tetralogy of Fallot (TOF)
defined 577
described 285–86
tetralogy of Fallot with pulmonary
atresia (TOF/PA), described 576
Texas, prenatal substance abuse
legislation 65
Texas Center for Fetal Surgery,
contact information 583
Texas Pediatric Surgical Associates,
publications
hydronephrosis 468n
spina bifida 403n

TGA *see* transposition of great
arteries
thalidomide
birth defect risks 80–81
pregnancy safety concerns 70
Thalomid (thalidomide) 80–81
theophylline, maternal
asthma 100
"There's Never Been a Better
Time to Quit" (American
Lung Association) 45n
thymus gland, isotretinoin 73
thyroid medications, pregnancy
safety concerns 69
tobacco use
placenta previa 174
preconception counseling 7
pregnancy 45–50
prenatal care 13, 14
toes, maternal tobacco use 49–50
TOF *see* tetralogy of Fallot
TOF/PA *see* tetralogy of Fallot with
pulmonary atresia
tonic-clonic seizure, defined 577
toot (slang) 62
torticollis, described 544
total anomalous pulmonary venous
connection, described 288–89
Toxoplasma gondii 151
toxoplasmosis
described 70
pregnancy 14, 37, 150–53
trachea, described 430
tracheoesophageal fistula (TEF),
described 430–31, 577
tracheomalacia, vascular rings 314
tracheostomy, cervical teratoma 552
transabdominal ultrasound,
described 24
transducer, described 24
transesophageal echocardiography,
patent foramen ovale 293
transient tachypnea, described 197
translocation, defined 577
transposition of great arteries (TGA)
defined 577
described 5, 286
transurethral puncture, ureterocele
500

transvaginal ultrasound, described 24

transverse limb deficiency, defined 573

TRAP sequence *see* acardiac twin

tremor, defined 577

trichomoniasis, pregnancy 139–40

tricuspid atresia
   defined 577
   described 286–87

trigonocephaly, described 331

trihexyphenidyl 376

triple screen, described 27–28

Triplet Connection, contact information 586

trisomy, defined 577

trisomy 13
   defined 578
   described 325
   omphalocele 442

trisomy 18
   defined 578
   described 325
   omphalocele 442

trisomy 21 *see* Down syndrome

truncus arteriosus
   defined 578
   described 288

TTTS *see* twin to twin transfusion syndrome

twins
   umbilical cord knots 180
   umbilical cord prolapse 179
   see also multiple births

twin to twin transfusion syndrome (TTTS)
   described 224
   overview 228–30

"Twin to Twin Transfusion Syndrome" (University of California) 228n, 232n

Tylenol (acetaminophen), pregnancy safety concerns 69

type 1 diabetes mellitus
   described 105
   pregnancy 107–9

type 2 diabetes mellitus
   described 105
   pregnancy 107–9

U

ultrasonogram *see* ultrasound

ultrasound
   amniotic fluid 164
   birth defect diagnosis 7
   cerebral palsy 371
   cervical teratoma 550
   congenital amputation 543
   defined 578
   hydrocephalus 319
   isotretinoin 74
   lissencephaly 327
   maternal cancer 102
   megaureter 495
   multiple gestations 223
   patent foramen ovale 293
   persistent pulmonary hypertension of newborn 308
   phenylketonuria 122
   porencephaly 329
   preeclampsia 117
   prenatal testing 23–25
   spina bifida 399
   twin pregnancy complications 228
   umbilical cord 177–78, 180–81
   ureterocele 499
   vesicoureteral reflux 503
   see also fetal echocardiography

umbilical cord
   alcohol use 53
   described 177
   urachal anomalies 505

umbilical cord abnormalities, overview 177–81

umbilical cord knots, described 180

umbilical cord prolapse, described 178–79

undescended testicles, described 510–12

"Unequal Placental Sharing" (University of California) 228n

United Cerebral Palsy Association, Inc., contact information 581

United Cerebral Palsy Research and Education Foundation, cerebral palsy prevention publication 391n

University of California, Fetal Treatment Center, contact information 583
University of California, Fetal Treatment Program, publications
    bowel obstruction 448n
    congenital diaphragmatic hernia 432n, 435n
    fetal intervention techniques 183n
    gastroschisis 437n
    omphalocele 441n
    sacrococcygeal teratoma 553n, 556n
    twin pregnancy complications 228n
    urinary tract obstruction 478n, 480n
University of California, San Diego Fetal Surgery Program, contact information 583
University of Missouri Children's Hospital, amniotic band syndrome publication 163n
upper limb deficiency, defined 573
upper pole nephrectomy, ureterocele 500
urachal anomalies, described 504–7
urachus, described 504
ureteral reimplantation, ectopic ureter 493
ureterocele, described 498–502
ureteropyelostomy
    ectopic ureter 493
    ureterocele 501
urinary incontinence, ectopic ureter 491
urinary tract disorders
    birth defects 478–507
    tests 473–75
urinary tract infections (UTI)
    prenatal diagnosis 7–8
    vesicoureteral reflux 502–4
urinary tract obstruction
    described 478–80
    fetal surgery 480–83
"Urinary Tract Obstruction: Learn More" (University of California) 478n
urine tests, prenatal testing 22, 25
urogenital sinus, described 517–18
USDA *see* US Department of Agriculture

US Department of Agriculture (USDA), listeriosis, pregnancy publication 147n
US Food and Drug Administration (FDA)
    drug safety rating system 69–70
    pregnancy registries Web site 70
    publications
        Paxil 78n
        thalidomide 80n
        x-rays, pregnancy 85n
"Using Illegal Drugs During Pregnancy" (American Pregnancy Association) 61n
Utah, prenatal substance abuse legislation 64

V

vaccinations
    hepatitis B 267–68
    preconception counseling 6
    pregnancy 82–84
    prenatal care 13
    varicella 129
"Vaccines and Pregnancy" (OTIS) 82n
vaginal agenesis, described 519–23
"Vaginal Anomalies: Urogenital Sinus" (American Urological Association Foundation) 517n
vanishing twin syndrome, multiple gestations 242
varicella (chickenpox)
    pregnancy 128–30
    prenatal testing 22
vasa previa, described 179
vascular lesions, described 299–305
vascular rings, overview 311–14
VCUG *see* voiding cystourethrogram
vegetarian diets, pregnancy 36
venous malformations, described 300–301
ventilators
    apnea of prematurity 207–8
    bronchopulmonary dysplasia 211
    congenital diaphragmatic hernia 433
    persistent pulmonary hypertension of newborn 309
    premature birth 201

ventricular, described 575
ventricular septal defect (VSD)
   defined 578
   described 283
vesicoureteral reflux (VUR)
   ectopic kidney 467
   hydronephrosis 469
   overview 502–4
Virginia, prenatal substance abuse
   legislation 64, 65
vision impairment, cerebral palsy 365
vitamin A 72, 75
vitamin B6, pregnancy safety
   concerns 69
vitamins
   diethylstilbestrol 71
   food sources *35*
   pregnancy 68
   spina bifida 397
   see also folic acid
vitrectomy, retinopathy of
   prematurity 218
voiding cystourethrogram (VCUG)
   ectopic ureter 490
   megaureter 496
   ureterocele 499
   vesicoureteral reflux 503
volvulus 451
VSD *see* ventricular septal defect
VUR *see* vesicoureteral reflux

W

weed (slang) 61
weight gain
   maternal tobacco use 46
   multiple gestations 225
   pregnancy 33–34, 39
Herman B. Wells Research Center,
   contact information 586
Wharton's jelly, described 177

"What I Need to Know about
   Hirschsprung Disease" (NIDDK)
   454n, 567n
"When Your Baby Has a Birth Defect"
   (Nemours Foundation) 269n
windpipe *see* trachea
Wisconsin, prenatal substance abuse
   legislation 65

X

X-linked disorders, prenatal testing
   19–20
x-rays
   bronchopulmonary dysplasia 212
   ectopic ureter 490
   Hirschsprung disease 456–57
   patent foramen ovale 292
   persistent pulmonary hypertension
      of newborn 308
   pregnancy 14, 85–87
   urachal anomalies 506
   ureterocele 499
   vascular rings 312–13
"X-Rays, Pregnancy and You" (FDA)
   85n

Y

yeast infections, group B
   streptococcus 265
"Your Child Has Been Diagnosed
   with Arthrogryposis" (Shriners
   Hospitals for Children) 532n

Z

zidovudine, pregnancy 70
zoster immune globulin (ZIG),
   varicella 129

Health Reference Series

COMPLETE CATALOG

List price $87 per volume. **School and library price $78 per volume.**

Adolescent Health Sourcebook, 2nd Edition

Basic Consumer Health Information about the Physical, Mental, and Emotional Growth and Development of Adolescents, Including Medical Care, Nutritional and Physical Activity Requirements, Puberty, Sexual Activity, Acne, Tanning, Body Piercing, Common Physical Illnesses and Disorders, Eating Disorders, Attention Deficit Hyperactivity Disorder, Depression, Bullying, Hazing, and Adolescent Injuries Related to Sports, Driving, and Work

Along with Substance Abuse Information about Nicotine, Alcohol, and Drug Use, a Glossary, and Directory of Additional Resources

Edited by Joyce Brennfleck Shannon. 683 pages. 2006. 0-7808-0943-2.

"It is written in clear, nontechnical language aimed at general readers. . . . Recommended for public libraries, community colleges, and other agencies serving health care consumers."
— *American Reference Books Annual, 2003*

"Recommended for school and public libraries. Parents and professionals dealing with teens will appreciate the easy-to-follow format and the clearly written text. This could become a 'must have' for every high school teacher." — *E-Streams, Jan '03*

"A good starting point for information related to common medical, mental, and emotional concerns of adolescents." — *School Library Journal, Nov '02*

"This book provides accurate information in an easy to access format. It addresses topics that parents and caregivers might not be aware of and provides practical, useable information."
— *Doody's Health Sciences Book Review Journal, Sep-Oct '02*

"Recommended reference source."
— *Booklist, American Library Association, Sep '02*

AIDS Sourcebook, 3rd Edition

Basic Consumer Health Information about Acquired Immune Deficiency Syndrome (AIDS) and Human Immunodeficiency Virus (HIV) Infection, Including Facts about Transmission, Prevention, Diagnosis, Treatment, Opportunistic Infections, and Other Complications, with a Section for Women and Children, Including Details about Associated Gynecological Concerns, Pregnancy, and Pediatric Care

Along with Updated Statistical Information, Reports on Current Research Initiatives, a Glossary, and Directories of Internet, Hotline, and Other Resources

Edited by Dawn D. Matthews. 664 pages. 2003. 0-7808-0631-X.

"The 3rd edition of the *AIDS Sourcebook*, part of Omnigraphics' *Health Reference Series*, is a welcome update. . . . This resource is highly recommended for academic and public libraries."
— *American Reference Books Annual, 2004*

"Excellent sourcebook. This continues to be a highly recommended book. There is no other book that provides as much information as this book provides."
— *AIDS Book Review Journal, Dec-Jan '00*

"Recommended reference source."
— *Booklist, American Library Association, Dec '99*

Alcoholism Sourcebook, 2nd Edition

Basic Consumer Health Information about Alcohol Use, Abuse, and Dependence, Featuring Facts about the Physical, Mental, and Social Health Effects of Alcohol Addiction, Including Alcoholic Liver Disease, Pancreatic Disease, Cardiovascular Disease, Neurological Disorders, and the Effects of Drinking during Pregnancy

Along with Information about Alcohol Treatment, Medications, and Recovery Programs, in Addition to Tips for Reducing the Prevalence of Underage Drinking, Statistics about Alcohol Use, a Glossary of Related Terms, and Directories of Resources for More Help and Information

Edited by Amy L. Sutton. 653 pages. 2006. 0-7808-0942-4.

"This title is one of the few reference works on alcoholism for general readers. For some readers this will be a welcome complement to the many self-help books on the market. Recommended for collections serving general readers and consumer health collections."
— *E-Streams, Mar '01*

"This book is an excellent choice for public and academic libraries."
— *American Reference Books Annual, 2001*

"Recommended reference source."
— *Booklist, American Library Association, Dec '00*

"Presents a wealth of information on alcohol use and abuse and its effects on the body and mind, treatment, and prevention." — *SciTech Book News, Dec '00*

"Important new health guide which packs in the latest consumer information about the problems of alcoholism." — *Reviewer's Bookwatch, Nov '00*

SEE ALSO *Drug Abuse Sourcebook, Substance Abuse Sourcebook*

Allergies Sourcebook, 2nd Edition

Basic Consumer Health Information about Allergic Disorders, Triggers, Reactions, and Related Symptoms, Including Anaphylaxis, Rhinitis, Sinusitis, Asthma, Dermatitis, Conjunctivitis, and Multiple Chemical Sensitivity

Along with Tips on Diagnosis, Prevention, and Treatment, Statistical Data, a Glossary, and a Directory of Sources for Further Help and Information

Edited by Annemarie S. Muth. 598 pages. 2002. 0-7808-0376-0.

"This book brings a great deal of useful material together. . . . This is an excellent addition to public and consumer health library collections."
— *American Reference Books Annual, 2003*

"This second edition would be useful to laypersons with little or advanced knowledge of the subject matter. This book would also serve as a resource for nursing and other health care professions students. It would be useful in public, academic, and hospital libraries with consumer health collections." — *E-Streams, Jul '02*

Alternative Medicine Sourcebook

SEE Complementary & Alternative Medicine Sourcebook, 3rd Edition

Alzheimer's Disease Sourcebook, 3rd Edition

Basic Consumer Health Information about Alzheimer's Disease, Other Dementias, and Related Disorders, Including Multi-Infarct Dementia, AIDS Dementia Complex, Dementia with Lewy Bodies, Huntington's Disease, Wernicke-Korsakoff Syndrome (Alcohol-Reated Dementia), Delirium, and Confusional States

Along with Information for People Newly Diagnosed with Alzheimer's Disease and Caregivers, Reports Detailing Current Research Efforts in Prevention, Diagnosis, and Treatment, Facts about Long-Term Care Issues, and Listings of Sources for Additional Information

Edited by Karen Bellenir. 645 pages. 2003. 0-7808-0666-2.

"This very informative and valuable tool will be a great addition to any library serving consumers, students and health care workers."
— *American Reference Books Annual, 2004*

"This is a valuable resource for people affected by dementias such as Alzheimer's. It is easy to navigate and includes important information and resources."
— *Doody's Review Service, Feb '04*

"Recommended reference source."
— *Booklist, American Library Association, Oct '99*

SEE ALSO Brain Disorders Sourcebook

Arthritis Sourcebook, 2nd Edition

Basic Consumer Health Information about Osteoarthritis, Rheumatoid Arthritis, Other Rheumatic Disorders, Infectious Forms of Arthritis, and Diseases with Symptoms Linked to Arthritis, Featuring Facts about Diagnosis, Pain Management, and Surgical Therapies

Along with Coping Strategies, Research Updates, a Glossary, and Resources for Additional Help and Information

Edited by Amy L. Sutton. 593 pages. 2004. 0-7808-0667-0.

"This easy-to-read volume is recommended for consumer health collections within public or academic libraries." — *E-Streams, May '05*

"As expected, this updated edition continues the excellent reputation of this series in providing sound, usable health information. . . . Highly recommended."
— *American Reference Books Annual, 2005*

"Excellent reference." — *The Bookwatch, Jan '05*

Asthma Sourcebook, 2nd Edition

Basic Consumer Health Information about the Causes, Symptoms, Diagnosis, and Treatment of Asthma in Infants, Children, Teenagers, and Adults, Including Facts about Different Types of Asthma, Common Co-Occurring Conditions, Asthma Management Plans, Triggers, Medications, and Medication Delivery Devices

Along with Asthma Statistics, Research Updates, a Glossary, a Directory of Asthma-Related Resources, and More

Edited by Karen Bellenir. 609 pages. 2006. 0-7808-0866-5.

"A worthwhile reference acquisition for public libraries and academic medical libraries whose readers desire a quick introduction to the wide range of asthma information." — *Choice, Association of College & Research Libraries, Jun '01*

"Recommended reference source."
— *Booklist, American Library Association, Feb '01*

"Highly recommended." — *The Bookwatch, Jan '01*

"There is much good information for patients and their families who deal with asthma daily."
— *American Medical Writers Association Journal, Winter '01*

"This informative text is recommended for consumer health collections in public, secondary school, and community college libraries and the libraries of universities with a large undergraduate population."
— *American Reference Books Annual, 2001*

Attention Deficit Disorder Sourcebook

Basic Consumer Health Information about Attention Deficit/Hyperactivity Disorder in Children and Adults, Including Facts about Causes, Symptoms, Diagnostic Criteria, and Treatment Options Such as Medications, Behavior Therapy, Coaching, and Homeopathy

Along with Reports on Current Research Initiatives, Legal Issues, and Government Regulations, and Featuring a Glossary of Related Terms, Internet Resources, and a List of Additional Reading Material

Edited by Dawn D. Matthews. 470 pages. 2002. 0-7808-0624-7.

"Recommended reference source."
— Booklist, American Library Association, Jan '03

"This book is recommended for all school libraries and the reference or consumer health sections of public libraries." — American Reference Books Annual, 2003

Back & Neck Sourcebook, 2nd Edition

Basic Consumer Health Information about Spinal Pain, Spinal Cord Injuries, and Related Disorders, Such as Degenerative Disk Disease, Osteoarthritis, Scoliosis, Sciatica, Spina Bifida, and Spinal Stenosis, and Featuring Facts about Maintaining Spinal Health, Self-Care, Pain Management, Rehabilitative Care, Chiropractic Care, Spinal Surgeries, and Complementary Therapies

Along with Suggestions for Preventing Back and Neck Pain, a Glossary of Related Terms, and a Directory of Resources

Edited by Amy L. Sutton. 633 pages. 2004. 0-7808-0738-3.

"Recommended . . . an easy to use, comprehensive medical reference book." — E-Streams, Sep '05

"The strength of this work is its basic, easy-to-read format. Recommended." — Reference and User Services Quarterly, American Library Association, Winter '97

Blood & Circulatory Disorders Sourcebook, 2nd Edition

Basic Consumer Health Information about the Blood and Circulatory System and Related Disorders, Such as Anemia and Other Hemoglobin Diseases, Cancer of the Blood and Associated Bone Marrow Disorders, Clotting and Bleeding Problems, and Conditions That Affect the Veins, Blood Vessels, and Arteries, Including Facts about the Donation and Transplantation of Bone Marrow, Stem Cells, and Blood and Tips for Keeping the Blood and Circulatory System Healthy

Along with a Glossary of Related Terms and Resources for Additional Help and Information

Edited by Amy L. Sutton. 659 pages. 2005. 0-7808-0746-4.

"Highly recommended pick for basic consumer health reference holdings at all levels."
— The Bookwatch, Aug '05

"Recommended reference source."
— Booklist, American Library Association, Feb '99

"An important reference sourcebook written in simple language for everyday, non-technical users. "
— Reviewer's Bookwatch, Jan '99

Brain Disorders Sourcebook, 2nd Edition

Basic Consumer Health Information about Acquired and Traumatic Brain Injuries, Infections of the Brain, Epilepsy and Seizure Disorders, Cerebral Palsy, and Degenerative Neurological Disorders, Including Amyotrophic Lateral Sclerosis (ALS), Dementias, Multiple Sclerosis, and More

Along with Information on the Brain's Structure and Function, Treatment and Rehabilitation Options, Reports on Current Research Initiatives, a Glossary of Terms Related to Brain Disorders and Injuries, and a Directory of Sources for Further Help and Information

Edited by Sandra J. Judd. 625 pages. 2005. 0-7808-0744-8.

"Highly recommended pick for basic consumer health reference holdings at all levels."
— The Bookwatch, Aug '05

"Belongs on the shelves of any library with a consumer health collection." — E-Streams, Mar '00

"Recommended reference source."
— Booklist, American Library Association, Oct '99

SEE ALSO Alzheimer's Disease Sourcebook

Breast Cancer Sourcebook, 2nd Edition

Basic Consumer Health Information about Breast Cancer, Including Facts about Risk Factors, Prevention, Screening and Diagnostic Methods, Treatment Options, Complementary and Alternative Therapies, Post-Treatment Concerns, Clinical Trials, Special Risk Populations, and New Developments in Breast Cancer Research

Along with Breast Cancer Statistics, a Glossary of Related Terms, and a Directory of Resources for Additional Help and Information

Edited by Sandra J. Judd. 595 pages. 2004. 0-7808-0668-9.

"This book will be an excellent addition to public, community college, medical, and academic libraries."
— American Reference Books Annual, 2006

"It would be a useful reference book in a library or on loan to women in a support group."
— Cancer Forum, Mar '03

"Recommended reference source."
— Booklist, American Library Association, Jan '02

"This reference source is highly recommended. It is quite informative, comprehensive and detailed in nature, and yet it offers practical advice in easy-to-read language. It could be thought of as the 'bible' of breast cancer for the consumer." — E-Streams, Jan '02

"From the pros and cons of different screening methods and results to treatment options, Breast Cancer Sourcebook provides the latest information on the subject."
— Library Bookwatch, Dec '01

"This thoroughgoing, very readable reference covers all aspects of breast health and cancer. . . . Readers will find

much to consider here. Recommended for all public and patient health collections."
— *Library Journal, Sep '01*

SEE ALSO *Cancer Sourcebook for Women, Women's Health Concerns Sourcebook*

■

Breastfeeding Sourcebook

Basic Consumer Health Information about the Benefits of Breastmilk, Preparing to Breastfeed, Breastfeeding as a Baby Grows, Nutrition, and More, Including Information on Special Situations and Concerns Such as Mastitis, Illness, Medications, Allergies, Multiple Births, Prematurity, Special Needs, and Adoption

Along with a Glossary and Resources for Additional Help and Information

Edited by Jenni Lynn Colson. 388 pages. 2002. 0-7808-0332-9.

"Particularly useful is the information about professional lactation services and chapters on breastfeeding when returning to work. . . . *Breastfeeding Sourcebook* will be useful for public libraries, consumer health libraries, and technical schools offering nurse assistant training, especially in areas where Internet access is problematic."
— *American Reference Books Annual, 2003*

SEE ALSO *Pregnancy & Birth Sourcebook*

■

Burns Sourcebook

Basic Consumer Health Information about Various Types of Burns and Scalds, Including Flame, Heat, Cold, Electrical, Chemical, and Sun Burns

Along with Information on Short-Term and Long-Term Treatments, Tissue Reconstruction, Plastic Surgery, Prevention Suggestions, and First Aid

Edited by Allan R. Cook. 604 pages. 1999. 0-7808-0204-7.

"This is an exceptional addition to the series and is highly recommended for all consumer health collections, hospital libraries, and academic medical centers."
— *E-Streams, Mar '00*

"This key reference guide is an invaluable addition to all health care and public libraries in confronting this ongoing health issue."
— *American Reference Books Annual, 2000*

"Recommended reference source."
— *Booklist, American Library Association, Dec '99*

SEE ALSO *Dermatological Disorders Sourcebook*

■

Cancer Sourcebook, 4th Edition

Basic Consumer Health Information about Major Forms and Stages of Cancer, Featuring Facts about Head and Neck Cancers, Lung Cancers, Gastrointestinal Cancers, Genitourinary Cancers, Lymphomas, Blood Cell Cancers, Endocrine Cancers, Skin Cancers, Bone Cancers, Sarcomas, and Others, and Including Information about Cancer Treatments and Therapies,

Identifying and Reducing Cancer Risks, and Strategies for Coping with Cancer and the Side Effects of Treatment

Along with a Cancer Glossary, Statistical and Demographic Data, and a Directory of Sources for Additional Help and Information

Edited by Karen Bellenir. 1,119 pages. 2003. 0-7808-0633-6.

"With cancer being the second leading cause of death for Americans, a prodigious work such as this one, which locates centrally so much cancer-related information, is clearly an asset to this nation's citizens and others."
— *Journal of the National Medical Association, 2004*

"This title is recommended for health sciences and public libraries with consumer health collections."
— *E-Streams, Feb '01*

". . . can be effectively used by cancer patients and their families who are looking for answers in a language they can understand. Public and hospital libraries should have it on their shelves."
— *American Reference Books Annual, 2001*

"Recommended reference source."
— *Booklist, American Library Association, Dec '00*

SEE ALSO *Breast Cancer Sourcebook, Cancer Sourcebook for Women, Pediatric Cancer Sourcebook, Prostate Cancer Sourcebook*

■

Cancer Sourcebook for Women, 3rd Edition

Basic Consumer Health Information about Leading Causes of Cancer in Women, Featuring Facts about Gynecologic Cancers and Related Concerns, Such as Breast Cancer, Cervical Cancer, Endometrial Cancer, Uterine Sarcoma, Vaginal Cancer, Vulvar Cancer, and Common Non-Cancerous Gynecologic Conditions, in Addition to Facts about Lung Cancer, Colorectal Cancer, and Thyroid Cancer in Women

Along with Information about Cancer Risk Factors, Screening and Prevention, Treatment Options, and Tips on Coping with Life after Cancer Treatment, a Glossary of Cancer Terms, and a Directory of Resources for Additional Help and Information

Edited by Amy L. Sutton. 715 pages. 2006. 0-7808-0867-3.

"An excellent addition to collections in public, consumer health, and women's health libraries."
— *American Reference Books Annual, 2003*

"Overall, the information is excellent, and complex topics are clearly explained. As a reference book for the consumer it is a valuable resource to assist them to make informed decisions about cancer and its treatments."
— *Cancer Forum, Nov '02*

"Highly recommended for academic and medical reference collections."
— *Library Bookwatch, Sep '02*

"This is a highly recommended book for any public or consumer library, being reader friendly and containing accurate and helpful information."
— *E-Streams, Aug '02*

■

Cardiovascular Diseases & Disorders Sourcebook, 3rd Edition

Basic Consumer Health Information about Heart and Vascular Diseases and Disorders, Such as Angina, Heart Attacks, Arrhythmias, Cardiomyopathy, Valve Disease, Atherosclerosis, and Aneurysms, with Information about Managing Cardiovascular Risk Factors and Maintaining Heart Health, Medications and Procedures Used to Treat Cardiovascular Disorders, and Concerns of Special Significance to Women

Along with Reports on Current Research Initiatives, a Glossary of Related Medical Terms, and a Directory of Sources for Further Help and Information

Edited by Sandra J. Judd. 713 pages. 2005. 0-7808-0739-1.

"This updated sourcebook is still the best first stop for comprehensive introductory information on cardiovascular diseases."
—*American Reference Books Annual, 2006*

"Recommended for public libraries and libraries supporting health care professionals."
—*E-Streams, Sep '05*

"This should be a standard health library reference."
—*The Bookwatch, Jun '05*

"Recommended reference source."
—*Booklist, American Library Association, Dec '00*

". . . comprehensive format provides an extensive overview on this subject."
—*Choice, Association of College & Research Libraries*

■

Caregiving Sourcebook

Basic Consumer Health Information for Caregivers, Including a Profile of Caregivers, Caregiving Responsibilities and Concerns, Tips for Specific Conditions, Care Environments, and the Effects of Caregiving

Along with Facts about Legal Issues, Financial Information, and Future Planning, a Glossary, and a Listing of Additional Resources

Edited by Joyce Brennfleck Shannon. 600 pages. 2001. 0-7808-0331-0.

"Essential for most collections."
—*Library Journal, Apr 1, 2002*

"An ideal addition to the reference collection of any public library. Health sciences information professionals may also want to acquire the *Caregiving Sourcebook* for their hospital or academic library for use as a ready reference tool by health care workers interested in aging and caregiving."
—*E-Streams, Jan '02*

"Recommended reference source."
—*Booklist, American Library Association, Oct '01*

Child Abuse Sourcebook

Basic Consumer Health Information about the Physical, Sexual, and Emotional Abuse of Children, with Additional Facts about Neglect, Munchausen Syndrome by Proxy (MSBP), Shaken Baby Syndrome, and Controversial Issues Related to Child Abuse, Such as Withholding Medical Care, Corporal Punishment, and Child Maltreatment in Youth Sports, and Featuring Facts about Child Protective Services, Foster Care, Adoption, Parenting Challenges, and Other Abuse Prevention Efforts

Along with a Glossary of Related Terms and Resources for Additional Help and Information

Edited by Dawn D. Matthews. 620 pages. 2004. 0-7808-0705-7.

"A valuable and highly recommended resource for school, academic and public libraries whether used on its own or as a starting point for more in-depth research."
—*E-Streams, Apr '05*

"Every week the news brings cases of child abuse or neglect, so it is useful to have a source that supplies so much helpful information. . . . Recommended. Public and academic libraries, and child welfare offices."
—*Choice, Association of College & Research Libraries, Mar '05*

"Packed with insights on all kinds of issues, from foster care and adoption to parenting and abuse prevention."
—*The Bookwatch, Nov '04*

SEE ALSO: *Domestic Violence Sourcebook, 2nd Edition*

■

Childhood Diseases & Disorders Sourcebook

Basic Consumer Health Information about Medical Problems Often Encountered in Pre-Adolescent Children, Including Respiratory Tract Ailments, Ear Infections, Sore Throats, Disorders of the Skin and Scalp, Digestive and Genitourinary Diseases, Infectious Diseases, Inflammatory Disorders, Chronic Physical and Developmental Disorders, Allergies, and More

Along with Information about Diagnostic Tests, Common Childhood Surgeries, and Frequently Used Medications, with a Glossary of Important Terms and Resource Directory

Edited by Chad T. Kimball. 662 pages. 2003. 0-7808-0458-9.

"This is an excellent book for new parents and should be included in all health care and public libraries."
—*American Reference Books Annual, 2004*

SEE ALSO: *Healthy Children Sourcebook*

■

Colds, Flu & Other Common Ailments Sourcebook

Basic Consumer Health Information about Common Ailments and Injuries, Including Colds, Coughs, the Flu, Sinus Problems, Headaches, Fever, Nausea and

Vomiting, Menstrual Cramps, Diarrhea, Constipation, Hemorrhoids, Back Pain, Dandruff, Dry and Itchy Skin, Cuts, Scrapes, Sprains, Bruises, and More

Along with Information about Prevention, Self-Care, Choosing a Doctor, Over-the-Counter Medications, Folk Remedies, and Alternative Therapies, and Including a Glossary of Important Terms and a Directory of Resources for Further Help and Information

Edited by Chad T. Kimball. 638 pages. 2001. 0-7808-0435-X.

"A good starting point for research on common illnesses. It will be a useful addition to public and consumer health library collections."
— *American Reference Books Annual, 2002*

"Will prove valuable to any library seeking to maintain a current, comprehensive reference collection of health resources. . . . Excellent reference."
— *The Bookwatch, Aug '01*

"Recommended reference source."
— *Booklist, American Library Association, Jul '01*

■

Communication Disorders Sourcebook

Basic Information about Deafness and Hearing Loss, Speech and Language Disorders, Voice Disorders, Balance and Vestibular Disorders, and Disorders of Smell, Taste, and Touch

Edited by Linda M. Ross. 533 pages. 1996. 0-7808-0077-X.

"This is skillfully edited and is a welcome resource for the layperson. It should be found in every public and medical library."   — *Booklist Health Sciences Supplement, American Library Association, Oct '97*

■

Complementary & Alternative Medicine Sourcebook, 3rd Edition

Basic Consumer Health Information about Complementary and Alternative Medical Therapies, Including Acupuncture, Ayurveda, Traditional Chinese Medicine, Herbal Medicine, Homeopathy, Naturopathy, Biofeedback, Hypnotherapy, Yoga, Art Therapy, Aromatherapy, Clinical Nutrition, Vitamin and Mineral Supplements, Chiropractic, Massage, Reflexology, Crystal Therapy, Therapeutic Touch, and More

Along with Facts about Alternative and Complementary Treatments for Specific Conditions Such as Cancer, Diabetes, Osteoarthritis, Chronic Pain, Menopause, Gastrointestinal Disorders, Headaches, and Mental Illness, a Glossary, and a Resource List for Additional Help and Information

Edited by Sandra J. Judd. 657 pages. 2006. 0-7808-0864-9.

"Recommended for public, high school, and academic libraries that have consumer health collections. Hospital libraries that also serve the public will find this to be a useful resource."   — *E-Streams, Feb '03*

"Recommended reference source."
— *Booklist, American Library Association, Jan '03*

"An important alternate health reference."
— *MBR Bookwatch, Oct '02*

"A great addition to the reference collection of every type of library." — *American Reference Books Annual, 2000*

■

Congenital Disorders Sourcebook, 2nd Edition

Basic Consumer Health Information about Nonhereditary Birth Defects and Disorders Related to Prematurity, Gestational Injuries, Congenital Infections, and Birth Complications, Including Heart Defects, Hydrocephalus, Spina Bifida, Cleft Lip and Palate, Cerebral Palsy, and More

Along with Facts about the Prevention of Birth Defects, Fetal Surgery and Other Treatment Options, Research Initiatives, a Glossary of Related Terms, and Resources for Additional Information and Support

Edited by Sandra J. Judd. 647 pages. 2006. 0-7808-0945-9.

"Recommended reference source."
— *Booklist, American Library Association, Oct '97*

SEE ALSO Pregnancy & Birth Sourcebook

■

Consumer Issues in Health Care Sourcebook

Basic Information about Health Care Fundamentals and Related Consumer Issues, Including Exams and Screening Tests, Physician Specialties, Choosing a Doctor, Using Prescription and Over-the-Counter Medications Safely, Avoiding Health Scams, Managing Common Health Risks in the Home, Care Options for Chronically or Terminally Ill Patients, and a List of Resources for Obtaining Help and Further Information

Edited by Karen Bellenir. 618 pages. 1998. 0-7808-0221-7.

"Both public and academic libraries will want to have a copy in their collection for readers who are interested in self-education on health issues."
— *American Reference Books Annual, 2000*

"The editor has researched the literature from government agencies and others, saving readers the time and effort of having to do the research themselves. Recommended for public libraries."
— *Reference and User Services Quarterly, American Library Association, Spring '99*

"Recommended reference source."
— *Booklist, American Library Association, Dec '98*

■

Contagious Diseases Sourcebook

Basic Consumer Health Information about Infectious Diseases Spread by Person-to-Person Contact through Direct Touch, Airborne Transmission, Sexual Contact, or Contact with Blood or Other Body Fluids, Including Hepatitis, Herpes, Influenza, Lice, Measles, Mumps, Pinworm, Ringworm, Severe Acute Respiratory Syndrome (SARS), Streptococcal Infections, Tuberculosis, and Others

Along with Facts about Disease Transmission, Antimicrobial Resistance, and Vaccines, with a Glossary and Directories of Resources for More Information

Edited by Karen Bellenir. 643 pages. 2004. 0-7808-0736-7.

"This easy-to-read volume is recommended for consumer health collections within public or academic libraries." — *E-Streams, May '05*

"This informative book is highly recommended for public libraries, consumer health collections, and secondary schools and undergraduate libraries." — *American Reference Books Annual, 2005*

"Excellent reference." — *The Bookwatch, Jan '05*

Contagious & Non-Contagious Infectious Diseases Sourcebook

Basic Information about Contagious Diseases like Measles, Polio, Hepatitis B, and Infectious Mononucleosis, and Non-Contagious Infectious Diseases like Tetanus and Toxic Shock Syndrome, and Diseases Occurring as Secondary Infections Such as Shingles and Reye Syndrome

Along with Vaccination, Prevention, and Treatment Information, and a Section Describing Emerging Infectious Disease Threats

Edited by Karen Bellenir and Peter D. Dresser. 566 pages. 1996. 0-7808-0075-3.

SEE ALSO Infectious Diseases Sourcebook

Death & Dying Sourcebook, 2nd Edition

Basic Consumer Health Information about End-of-Life Care and Related Perspectives and Ethical Issues, Including End-of-Life Symptoms and Treatments, Pain Management, Quality-of-Life Concerns, the Use of Life Support, Patients' Rights and Privacy Issues, Advance Directives, Physician-Assisted Suicide, Caregiving, Organ and Tissue Donation, Autopsies, Funeral Arrangements, and Grief

Along with Statistical Data, Information about the Leading Causes of Death, a Glossary, and Directories of Support Groups and Other Resources

Edited by Joyce Brennfleck Shannon. 653 pages. 2006. 0-7808-0871-1.

"Public libraries, medical libraries, and academic libraries will all find this sourcebook a useful addition to their collections." — *American Reference Books Annual, 2001*

"An extremely useful resource for those concerned with death and dying in the United States." — *Respiratory Care, Nov '00*

"Recommended reference source." — *Booklist, American Library Association, Aug '00*

"This book is a definite must for all those involved in end-of-life care." — *Doody's Review Service, 2000*

Dental Care & Oral Health Sourcebook, 2nd Edition

Basic Consumer Health Information about Dental Care, Including Oral Hygiene, Dental Visits, Pain Management, Cavities, Crowns, Bridges, Dental Implants, and Fillings, and Other Oral Health Concerns, Such as Gum Disease, Bad Breath, Dry Mouth, Genetic and Developmental Abnormalities, Oral Cancers, Orthodontics, and Temporomandibular Disorders

Along with Updates on Current Research in Oral Health, a Glossary, a Directory of Dental and Oral Health Organizations, and Resources for People with Dental and Oral Health Disorders

Edited by Amy L. Sutton. 609 pages. 2003. 0-7808-0634-4.

"This book could serve as a turning point in the battle to educate consumers in issues concerning oral health." — *American Reference Books Annual, 2004*

"Unique source which will fill a gap in dental sources for patients and the lay public. A valuable reference tool even in a library with thousands of books on dentistry. Comprehensive, clear, inexpensive, and easy to read and use. It fills an enormous gap in the health care literature." — *Reference & User Services Quarterly, American Library Association, Summer '98*

"Recommended reference source." — *Booklist, American Library Association, Dec '97*

Depression Sourcebook

Basic Consumer Health Information about Unipolar Depression, Bipolar Disorder, Postpartum Depression, Seasonal Affective Disorder, and Other Types of Depression in Children, Adolescents, Women, Men, the Elderly, and Other Selected Populations

Along with Facts about Causes, Risk Factors, Diagnostic Criteria, Treatment Options, Coping Strategies, Suicide Prevention, a Glossary, and a Directory of Sources for Additional Help and Information

Edited by Karen Belleni. 602 pages. 2002. 0-7808-0611-5.

"*Depression Sourcebook* is of a very high standard. Its purpose, which is to serve as a reference source to the lay reader, is very well served." — *Journal of the National Medical Association, 2004*

"Invaluable reference for public and school library collections alike." — *Library Bookwatch, Apr '03*

"Recommended for purchase." — *American Reference Books Annual, 2003*

Dermatological Disorders Sourcebook, 2nd Edition

Basic Consumer Health Information about Conditions and Disorders Affecting the Skin, Hair, and Nails, Such as Acne, Rosacea, Rashes, Dermatitis, Pigmentation Disorders, Birthmarks, Skin Cancer, Skin Injuries, Psoriasis, Scleroderma, and Hair Loss, Including Facts about Medications and Treatments for Dermatological

Disorders and Tips for Maintaining Healthy Skin, Hair, and Nails

Along with Information about How Aging Affects the Skin, a Glossary of Related Terms, and a Directory of Resources for Additional Help and Information

Edited by Amy L. Sutton. 645 pages. 2005. 0-7808-0795-2.

". . . comprehensive, easily read reference book."
—Doody's Health Sciences Book Reviews, Oct '97

SEE ALSO Burns Sourcebook

■

Diabetes Sourcebook, 3rd Edition

Basic Consumer Health Information about Type 1 Diabetes (Insulin-Dependent or Juvenile-Onset Diabetes), Type 2 Diabetes (Noninsulin-Dependent or Adult-Onset Diabetes), Gestational Diabetes, Impaired Glucose Tolerance (IGT), and Related Complications, Such as Amputation, Eye Disease, Gum Disease, Nerve Damage, and End-Stage Renal Disease, Including Facts about Insulin, Oral Diabetes Medications, Blood Sugar Testing, and the Role of Exercise and Nutrition in the Control of Diabetes

Along with a Glossary and Resources for Further Help and Information

Edited by Dawn D. Matthews. 622 pages. 2003. 0-7808-0629-8.

"This edition is even more helpful than earlier versions. . . . It is a truly valuable tool for anyone seeking readable and authoritative information on diabetes."
— American Reference Books Annual, 2004

"An invaluable reference." — Library Journal, May '00

Selected as one of the 250 "Best Health Sciences Books of 1999." — Doody's Rating Service, Mar-Apr '00

"Provides useful information for the general public."
— Healthlines, University of Michigan Health Management Research Center, Sep/Oct '99

". . . provides reliable mainstream medical information . . . belongs on the shelves of any library with a consumer health collection." — E-Streams, Sep '99

"Recommended reference source."
— Booklist, American Library Association, Feb '99

■

Diet & Nutrition Sourcebook, 3rd Edition

Basic Consumer Health Information about Dietary Guidelines and the Food Guidance System, Recommended Daily Nutrient Intakes, Serving Proportions, Weight Control, Vitamins and Supplements, Nutrition Issues for Different Life Stages and Lifestyles, and the Needs of People with Specific Medical Concerns, Including Cancer, Celiac Disease, Diabetes, Eating Disorders, Food Allergies, and Cardiovascular Disease

Along with Facts about Federal Nutrition Support Programs, a Glossary of Nutrition and Dietary Terms, and Directories of Additional Resources for More Information about Nutrition

Edited by Joyce Brennfleck Shannon. 633 pages. 2006. 0-7808-0800-2.

"This book is an excellent source of basic diet and nutrition information." — Booklist Health Sciences Supplement, American Library Association, Dec '00

"This reference document should be in any public library, but it would be a very good guide for beginning students in the health sciences. If the other books in this publisher's series are as good as this, they should all be in the health sciences collections."
—American Reference Books Annual, 2000

"This book is an excellent general nutrition reference for consumers who desire to take an active role in their health care for prevention. Consumers of all ages who select this book can feel confident they are receiving current and accurate information." — Journal of Nutrition for the Elderly, Vol. 19, No. 4, 2000

SEE ALSO Digestive Diseases & Disorders Sourcebook, Eating Disorders Sourcebook, Gastrointestinal Diseases & Disorders Sourcebook, Vegetarian Sourcebook

■

Digestive Diseases & Disorders Sourcebook

Basic Consumer Health Information about Diseases and Disorders that Impact the Upper and Lower Digestive System, Including Celiac Disease, Constipation, Crohn's Disease, Cyclic Vomiting Syndrome, Diarrhea, Diverticulosis and Diverticulitis, Gallstones, Heartburn, Hemorrhoids, Hernias, Indigestion (Dyspepsia), Irritable Bowel Syndrome, Lactose Intolerance, Ulcers, and More

Along with Information about Medications and Other Treatments, Tips for Maintaining a Healthy Digestive Tract, a Glossary, and Directory of Digestive Diseases Organizations

Edited by Karen Bellenir. 335 pages. 2000. 0-7808-0327-2.

"This title would be an excellent addition to all public or patient-research libraries."
— American Reference Books Annual, 2001

"This title is recommended for public, hospital, and health sciences libraries with consumer health collections." — E-Streams, Jul-Aug '00

"Recommended reference source."
— Booklist, American Library Association, May '00

SEE ALSO Eating Disorders Sourcebook, Gastrointestinal Diseases & Disorders Sourcebook

■

Disabilities Sourcebook

Basic Consumer Health Information about Physical and Psychiatric Disabilities, Including Descriptions of Major Causes of Disability, Assistive and Adaptive Aids, Workplace Issues, and Accessibility Concerns

Along with Information about the Americans with Disabilities Act, a Glossary, and Resources for Additional Help and Information

Edited by Dawn D. Matthews. 616 pages. 2000. 0-7808-0389-2.

"It is a must for libraries with a consumer health section." — *American Reference Books Annual, 2002*

"A much needed addition to the Omnigraphics Health Reference Series. A current reference work to provide people with disabilities, their families, caregivers or those who work with them, a broad range of information in one volume, has not been available until now. . . . It is recommended for all public and academic library reference collections." — *E-Streams, May '01*

"An excellent source book in easy-to-read format covering many current topics; highly recommended for all libraries." — *Choice, Association of College & Research Libraries, Jan '01*

"Recommended reference source." —*Booklist, American Library Association, Jul '00*

■

Domestic Violence Sourcebook, 2nd Edition

Basic Consumer Health Information about the Causes and Consequences of Abusive Relationships, Including Physical Violence, Sexual Assault, Battery, Stalking, and Emotional Abuse, and Facts about the Effects of Violence on Women, Men, Young Adults, and the Elderly, with Reports about Domestic Violence in Selected Populations, and Featuring Facts about Medical Care, Victim Assistance and Protection, Prevention Strategies, Mental Health Services, and Legal Issues

Along with a Glossary of Related Terms and Resources for Additional Help and Information

Edited by Dawn D. Matthews. 628 pages. 2004. 0-7808-0669-7.

"Educators, clergy, medical professionals, police, and victims and their families will benefit from this realistic and easy-to-understand resource." — *American Reference Books Annual, 2005*

"Recommended for all collections supporting consumer health information. It should also be considered for any collection needing general, readable information on domestic violence." — *E-Streams, Jan '05*

"This sourcebook complements other books in its field, providing a one-stop resource . . . Recommended." —*Choice, Association of College & Research Libraries, Jan '05*

"Interested lay persons should find the book extremely beneficial. . . . A copy of *Domestic Violence and Child Abuse Sourcebook* should be in every public library in the United States." — *Social Science & Medicine, No. 56, 2003*

"This is important information. The Web has many resources but this sourcebook fills an important societal need. I am not aware of any other resources of this type." — *Doody's Review Service, Sep '01*

"Recommended reference source." —*Booklist, American Library Association, Apr '01*

"Important pick for college-level health reference libraries." — *The Bookwatch, Mar '01*

"Because this problem is so widespread and because this book includes a lot of issues within one volume, this work is recommended for all public libraries." — *American Reference Books Annual, 2001*

SEE ALSO *Child Abuse Sourcebook*

■

Drug Abuse Sourcebook, 2nd Edition

Basic Consumer Health Information about Illicit Substances of Abuse and the Misuse of Prescription and Over-the-Counter Medications, Including Depressants, Hallucinogens, Inhalants, Marijuana, Stimulants, and Anabolic Steroids

Along with Facts about Related Health Risks, Treatment Programs, Prevention Programs, a Glossary of Abuse and Addiction Terms, a Glossary of Drug-Related Street Terms, and a Directory of Resources for More Information

Edited by Catherine Ginther. 607 pages. 2004. 0-7808-0740-5.

"Commendable for organizing useful, normally scattered government and association-produced data into a logical sequence." — *American Reference Books Annual, 2006*

"This easy-to-read volume is recommended for consumer health collections within public or academic libraries." — *E-Streams, Sep '05*

"An excellent library reference." — *The Bookwatch, May '05*

"Containing a wealth of information, this book will be useful to the college student just beginning to explore the topic of substance abuse. This resource belongs in libraries that serve a lower-division undergraduate or community college clientele as well as the general public." — *Choice, Association of College & Research Libraries, Jun '01*

"Recommended reference source." —*Booklist, American Library Association, Feb '01*

SEE ALSO *Alcoholism Sourcebook, Substance Abuse Sourcebook*

■

Ear, Nose & Throat Disorders Sourcebook, 2nd Edition

Basic Consumer Health Information about Disorders of the Ears, Hearing Loss, Vestibular Disorders, Nasal and Sinus Problems, Throat and Vocal Cord Disorders, and Otolaryngologic Cancers, Including Facts about Ear Infections and Injuries, Genetic and Congenital Deafness, Sensorineural Hearing Disorders, Tinnitus, Vertigo, Ménière Disease, Rhinitis, Sinusitis, Snoring, Sore Throats, Hoarseness, and More

Along with Reports on Current Research Initiatives, a Glossary of Related Medical Terms, and a Directory of Sources for Further Help and Information

Edited by Sandra J. Judd. 659 pages. 2006. 0-7808-0872-X.

"Overall, this sourcebook is helpful for the consumer seeking information on ENT issues. It is recommended for public libraries."
—American Reference Books Annual, 1999

"Recommended reference source."
—Booklist, American Library Association, Dec '98

■

Eating Disorders Sourcebook

Basic Consumer Health Information about Eating Disorders, Including Information about Anorexia Nervosa, Bulimia Nervosa, Binge Eating, Body Dysmorphic Disorder, Pica, Laxative Abuse, and Night Eating Syndrome

Along with Information about Causes, Adverse Effects, and Treatment and Prevention Issues, and Featuring a Section on Concerns Specific to Children and Adolescents, a Glossary, and Resources for Further Help and Information

Edited by Dawn D. Matthews. 322 pages. 2001. 0-7808-0335-3.

"Recommended for health science libraries that are open to the public, as well as hospital libraries. This book is a good resource for the consumer who is concerned about eating disorders." —E-Streams, Mar '02

"This volume is another convenient collection of excerpted articles. Recommended for school and public library patrons; lower-division undergraduates; and two-year technical program students."
—Choice, Association of College & Research Libraries, Jan '02

"Recommended reference source."
—Booklist, American Library Association, Oct '01

SEE ALSO Diet & Nutrition Sourcebook, Digestive Diseases & Disorders Sourcebook, Gastrointestinal Diseases & Disorders Sourcebook

■

Emergency Medical Services Sourcebook

Basic Consumer Health Information about Preventing, Preparing for, and Managing Emergency Situations, When and Who to Call for Help, What to Expect in the Emergency Room, the Emergency Medical Team, Patient Issues, and Current Topics in Emergency Medicine

Along with Statistical Data, a Glossary, and Sources of Additional Help and Information

Edited by Jenni Lynn Colson. 494 pages. 2002. 0-7808-0420-1.

"Handy and convenient for home, public, school, and college libraries. Recommended."
— Choice, Association of College & Research Libraries, Apr '03

"This reference can provide the consumer with answers to most questions about emergency care in the United States, or it will direct them to a resource where the answer can be found."
—American Reference Books Annual, 2003

"Recommended reference source."
— Booklist, American Library Association, Feb '03

■

Endocrine & Metabolic Disorders Sourcebook

Basic Information for the Layperson about Pancreatic and Insulin-Related Disorders Such as Pancreatitis, Diabetes, and Hypoglycemia; Adrenal Gland Disorders Such as Cushing's Syndrome, Addison's Disease, and Congenital Adrenal Hyperplasia; Pituitary Gland Disorders Such as Growth Hormone Deficiency, Acromegaly, and Pituitary Tumors; Thyroid Disorders Such as Hypothyroidism, Graves' Disease, Hashimoto's Disease, and Goiter; Hyperparathyroidism; and Other Diseases and Syndromes of Hormone Imbalance or Metabolic Dysfunction

Along with Reports on Current Research Initiatives

Edited by Linda M. Shin. 574 pages. 1998. 0-7808-0207-1.

"Omnigraphics has produced another needed resource for health information consumers."
—American Reference Books Annual, 2000

"Recommended reference source."
— Booklist, American Library Association, Dec '98

■

Environmental Health Sourcebook, 2nd Edition

Basic Consumer Health Information about the Environment and Its Effect on Human Health, Including the Effects of Air Pollution, Water Pollution, Hazardous Chemicals, Food Hazards, Radiation Hazards, Biological Agents, Household Hazards, Such as Radon, Asbestos, Carbon Monoxide, and Mold, and Information about Associated Diseases and Disorders, Including Cancer, Allergies, Respiratory Problems, and Skin Disorders

Along with Information about Environmental Concerns for Specific Populations, a Glossary of Related Terms, and Resources for Further Help and Information

Edited by Dawn D. Matthews. 673 pages. 2003. 0-7808-0632-8.

"This recently updated edition continues the level of quality and the reputation of the numerous other volumes in Omnigraphics' Health Reference Series."
—American Reference Books Annual, 2004

"An excellent updated edition."
—The Bookwatch, Oct '03

"Recommended reference source."
—Booklist, American Library Association, Sep '98

"This book will be a useful addition to anyone's library." —Choice Health Sciences Supplement, Association of College & Research Libraries, May '98

Environmentally Induced Disorders Sourcebook

SEE *Environmental Health Sourcebook, 2nd Edition*

Ethnic Diseases Sourcebook

Basic Consumer Health Information for Ethnic and Racial Minority Groups in the United States, Including General Health Indicators and Behaviors, Ethnic Diseases, Genetic Testing, the Impact of Chronic Diseases, Women's Health, Mental Health Issues, and Preventive Health Care Services

Along with a Glossary and a Listing of Additional Resources

Edited by Joyce Brennfleck Shannon. 664 pages. 2001. 0-7808-0336-1.

Eye Care Sourcebook, 2nd Edition

Basic Consumer Health Information about Eye Care and Eye Disorders, Including Facts about the Diagnosis, Prevention, and Treatment of Common Refractive Problems Such as Myopia, Hyperopia, Astigmatism, and Presbyopia, and Eye Diseases, Including Glaucoma, Cataract, Age-Related Macular Degeneration, and Diabetic Retinopathy

Along with a Section on Vision Correction and Refractive Surgeries, Including LASIK and LASEK, a Glossary, and Directories of Resources for Additional Help and Information

Edited by Amy L. Sutton. 543 pages. 2003. 0-7808-0635-2.

Family Planning Sourcebook

Basic Consumer Health Information about Planning for Pregnancy and Contraception, Including Traditional Methods, Barrier Methods, Hormonal Methods, Permanent Methods, Future Methods, Emergency Contraception, and Birth Control Choices for Women at Each Stage of Life

Along with Statistics, a Glossary, and Sources of Additional Information

Edited by Amy Marcaccio Keyzer. 520 pages. 2001. 0-7808-0379-5.

SEE ALSO *Pregnancy & Birth Sourcebook*

Fitness & Exercise Sourcebook, 3rd Edition

Basic Consumer Health Information about the Physical and Mental Benefits of Fitness, Including Cardiorespiratory Endurance, Muscular Strength, Muscular Endurance, and Flexibility, with Facts about Sports Nutrition and Exercise-Related Injuries and Tips about Physical Activity and Exercises for People of All Ages and for People with Health Concerns

Along with Advice on Selecting and Using Exercise Equipment, Maintaining Exercise Motivation, a Glossary of Related Terms, and a Directory of Resources for More Help and Information

Edited by Amy L. Sutton. 625 pages. 2007. 0-7808-0946-7.

Food & Animal Borne Diseases Sourcebook

Basic Information about Diseases That Can Be Spread to Humans through the Ingestion of Contaminated Food or Water or by Contact with Infected Animals and Insects, Such as Botulism, E. Coli, Hepatitis A, Trichinosis, Lyme Disease, and Rabies

Along with Information Regarding Prevention and Treatment Methods, and Including a Special Section for International Travelers Describing Diseases Such as Cholera, Malaria, Travelers' Diarrhea, and Yellow Fever, and Offering Recommendations for Avoiding Illness

Edited by Karen Bellenir and Peter D. Dresser. 535 pages. 1995. 0-7808-0033-8.

"Targeting general readers and providing them with a single, comprehensive source of information on selected topics, this book continues, with the excellent caliber of its predecessors, to catalog topical information on health matters of general interest. Readable and thorough, this valuable resource is highly recommended for all libraries."
— Academic Library Book Review, Summer '96

"A comprehensive collection of authoritative information." — Emergency Medical Services, Oct '95

Food Safety Sourcebook

Basic Consumer Health Information about the Safe Handling of Meat, Poultry, Seafood, Eggs, Fruit Juices, and Other Food Items, and Facts about Pesticides, Drinking Water, Food Safety Overseas, and the Onset, Duration, and Symptoms of Foodborne Illnesses, Including Types of Pathogenic Bacteria, Parasitic Protozoa, Worms, Viruses, and Natural Toxins

Along with the Role of the Consumer, the Food Handler, and the Government in Food Safety; a Glossary, and Resources for Additional Help and Information

Edited by Dawn D. Matthews. 339 pages. 1999. 0-7808-0326-4.

"This book is recommended for public libraries and universities with home economic and food science programs." — E-Streams, Nov '00

"Recommended reference source."
— Booklist, American Library Association, May '00

"This book takes the complex issues of food safety and foodborne pathogens and presents them in an easily understood manner. [It does] an excellent job of covering a large and often confusing topic."
— American Reference Books Annual, 2000

Forensic Medicine Sourcebook

Basic Consumer Information for the Layperson about Forensic Medicine, Including Crime Scene Investigation, Evidence Collection and Analysis, Expert Testimony, Computer-Aided Criminal Identification, Digital Imaging in the Courtroom, DNA Profiling, Accident Reconstruction, Autopsies, Ballistics, Drugs and Explosives Detection, Latent Fingerprints, Product Tampering, and Questioned Document Examination

Along with Statistical Data, a Glossary of Forensics Terminology, and Listings of Sources for Further Help and Information

Edited by Annemarie S. Muth. 574 pages. 1999. 0-7808-0232-2.

"Given the expected widespread interest in its content and its easy to read style, this book is recommended for most public and all college and university libraries."
— E-Streams, Feb '01

"Recommended for public libraries."
— Reference & User Services Quarterly, American Library Association, Spring 2000

"Recommended reference source."
— Booklist, American Library Association, Feb '00

"A wealth of information, useful statistics, references are up-to-date and extremely complete. This wonderful collection of data will help students who are interested in a career in any type of forensic field. It is a great resource for attorneys who need information about types of expert witnesses needed in a particular case. It also offers useful information for fiction and nonfiction writers whose work involves a crime. A fascinating compilation. All levels."
— Choice, Association of College & Research Libraries, Jan '00

"There are several items that make this book attractive to consumers who are seeking certain forensic data. . . . This is a useful current source for those seeking general forensic medical answers."
— American Reference Books Annual, 2000

Gastrointestinal Diseases & Disorders Sourcebook, 2nd Edition

Basic Consumer Health Information about the Upper and Lower Gastrointestinal (GI) Tract, Including the Esophagus, Stomach, Intestines, Rectum, Liver, and Pancreas, with Facts about Gastroesophageal Reflux Disease, Gastritis, Hernias, Ulcers, Celiac Disease, Diverticulitis, Irritable Bowel Syndrome, Hemorrhoids, Gastrointestinal Cancers, and Other Diseases and Disorders Related to the Digestive Process

Along with Information about Commonly Used Diagnostic and Surgical Procedures, Statistics, Reports on Current Research Initiatives and Clinical Trials, a Glossary, and Resources for Additional Help and Information

Edited by Sandra J. Judd. 681 pages. 2006. 0-7808-0798-7.

". . . very readable form. The successful editorial work that brought this material together into a useful and understandable reference makes accessible to all readers information that can help them more effectively understand and obtain help for digestive tract problems."
— Choice, Association of College & Research Libraries, Feb '97

SEE ALSO *Diet & Nutrition Sourcebook, Digestive Diseases & Disorders, Eating Disorders Sourcebook*

■

Genetic Disorders Sourcebook, 3rd Edition

Basic Consumer Health Information about Hereditary Diseases and Disorders, Including Facts about the Human Genome, Genetic Inheritance Patterns, Disorders Associated with Specific Genes, Such as Sickle Cell Disease, Hemophilia, and Cystic Fibrosis, Chromosome Disorders, Such as Down Syndrome, Fragile X Syndrome, and Turner Syndrome, and Complex Diseases and Disorders Resulting from the Interaction of Environmental and Genetic Factors, Such as Allergies, Cancer, and Obesity

Along with Facts about Genetic Testing, Suggestions for Parents of Children with Special Needs, Reports on Current Research Initiatives, a Glossary of Genetic Terminology, and Resources for Additional Help and Information

Edited by Karen Bellenir. 777 pages. 2004. 0-7808-0742-1.

"This text is recommended for any library with an interest in providing consumer health resources."
— *E-Streams, Aug '05*

"This is a valuable resource for anyone wishing to have an understandable description of any of the topics or disorders included. The editor succeeds in making complex genetic issues understandable."
— *Doody's Book Review Service, May '05*

"A good acquisition for public libraries."
— *American Reference Books Annual, 2005*

"Excellent reference." — *The Bookwatch, Jan '05*

"Recommended reference source."
— *Booklist, American Library Association, Apr '01*

"Important pick for college-level health reference libraries." — *The Bookwatch, Mar '01*

■

Head Trauma Sourcebook

Basic Information for the Layperson about Open-Head and Closed-Head Injuries, Treatment Advances, Recovery, and Rehabilitation

Along with Reports on Current Research Initiatives

Edited by Karen Bellenir. 414 pages. 1997. 0-7808-0208-X.

■

Headache Sourcebook

Basic Consumer Health Information about Migraine, Tension, Cluster, Rebound and Other Types of Headaches, with Facts about the Cause and Prevention of Headaches, the Effects of Stress and the Environment, Headaches during Pregnancy and Menopause, and Childhood Headaches

Along with a Glossary and Other Resources for Additional Help and Information

Edited by Dawn D. Matthews. 362 pages. 2002. 0-7808-0337-X.

"Highly recommended for academic and medical reference collections." — *Library Bookwatch, Sep '02*

■

Health Insurance Sourcebook

Basic Information about Managed Care Organizations, Traditional Fee-for-Service Insurance, Insurance Portability and Pre-Existing Conditions Clauses, Medicare, Medicaid, Social Security, and Military Health Care

Along with Information about Insurance Fraud

Edited by Wendy Wilcox. 530 pages. 1997. 0-7808-0222-5.

"Particularly useful because it brings much of this information together in one volume. This book will be a handy reference source in the health sciences library, hospital library, college and university library, and medium to large public library."
— *Medical Reference Services Quarterly, Fall '98*

Awarded "Books of the Year Award"
— *American Journal of Nursing, 1997*

"The layout of the book is particularly helpful as it provides easy access to reference material. A most useful addition to the vast amount of information about health insurance. The use of data from U.S. government agencies is most commendable. Useful in a library or learning center for healthcare professional students."
— *Doody's Health Sciences Book Reviews, Nov '97*

■

Healthy Aging Sourcebook

Basic Consumer Health Information about Maintaining Health through the Aging Process, Including Advice on Nutrition, Exercise, and Sleep, Help in Making Decisions about Midlife Issues and Retirement, and Guidance Concerning Practical and Informed Choices in Health Consumerism

Along with Data Concerning the Theories of Aging, Different Experiences in Aging by Minority Groups, and Facts about Aging Now and Aging in the Future; and Featuring a Glossary, a Guide to Consumer Help, Additional Suggested Reading, and Practical Resource Directory

Edited by Jenifer Swanson. 536 pages. 1999. 0-7808-0390-6.

"Recommended reference source."
— *Booklist, American Library Association, Feb '00*

SEE ALSO *Physical & Mental Issues in Aging Sourcebook*

■

Healthy Children Sourcebook

Basic Consumer Health Information about the Physical and Mental Development of Children between the Ages of 3 and 12, Including Routine Health Care, Preventative Health Services, Safety and First Aid, Healthy Sleep, Dental Care, Nutrition, and Fitness, and Featuring Parenting Tips on Such Topics as Bed-

wetting, Choosing Day Care, Monitoring TV and Other Media, and Establishing a Foundation for Substance Abuse Prevention

Along with a Glossary of Commonly Used Pediatric Terms and Resources for Additional Help and Information.

Edited by Chad T. Kimball. 647 pages. 2003. 0-7808-0247-0.

"It is hard to imagine that any other single resource exists that would provide such a comprehensive guide of timely information on health promotion and disease prevention for children aged 3 to 12."
—American Reference Books Annual, 2004

"The strengths of this book are many. It is clearly written, presented and structured."
—Journal of the National Medical Association, 2004

SEE ALSO Childhood Diseases & Disorders Sourcebook

■

Healthy Heart Sourcebook for Women

Basic Consumer Health Information about Cardiac Issues Specific to Women, Including Facts about Major Risk Factors and Prevention, Treatment and Control Strategies, and Important Dietary Issues

Along with a Special Section Regarding the Pros and Cons of Hormone Replacement Therapy and Its Impact on Heart Health, and Additional Help, Including Recipes, a Glossary, and a Directory of Resources

Edited by Dawn D. Matthews. 336 pages. 2000. 0-7808-0329-9.

"A good reference source and recommended for all public, academic, medical, and hospital libraries."
—Medical Reference Services Quarterly, Summer '01

"Because of the lack of information specific to women on this topic, this book is recommended for public libraries and consumer libraries."
—American Reference Books Annual, 2001

"Contains very important information about coronary artery disease that all women should know. The information is current and presented in an easy-to-read format. The book will make a good addition to any library."
—American Medical Writers Association Journal, Summer '00

"Important, basic reference."
—Reviewer's Bookwatch, Jul '00

SEE ALSO Cardiovascular Diseases & Disorders Sourcebook, Women's Health Concerns Sourcebook

■

Heart Diseases & Disorders Sourcebook

SEE Cardiovascular Diseases & Disorders Sourcebook, 3rd Edition

Hepatitis Sourcebook

Basic Consumer Health Information about Hepatitis A, Hepatitis B, Hepatitis C, and Other Forms of Hepatitis, Including Autoimmune Hepatitis, Alcoholic Hepatitis, Nonalcoholic Steatohepatitis, and Toxic Hepatitis, with Facts about Risk Factors, Screening Methods, Diagnostic Tests, and Treatment Options

Along with Information on Liver Health, Tips for People Living with Chronic Hepatitis, Reports on Current Research Initiatives, a Glossary of Terms Related to Hepatitis, and a Directory of Sources for Further Help and Information

Edited by Sandra J. Judd. 597 pages. 2005. 0-7808-0749-9.

"Highly recommended."
—American Reference Books Annual, 2006

■

Household Safety Sourcebook

Basic Consumer Health Information about Household Safety, Including Information about Poisons, Chemicals, Fire, and Water Hazards in the Home

Along with Advice about the Safe Use of Home Maintenance Equipment, Choosing Toys and Nursery Furniture, Holiday and Recreation Safety, a Glossary, and Resources for Further Help and Information

Edited by Dawn D. Matthews. 606 pages. 2002. 0-7808-0338-8.

"This work will be useful in public libraries with large consumer health and wellness departments."
—American Reference Books Annual, 2003

"As a sourcebook on household safety this book meets its mark. It is encyclopedic in scope and covers a wide range of safety issues that are commonly seen in the home."
—E-Streams, Jul '02

■

Hypertension Sourcebook

Basic Consumer Health Information about the Causes, Diagnosis, and Treatment of High Blood Pressure, with Facts about Consequences, Complications, and Co-Occurring Disorders, Such as Coronary Heart Disease, Diabetes, Stroke, Kidney Disease, and Hypertensive Retinopathy, and Issues in Blood Pressure Control, Including Dietary Choices, Stress Management, and Medications

Along with Reports on Current Research Initiatives and Clinical Trials, a Glossary, and Resources for Additional Help and Information

Edited by Dawn D. Matthews and Karen Bellenir. 613 pages. 2004. 0-7808-0674-3.

"Academic, public, and medical libraries will want to add the Hypertension Sourcebook to their collections."
—E-Streams, Aug '05

"The strength of this source is the wide range of information given about hypertension."
—American Reference Books Annual, 2005

Immune System Disorders Sourcebook, 2nd Edition

Basic Consumer Health Information about Disorders of the Immune System, Including Immune System Function and Response, Diagnosis of Immune Disorders, Information about Inherited Immune Disease, Acquired Immune Disease, and Autoimmune Diseases, Including Primary Immune Deficiency, Acquired Immunodeficiency Syndrome (AIDS), Lupus, Multiple Sclerosis, Type 1 Diabetes, Rheumatoid Arthritis, and Graves' Disease

Along with Treatments, Tips for Coping with Immune Disorders, a Glossary, and a Directory of Additional Resources.

Edited by Joyce Brennfleck Shannon. 671 pages. 2005. 0-7808-0748-0

"Highly recommended for academic and public libraries." — *American Reference Books Annual, 2006*

"The updated second edition is a 'must' for any consumer health library seeking a solid resource covering the treatments, symptoms, and options for immune disorder sufferers. . . . An excellent guide."
— *MBR Bookwatch, Jan '06*

Infant & Toddler Health Sourcebook

Basic Consumer Health Information about the Physical and Mental Development of Newborns, Infants, and Toddlers, Including Neonatal Concerns, Nutrition Recommendations, Immunization Schedules, Common Pediatric Disorders, Assessments and Milestones, Safety Tips, and Advice for Parents and Other Caregivers

Along with a Glossary of Terms and Resource Listings for Additional Help

Edited by Jenifer Swanson. 585 pages. 2000. 0-7808-0246-2.

"As a reference for the general public, this would be useful in any library." — *E-Streams, May '01*

"Recommended reference source."
— *Booklist, American Library Association, Feb '01*

"This is a good source for general use."
— *American Reference Books Annual, 2001*

Infectious Diseases Sourcebook

Basic Consumer Health Information about Non-Contagious Bacterial, Viral, Prion, Fungal, and Parasitic Diseases Spread by Food and Water, Insects and Animals, or Environmental Contact, Including Botulism, E. Coli, Encephalitis, Legionnaires' Disease, Lyme Disease, Malaria, Plague, Rabies, Salmonella, Tetanus, and Others, and Facts about Newly Emerging Diseases, Such as Hantavirus, Mad Cow Disease, Monkeypox, and West Nile Virus

Along with Information about Preventing Disease Transmission, the Threat of Bioterrorism, and Current

Research Initiatives, with a Glossary and Directory of Resources for More Information

Edited by Karen Bellenir. 634 pages. 2004. 0-7808-0675-1.

"This reference continues the excellent tradition of the *Health Reference Series* **in consolidating a wealth of information on a selected topic into a format that is easy to use and accessible to the general public."**
— *American Reference Books Annual, 2005*

"Recommended for public and academic libraries."
— *E-Streams, Jan '05*

Injury & Trauma Sourcebook

Basic Consumer Health Information about the Impact of Injury, the Diagnosis and Treatment of Common and Traumatic Injuries, Emergency Care, and Specific Injuries Related to Home, Community, Workplace, Transportation, and Recreation

Along with Guidelines for Injury Prevention, a Glossary, and a Directory of Additional Resources

Edited by Joyce Brennfleck Shannon. 696 pages. 2002. 0-7808-0421-X.

"This publication is the most comprehensive work of its kind about injury and trauma."
— *American Reference Books Annual, 2003*

"This sourcebook provides concise, easily readable, basic health information about injuries. . . . This book is well organized and an easy to use reference resource suitable for hospital, health sciences and public libraries with consumer health collections."
— *E-Streams, Nov '02*

"Practitioners should be aware of guides such as this in order to facilitate their use by patients and their families." — *Doody's Health Sciences Book Review Journal, Sep-Oct '02*

"Recommended reference source."
— *Booklist, American Library Association, Sep '02*

"Highly recommended for academic and medical reference collections." — *Library Bookwatch, Sep '02*

Kidney & Urinary Tract Diseases & Disorders Sourcebook

SEE Urinary Tract & Kidney Diseases & Disorders Sourcebook, 2nd Edition

---

Learning Disabilities Sourcebook, 2nd Edition

Basic Consumer Health Information about Learning Disabilities, Including Dyslexia, Developmental Speech and Language Disabilities, Non-Verbal Learning Disorders, Developmental Arithmetic Disorder, Developmental Writing Disorder, and Other Conditions That Impede Learning Such as Attention Deficit/ Hyperac-

tivity Disorder, Brain Injury, Hearing Impairment, Klinefelter Syndrome, Dyspraxia, and Tourette's Syndrome

Along with Facts about Educational Issues and Assistive Technology, Coping Strategies, a Glossary of Related Terms, and Resources for Further Help and Information

Edited by Dawn D. Matthews. 621 pages. 2003. 0-7808-0626-3.

"The second edition of Learning Disabilities Sourcebook far surpasses the earlier edition in that it is more focused on information that will be useful as a consumer health resource."
—American Reference Books Annual, 2004

"Teachers as well as consumers will find this an essential guide to understanding various syndromes and their latest treatments. [An] invaluable reference for public and school library collections alike."
—Library Bookwatch, Apr '03

Named "Outstanding Reference Book of 1999."
—New York Public Library, Feb 2000

"An excellent candidate for inclusion in a public library reference section. It's a great source of information. Teachers will also find the book useful. Definitely worth reading."
—Journal of Adolescent & Adult Literacy, Feb 2000

"Readable . . . provides a solid base of information regarding successful techniques used with individuals who have learning disabilities, as well as practical suggestions for educators and family members. Clear language, concise descriptions, and pertinent information for contacting multiple resources add to the strength of this book as a useful tool."   —Choice, Association of College & Research Libraries, Feb '99

"Recommended reference source."
—Booklist, American Library Association, Sep '98

"A useful resource for libraries and for those who don't have the time to identify and locate the individual publications."   —Disability Resources Monthly, Sep '98

■

Leukemia Sourcebook

Basic Consumer Health Information about Adult and Childhood Leukemias, Including Acute Lymphocytic Leukemia (ALL), Chronic Lymphocytic Leukemia (CLL), Acute Myelogenous Leukemia (AML), Chronic Myelogenous Leukemia (CML), and Hairy Cell Leukemia, and Treatments Such as Chemotherapy, Radiation Therapy, Peripheral Blood Stem Cell and Marrow Transplantation, and Immunotherapy

Along with Tips for Life During and After Treatment, a Glossary, and Directories of Additional Resources

Edited by Joyce Brennfleck Shannon. 587 pages. 2003. 0-7808-0627-1.

"Unlike other medical books for the layperson, . . . the language does not talk down to the reader. . . . This volume is highly recommended for all libraries."
—American Reference Books Annual, 2004

"'. . . a fine title which ranges from diagnosis to alternative treatments, staging, and tips for life during and after diagnosis."   —The Bookwatch, Dec '03

■

Liver Disorders Sourcebook

Basic Consumer Health Information about the Liver and How It Works; Liver Diseases, Including Cancer, Cirrhosis, Hepatitis, and Toxic and Drug Related Diseases; Tips for Maintaining a Healthy Liver; Laboratory Tests, Radiology Tests, and Facts about Liver Transplantation

Along with a Section on Support Groups, a Glossary, and Resource Listings

Edited by Joyce Brennfleck Shannon. 591 pages. 2000. 0-7808-0383-3.

"A valuable resource."
—American Reference Books Annual, 2001

"This title is recommended for health sciences and public libraries with consumer health collections."
—E-Streams, Oct '00

"Recommended reference source."
—Booklist, American Library Association, Jun '00

■

Lung Disorders Sourcebook

Basic Consumer Health Information about Emphysema, Pneumonia, Tuberculosis, Asthma, Cystic Fibrosis, and Other Lung Disorders, Including Facts about Diagnostic Procedures, Treatment Strategies, Disease Prevention Efforts, and Such Risk Factors as Smoking, Air Pollution, and Exposure to Asbestos, Radon, and Other Agents

Along with a Glossary and Resources for Additional Help and Information

Edited by Dawn D. Matthews. 678 pages. 2002. 0-7808-0339-6.

"This title is a great addition for public and school libraries because it provides concise health information on the lungs."
—American Reference Books Annual, 2003

"Highly recommended for academic and medical reference collections."   —Library Bookwatch, Sep '02

SEE ALSO Respiratory Diseases & Disorders Sourcebook

■

Medical Tests Sourcebook, 2nd Edition

Basic Consumer Health Information about Medical Tests, Including Age-Specific Health Tests, Important Health Screenings and Exams, Home-Use Tests, Blood and Specimen Tests, Electrical Tests, Scope Tests, Genetic Testing, and Imaging Tests, Such as X-Rays, Ultrasound, Computed Tomography, Magnetic Resonance Imaging, Angiography, and Nuclear Medicine

636

Along with a Glossary and Directory of Additional Resources

Edited by Joyce Brennfleck Shannon. 654 pages. 2004. 0-7808-0670-0.

"Recommended for hospital and health sciences libraries with consumer health collections."
— *E-Streams, Mar '00*

"This is an overall excellent reference with a wealth of general knowledge that may aid those who are reluctant to get vital tests performed."
— *Today's Librarian, Jan '00*

"A valuable reference guide."
— *American Reference Books Annual, 2000*

■

Men's Health Concerns Sourcebook, 2nd Edition

Basic Consumer Health Information about the Medical and Mental Concerns of Men, Including Theories about the Shorter Male Lifespan, the Leading Causes of Death and Disability, Physical Concerns of Special Significance to Men, Reproductive and Sexual Concerns, Sexually Transmitted Diseases, Men's Mental and Emotional Health, and Lifestyle Choices That Affect Wellness, Such as Nutrition, Fitness, and Substance Use

Along with a Glossary of Related Terms and a Directory of Organizational Resources in Men's Health

Edited by Robert Aquinas McNally. 644 pages. 2004. 0-7808-0671-9.

"A very accessible reference for non-specialist general readers and consumers." — *The Bookwatch, Jun '04*

"This comprehensive resource and the series are highly recommended."
— *American Reference Books Annual, 2000*

"Recommended reference source."
— *Booklist, American Library Association, Dec '98*

■

Mental Health Disorders Sourcebook, 3rd Edition

Basic Consumer Health Information about Mental and Emotional Health and Mental Illness, Including Facts about Depression, Bipolar Disorder, and Other Mood Disorders, Phobias, Post-Traumatic Stress Disorder (PTSD), Obsessive-Compulsive Disorder, and Other Anxiety Disorders, Impulse Control Disorders, Eating Disorders, Personality Disorders, and Psychotic Disorders, Including Schizophrenia and Dissociative Disorders

Along with Statistical Information, a Special Section Concerning Mental Health Issues in Children and Adolescents, a Glossary, and Directories of Resources for Additional Help and Information

Edited by Karen Bellenir. 661 pages. 2005. 0-7808-0747-2.

"Recommended for public libraries and academic libraries with an undergraduate program in psychology."
— *American Reference Books Annual, 2006*

"Recommended reference source."
— *Booklist, American Library Association, Jun '00*

■

Mental Retardation Sourcebook

Basic Consumer Health Information about Mental Retardation and Its Causes, Including Down Syndrome, Fetal Alcohol Syndrome, Fragile X Syndrome, Genetic Conditions, Injury, and Environmental Sources

Along with Preventive Strategies, Parenting Issues, Educational Implications, Health Care Needs, Employment and Economic Matters, Legal Issues, a Glossary, and a Resource Listing for Additional Help and Information

Edited by Joyce Brennfleck Shannon. 642 pages. 2000. 0-7808-0377-9.

"Public libraries will find the book useful for reference and as a beginning research point for students, parents, and caregivers."
— *American Reference Books Annual, 2001*

"The strength of this work is that it compiles many basic fact sheets and addresses for further information in one volume. It is intended and suitable for the general public. This sourcebook is relevant to any collection providing health information to the general public."
— *E-Streams, Nov '00*

"From preventing retardation to parenting and family challenges, this covers health, social and legal issues and will prove an invaluable overview."
— *Reviewer's Bookwatch, Jul '00*

■

Movement Disorders Sourcebook

Basic Consumer Health Information about Neurological Movement Disorders, Including Essential Tremor, Parkinson's Disease, Dystonia, Cerebral Palsy, Huntington's Disease, Myasthenia Gravis, Multiple Sclerosis, and Other Early-Onset and Adult-Onset Movement Disorders, Their Symptoms and Causes, Diagnostic Tests, and Treatments

Along with Mobility and Assistive Technology Information, a Glossary, and a Directory of Additional Resources

Edited by Joyce Brennfleck Shannon. 655 pages. 2003. 0-7808-0628-X.

". . . a good resource for consumers and recommended for public, community college and undergraduate libraries." — *American Reference Books Annual, 2004*

■

Muscular Dystrophy Sourcebook

Basic Consumer Health Information about Congenital, Childhood-Onset, and Adult-Onset Forms of Muscular Dystrophy, Such as Duchenne, Becker, Emery-Dreifuss, Distal, Limb-Girdle, Facioscapulohumeral (FSHD), Myotonic, and Ophthalmoplegic Muscular Dystro-

phies, Including Facts about Diagnostic Tests, Medical and Physical Therapies, Management of Co-Occurring Conditions, and Parenting Guidelines

Along with Practical Tips for Home Care, a Glossary, and Directories of Additional Resources

Edited by Joyce Brennfleck Shannon. 577 pages. 2004. 0-7808-0676-X.

"This book is highly recommended for public and academic libraries as well as health care offices that support the information needs of patients and their families."
— *E-Streams, Apr '05*

"Excellent reference." — *The Bookwatch, Jan '05*

▪

Obesity Sourcebook

Basic Consumer Health Information about Diseases and Other Problems Associated with Obesity, and Including Facts about Risk Factors, Prevention Issues, and Management Approaches

Along with Statistical and Demographic Data, Information about Special Populations, Research Updates, a Glossary, and Source Listings for Further Help and Information

Edited by Wilma Caldwell and Chad T. Kimball. 376 pages. 2001. 0-7808-0333-7.

"The book synthesizes the reliable medical literature on obesity into one easy-to-read and useful resource for the general public."
— *American Reference Books Annual, 2002*

"This is a very useful resource book for the lay public."
— *Doody's Review Service, Nov '01*

"Well suited for the health reference collection of a public library or an academic health science library that serves the general population." — *E-Streams, Sep '01*

"Recommended reference source."
— *Booklist, American Library Association, Apr '01*

"Recommended pick both for specialty health library collections and any general consumer health reference collection." — *The Bookwatch, Apr '01*

▪

Ophthalmic Disorders Sourcebook

SEE *Eye Care Sourcebook, 2nd Edition*

▪

Oral Health Sourcebook

SEE *Dental Care & Oral Health Sourcebook, 2nd Edition*

▪

Osteoporosis Sourcebook

Basic Consumer Health Information about Primary and Secondary Osteoporosis and Juvenile Osteoporosis and Related Conditions, Including Fibrous Dysplasia,

Gaucher Disease, Hyperthyroidism, Hypophosphatasia, Myeloma, Osteopetrosis, Osteogenesis Imperfecta, and Paget's Disease

Along with Information about Risk Factors, Treatments, Traditional and Non-Traditional Pain Management, a Glossary of Related Terms, and a Directory of Resources

Edited by Allan R. Cook. 584 pages. 2001. 0-7808-0239-X.

"This would be a book to be kept in a staff or patient library. The targeted audience is the layperson, but the therapist who needs a quick bit of information on a particular topic will also find the book useful."
— *Physical Therapy, Jan '02*

"This resource is recommended as a great reference source for public, health, and academic libraries, and is another triumph for the editors of Omnigraphics."
— *American Reference Books Annual, 2002*

"Recommended for all public libraries and general health collections, especially those supporting patient education or consumer health programs."
— *E-Streams, Nov '01*

"Will prove valuable to any library seeking to maintain a current, comprehensive reference collection of health resources. . . . From prevention to treatment and associated conditions, this provides an excellent survey."
— *The Bookwatch, Aug '01*

"Recommended reference source."
— *Booklist, American Library Association, Jul '01*

SEE ALSO *Healthy Aging Sourcebook, Physical & Mental Issues in Aging Sourcebook, Women's Health Concerns Sourcebook*

▪

Pain Sourcebook, 2nd Edition

Basic Consumer Health Information about Specific Forms of Acute and Chronic Pain, Including Muscle and Skeletal Pain, Nerve Pain, Cancer Pain, and Disorders Characterized by Pain, Such as Fibromyalgia, Shingles, Angina, Arthritis, and Headaches

Along with Information about Pain Medications and Management Techniques, Complementary and Alternative Pain Relief Options, Tips for People Living with Chronic Pain, a Glossary, and a Directory of Sources for Further Information

Edited by Karen Bellenir. 670 pages. 2002. 0-7808-0612-3.

"A source of valuable information. . . . This book offers help to nonmedical people who need information about pain and pain management. It is also an excellent reference for those who participate in patient education."
— *Doody's Review Service, Sep '02*

"Highly recommended for academic and medical reference collections." — *Library Bookwatch, Sep '02*

"The text is readable, easily understood, and well indexed. This excellent volume belongs in all patient education libraries, consumer health sections of public libraries, and many personal collections."
— *American Reference Books Annual, 1999*

"The information is basic in terms of scholarship and is appropriate for general readers. Written in journalistic style . . . intended for non-professionals. Quite thorough in its coverage of different pain conditions and summarizes the latest clinical information regarding pain treatment."
— *Choice, Association of College and Research Libraries, Jun '98*

"Recommended reference source."
— *Booklist, American Library Association, Mar '98*

■

Pediatric Cancer Sourcebook

Basic Consumer Health Information about Leukemias, Brain Tumors, Sarcomas, Lymphomas, and Other Cancers in Infants, Children, and Adolescents, Including Descriptions of Cancers, Treatments, and Coping Strategies

Along with Suggestions for Parents, Caregivers, and Concerned Relatives, a Glossary of Cancer Terms, and Resource Listings

Edited by Edward J. Prucha. 587 pages. 1999. 0-7808-0245-4.

"An excellent source of information. Recommended for public, hospital, and health science libraries with consumer health collections." — *E-Streams, Jun '00*

"Recommended reference source."
— *Booklist, American Library Association, Feb '00*

"A valuable addition to all libraries specializing in health services and many public libraries."
— *American Reference Books Annual, 2000*

SEE ALSO Childhood Diseases & Disorders Sourcebook, Healthy Children Sourcebook

■

Physical & Mental Issues in Aging Sourcebook

Basic Consumer Health Information on Physical and Mental Disorders Associated with the Aging Process, Including Concerns about Cardiovascular Disease, Pulmonary Disease, Oral Health, Digestive Disorders, Musculoskeletal and Skin Disorders, Metabolic Changes, Sexual and Reproductive Issues, and Changes in Vision, Hearing, and Other Senses

Along with Data about Longevity and Causes of Death, Information on Acute and Chronic Pain, Descriptions of Mental Concerns, a Glossary of Terms, and Resource Listings for Additional Help

Edited by Jenifer Swanson. 660 pages. 1999. 0-7808-0233-0.

"This is a treasure of health information for the layperson." — *Choice Health Sciences Supplement, Association of College & Research Libraries, May '00*

"Recommended for public libraries."
— *American Reference Books Annual, 2000*

"Recommended reference source."
— *Booklist, American Library Association, Oct '99*

SEE ALSO Healthy Aging Sourcebook

Podiatry Sourcebook

Basic Consumer Health Information about Foot Conditions, Diseases, and Injuries, Including Bunions, Corns, Calluses, Athlete's Foot, Plantar Warts, Hammertoes and Clawtoes, Clubfoot, Heel Pain, Gout, and More

Along with Facts about Foot Care, Disease Prevention, Foot Safety, Choosing a Foot Care Specialist, a Glossary of Terms, and Resource Listings for Additional Information

Edited by M. Lisa Weatherford. 380 pages. 2001. 0-7808-0215-2.

"Recommended reference source."
— *Booklist, American Library Association, Feb '02*

"There is a lot of information presented here on a topic that is usually only covered sparingly in most larger comprehensive medical encyclopedias."
— *American Reference Books Annual, 2002*

■

Pregnancy & Birth Sourcebook, 2nd Edition

Basic Consumer Health Information about Conception and Pregnancy, Including Facts about Fertility, Infertility, Pregnancy Symptoms and Complications, Fetal Growth and Development, Labor, Delivery, and the Postpartum Period, as Well as Information about Maintaining Health and Wellness during Pregnancy and Caring for a Newborn

Along with Information about Public Health Assistance for Low-Income Pregnant Women, a Glossary, and Directories of Agencies and Organizations Providing Help and Support

Edited by Amy L. Sutton. 626 pages. 2004. 0-7808-0672-7.

"Will appeal to public and school reference collections strong in medicine and women's health. . . . Deserves a spot on any medical reference shelf."
— *The Bookwatch, Jul '04*

"A well-organized handbook. Recommended."
— *Choice, Association of College & Research Libraries, Apr '98*

"Recommended reference source."
— *Booklist, American Library Association, Mar '98*

"Recommended for public libraries."
— *American Reference Books Annual, 1998*

SEE ALSO Breastfeeding Sourcebook, Congenital Disorders Sourcebook, Family Planning Sourcebook

■

Prostate Cancer Sourcebook

Basic Consumer Health Information about Prostate Cancer, Including Information about the Associated Risk Factors, Detection, Diagnosis, and Treatment of Prostate Cancer

Along with Information on Non-Malignant Prostate Conditions, and Featuring a Section Listing Support and Treatment Centers and a Glossary of Related Terms

Edited by Dawn D. Matthews. 358 pages. 2001. 0-7808-0324-8.

"Recommended reference source."
— *Booklist, American Library Association, Jan '02*

"A valuable resource for health care consumers seeking information on the subject. . . . All text is written in a clear, easy-to-understand language that avoids technical jargon. Any library that collects consumer health resources would strengthen their collection with the addition of the Prostate Cancer Sourcebook."
— *American Reference Books Annual, 2002*

SEE ALSO Men's Health Concerns Sourcebook

■

Prostate & Urological Disorders Sourcebook

Basic Consumer Health Information about Urogenital and Sexual Disorders in Men, Including Prostate and Other Andrological Cancers, Prostatitis, Benign Prostatic Hyperplasia, Testicular and Penile Trauma, Cryptorchidism, Peyronie Disease, Erectile Dysfunction, and Male Factor Infertility, and Facts about Commonly Used Tests and Procedures, Such as Prostatectomy, Vasectomy, Vasectomy Reversal, Penile Implants, and Semen Analysis

Along with a Glossary of Andrological Terms and a Directory of Resources for Additional Information

Edited by Karen Bellenir. 631 pages. 2005. 0-7808-0797-9.

■

Public Health Sourcebook

Basic Information about Government Health Agencies, Including National Health Statistics and Trends, Healthy People 2000 Program Goals and Objectives, the Centers for Disease Control and Prevention, the Food and Drug Administration, and the National Institutes of Health

Along with Full Contact Information for Each Agency

Edited by Wendy Wilcox. 698 pages. 1998. 0-7808-0220-9.

"Recommended reference source."
— *Booklist, American Library Association, Sep '98*

"This consumer guide provides welcome assistance in navigating the maze of federal health agencies and their data on public health concerns."
— *SciTech Book News, Sep '98*

■

Reconstructive & Cosmetic Surgery Sourcebook

Basic Consumer Health Information on Cosmetic and Reconstructive Plastic Surgery, Including Statistical Information about Different Surgical Procedures, Things to Consider Prior to Surgery, Plastic Surgery Techniques and Tools, Emotional and Psychological Considerations, and Procedure-Specific Information

Along with a Glossary of Terms and a Listing of Resources for Additional Help and Information

Edited by M. Lisa Weatherford. 374 pages. 2001. 0-7808-0214-4.

"An excellent reference that addresses cosmetic and medically necessary reconstructive surgeries. . . . The style of the prose is calm and reassuring, discussing the many positive outcomes now available due to advances in surgical techniques."
— *American Reference Books Annual, 2002*

"Recommended for health science libraries that are open to the public, as well as hospital libraries that are open to the patients. This book is a good resource for the consumer interested in plastic surgery."
— *E-Streams, Dec '01*

"Recommended reference source."
— *Booklist, American Library Association, Jul '01*

■

Rehabilitation Sourcebook

Basic Consumer Health Information about Rehabilitation for People Recovering from Heart Surgery, Spinal Cord Injury, Stroke, Orthopedic Impairments, Amputation, Pulmonary Impairments, Traumatic Injury, and More, Including Physical Therapy, Occupational Therapy, Speech/Language Therapy, Massage Therapy, Dance Therapy, Art Therapy, and Recreational Therapy

Along with Information on Assistive and Adaptive Devices, a Glossary, and Resources for Additional Help and Information

Edited by Dawn D. Matthews. 531 pages. 1999. 0-7808-0236-5.

"This is an excellent resource for public library reference and health collections."
— *American Reference Books Annual, 2001*

"Recommended reference source."
— *Booklist, American Library Association, May '00*

■

Respiratory Diseases & Disorders Sourcebook

Basic Information about Respiratory Diseases and Disorders, Including Asthma, Cystic Fibrosis, Pneumonia, the Common Cold, Influenza, and Others, Featuring Facts about the Respiratory System, Statistical and Demographic Data, Treatments, Self-Help Management Suggestions, and Current Research Initiatives

Edited by Allan R. Cook and Peter D. Dresser. 771 pages. 1995. 0-7808-0037-0.

"Designed for the layperson and for patients and their families coping with respiratory illness. . . . an extensive array of information on diagnosis, treatment, management, and prevention of respiratory illnesses for the general reader."
— *Choice, Association of College & Research Libraries, Jun '96*

"A highly recommended text for all collections. It is a comforting reminder of the power of knowledge that good books carry between their covers."
— *Academic Library Book Review, Spring '96*

"A comprehensive collection of authoritative information presented in a nontechnical, humanitarian style for patients, families, and caregivers."
— *Association of Operating Room Nurses, Sep/Oct '95*

SEE ALSO *Lung Disorders Sourcebook*

Sexually Transmitted Diseases Sourcebook, 3rd Edition

Basic Consumer Health Information about Chlamydial Infections, Gonorrhea, Hepatitis, Herpes, HIV/AIDS, Human Papillomavirus, Pubic Lice, Scabies, Syphilis, Trichomoniasis, Vaginal Infections, and Other Sexually Transmitted Diseases, Including Facts about Risk Factors, Symptoms, Diagnosis, Treatment, and the Prevention of Sexually Transmitted Infections

Along with Updates on Current Research Initiatives, a Glossary of Related Terms, and Resources for Additional Help and Information

Edited by Amy L. Sutton. 629 pages. 2006. 0-7808-0824-X.

"Recommended for consumer health collections in public libraries, and secondary school and community college libraries."
— *American Reference Books Annual, 2002*

"Every school and public library should have a copy of this comprehensive and user-friendly reference book."
— *Choice, Association of College & Research Libraries, Sep '01*

"This is a highly recommended book. This is an especially important book for all school and public libraries."
— *AIDS Book Review Journal, Jul-Aug '01*

"Recommended reference source."
— *Booklist, American Library Association, Apr '01*

Skin Disorders Sourcebook

SEE *Dermatological Disorders Sourcebook, 2nd Edition*

Sleep Disorders Sourcebook, 2nd Edition

Basic Consumer Health Information about Sleep and Sleep Disorders, Including Insomnia, Sleep Apnea, Restless Legs Syndrome, Narcolepsy, Parasomnias, and Other Health Problems That Affect Sleep, Plus Facts about Diagnostic Procedures, Treatment Strategies, Sleep Medications, and Tips for Improving Sleep Quality

Along with a Glossary of Related Terms and Resources for Additional Help and Information

Edited by Amy L. Sutton. 567 pages. 2005. 0-7808-0743-X.

"This book will be useful for just about everybody, especially the 40 million Americans with sleep disorders."
— *American Reference Books Annual, 2006*

"Recommended for public libraries and libraries supporting health care professionals." — *E-Streams, Sep '05*

". . . key medical library acquisition."
— *The Bookwatch, Jun '05*

Smoking Concerns Sourcebook

Basic Consumer Health Information about Nicotine Addiction and Smoking Cessation, Featuring Facts about the Health Effects of Tobacco Use, Including Lung and Other Cancers, Heart Disease, Stroke, and Respiratory Disorders, Such as Emphysema and Chronic Bronchitis

Along with Information about Smoking Prevention Programs, Suggestions for Achieving and Maintaining a Smoke-Free Lifestyle, Statistics about Tobacco Use, Reports on Current Research Initiatives, a Glossary of Related Terms, and Directories of Resources for Additional Help and Information

Edited by Karen Bellenir. 621 pages. 2004. 0-7808-0323-X.

"Provides everything needed for the student or general reader seeking practical details on the effects of tobacco use." — *The Bookwatch, Mar '05*

"Public libraries and consumer health care libraries will find this work useful."
— *American Reference Books Annual, 2005*

Sports Injuries Sourcebook, 2nd Edition

Basic Consumer Health Information about the Diagnosis, Treatment, and Rehabilitation of Common Sports-Related Injuries in Children and Adults

Along with Suggestions for Conditioning and Training, Information and Prevention Tips for Injuries Frequently Associated with Specific Sports and Special Populations, a Glossary, and a Directory of Additional Resources

Edited by Joyce Brennfleck Shannon. 614 pages. 2002. 0-7808-0604-2.

"This is an excellent reference for consumers and it is recommended for public, community college, and undergraduate libraries."
— *American Reference Books Annual, 2003*

"Recommended reference source."
— *Booklist, American Library Association, Feb '03*

Stress-Related Disorders Sourcebook

Basic Consumer Health Information about Stress and Stress-Related Disorders, Including Stress Origins and Signals, Environmental Stress at Work and Home, Mental and Emotional Stress Associated with Depression, Post-Traumatic Stress Disorder, Panic Disorder, Suicide, and the Physical Effects of Stress on the Cardiovascular, Immune, and Nervous Systems

Along with Stress Management Techniques, a Glossary, and a Listing of Additional Resources

Edited by Joyce Brennfleck Shannon. 610 pages. 2002. 0-7808-0560-7.

"Well written for a general readership, the *Stress-Related Disorders Sourcebook* is a useful addition to the health reference literature."
— *American Reference Books Annual, 2003*

"I am impressed by the amount of information. It offers a thorough overview of the causes and consequences of stress for the layperson. . . . A well-done and thorough reference guide for professionals and nonprofessionals alike." — *Doody's Review Service, Dec '02*

■

Stroke Sourcebook

Basic Consumer Health Information about Stroke, Including Ischemic, Hemorrhagic, Transient Ischemic Attack (TIA), and Pediatric Stroke, Stroke Triggers and Risks, Diagnostic Tests, Treatments, and Rehabilitation Information

Along with Stroke Prevention Guidelines, Legal and Financial Information, a Glossary, and a Directory of Additional Resources

Edited by Joyce Brennfleck Shannon. 606 pages. 2003. 0-7808-0630-1.

"This volume is highly recommended and should be in every medical, hospital, and public library."
— *American Reference Books Annual, 2004*

"Highly recommended for the amount and variety of topics and information covered." — *Choice, Nov '03*

■

Substance Abuse Sourcebook

Basic Health-Related Information about the Abuse of Legal and Illegal Substances Such as Alcohol, Tobacco, Prescription Drugs, Marijuana, Cocaine, and Heroin; and Including Facts about Substance Abuse Prevention Strategies, Intervention Methods, Treatment and Recovery Programs, and a Section Addressing the Special Problems Related to Substance Abuse during Pregnancy

Edited by Karen Bellenir. 573 pages. 1996. 0-7808-0038-9.

"A valuable addition to any health reference section. Highly recommended."
— *The Book Report, Mar/Apr '97*

". . . a comprehensive collection of substance abuse information that's both highly readable and compact. Families and caregivers of substance abusers will find the information enlightening and helpful, while teachers, social workers and journalists should benefit from the concise format. Recommended."
— *Drug Abuse Update, Winter '96/'97*

SEE ALSO *Alcoholism Sourcebook, Drug Abuse Sourcebook*

Surgery Sourcebook

Basic Consumer Health Information about Inpatient and Outpatient Surgeries, Including Cardiac, Vascular, Orthopedic, Ocular, Reconstructive, Cosmetic, Gynecologic, and Ear, Nose, and Throat Procedures and More

Along with Information about Operating Room Policies and Instruments, Laser Surgery Techniques, Hospital Errors, Statistical Data, a Glossary, and Listings of Sources for Further Help and Information

Edited by Annemarie S. Muth and Karen Bellenir. 596 pages. 2002. 0-7808-0380-9.

"Large public libraries and medical libraries would benefit from this material in their reference collections."
— *American Reference Books Annual, 2004*

"Invaluable reference for public and school library collections alike." — *Library Bookwatch, Apr '03*

■

Thyroid Disorders Sourcebook

Basic Consumer Health Information about Disorders of the Thyroid and Parathyroid Glands, Including Hypothyroidism, Hyperthyroidism, Graves Disease, Hashimoto Thyroiditis, Thyroid Cancer, and Parathyroid Disorders, Featuring Facts about Symptoms, Risk Factors, Tests, and Treatments

Along with Information about the Effects of Thyroid Imbalance on Other Body Systems, Environmental Factors That Affect the Thyroid Gland, a Glossary, and a Directory of Additional Resources

Edited by Joyce Brennfleck Shannon. 599 pages. 2005. 0-7808-0745-6.

"Recommended for consumer health collections."
— *American Reference Books Annual, 2006*

"Highly recommended pick for basic consumer health reference holdings at all levels."
— *The Bookwatch, Aug '05*

■

Transplantation Sourcebook

Basic Consumer Health Information about Organ and Tissue Transplantation, Including Physical and Financial Preparations, Procedures and Issues Relating to Specific Solid Organ and Tissue Transplants, Rehabilitation, Pediatric Transplant Information, the Future of Transplantation, and Organ and Tissue Donation

Along with a Glossary and Listings of Additional Resources

Edited by Joyce Brennfleck Shannon. 628 pages. 2002. 0-7808-0322-1.

"Along with these advances [in transplantation technology] have come a number of daunting questions for potential transplant patients, their families, and their health care providers. This reference text is the best single tool to address many of these questions. . . . It will be a much-needed addition to the reference collections in health care, academic, and large public libraries."
— *American Reference Books Annual, 2003*

"Recommended for libraries with an interest in offering consumer health information." — E-Streams, Jul '02

"This is a unique and valuable resource for patients facing transplantation and their families."
— Doody's Review Service, Jun '02

■

Traveler's Health Sourcebook

Basic Consumer Health Information for Travelers, Including Physical and Medical Preparations, Transportation Health and Safety, Essential Information about Food and Water, Sun Exposure, Insect and Snake Bites, Camping and Wilderness Medicine, and Travel with Physical or Medical Disabilities

Along with International Travel Tips, Vaccination Recommendations, Geographical Health Issues, Disease Risks, a Glossary, and a Listing of Additional Resources

Edited by Joyce Brennfleck Shannon. 613 pages. 2000. 0-7808-0384-1.

"Recommended reference source."
— Booklist, American Library Association, Feb '01

"This book is recommended for any public library, any travel collection, and especially any collection for the physically disabled."
— American Reference Books Annual, 2001

SEE ALSO Worldwide Health Sourcebook

■

Urinary Tract & Kidney Diseases & Disorders Sourcebook, 2nd Edition

Basic Consumer Health Information about the Urinary System, Including the Bladder, Urethra, Ureters, and Kidneys, with Facts about Urinary Tract Infections, Incontinence, Congenital Disorders, Kidney Stones, Cancers of the Urinary Tract and Kidneys, Kidney Failure, Dialysis, and Kidney Transplantation

Along with Statistical and Demographic Information, Reports on Current Research in Kidney and Urologic Health, a Summary of Commonly Used Diagnostic Tests, a Glossary of Related Terms, and a Directory of Resources for Additional Help and Information

Edited by Ivy L. Alexander. 649 pages. 2005. 0-7808-0750-2.

"A good choice for a consumer health information library or for a medical library needing information to refer to their patients."
— American Reference Books Annual, 2006

■

Vegetarian Sourcebook

Basic Consumer Health Information about Vegetarian Diets, Lifestyle, and Philosophy, Including Definitions of Vegetarianism and Veganism, Tips about Adopting Vegetarianism, Creating a Vegetarian Pantry, and Meeting Nutritional Needs of Vegetarians, with Facts Regarding Vegetarianism's Effect on Pregnant and Lactating Women, Children, Athletes, and Senior Citizens

Along with a Glossary of Commonly Used Vegetarian Terms and Resources for Additional Help and Information

Edited by Chad T. Kimball. 360 pages. 2002. 0-7808-0439-2.

"Organizes into one concise volume the answers to the most common questions concerning vegetarian diets and lifestyles. This title is recommended for public and secondary school libraries." — E-Streams, Apr '03

"Invaluable reference for public and school library collections alike." — Library Bookwatch, Apr '03

"The articles in this volume are easy to read and come from authoritative sources. The book does not necessarily support the vegetarian diet but instead provides the pros and cons of this important decision. The Vegetarian Sourcebook is recommended for public libraries and consumer health libraries."
— American Reference Books Annual, 2003

SEE ALSO Diet & Nutrition Sourcebook

■

Women's Health Concerns Sourcebook, 2nd Edition

Basic Consumer Health Information about the Medical and Mental Concerns of Women, Including Maintaining Health and Wellness, Gynecological Concerns, Breast Health, Sexuality and Reproductive Issues, Menopause, Cancer in Women, Leading Causes of Death and Disability among Women, Physical Concerns of Special Significance to Women, and Women's Mental and Emotional Health

Along with a Glossary of Related Terms and Directories of Resources for Additional Help and Information

Edited by Amy L. Sutton. 746 pages. 2004. 0-7808-0673-5.

"This is a useful reference book, which makes the reader knowledgeable about several issues that concern women's health. It is recommended for public libraries and home library collections." — E-Streams, May '05

"A useful addition to public and consumer health library collections."
— American Reference Books Annual, 2005

"A highly recommended title."
— The Bookwatch, May '04

"Handy compilation. There is an impressive range of diseases, devices, disorders, procedures, and other physical and emotional issues covered . . . well organized, illustrated, and indexed." — Choice, Association of College & Research Libraries, Jan '98

SEE ALSO Breast Cancer Sourcebook, Cancer Sourcebook for Women, Healthy Heart Sourcebook for Women, Osteoporosis Sourcebook

Workplace Health & Safety Sourcebook

Basic Consumer Health Information about Workplace Health and Safety, Including the Effect of Workplace Hazards on the Lungs, Skin, Heart, Ears, Eyes, Brain, Reproductive Organs, Musculoskeletal System, and Other Organs and Body Parts

Along with Information about Occupational Cancer, Personal Protective Equipment, Toxic and Hazardous Chemicals, Child Labor, Stress, and Workplace Violence

Edited by Chad T. Kimball. 626 pages. 2000. 0-7808-0231-4.

"As a reference for the general public, this would be useful in any library." —*E-Streams, Jun '01*

"Provides helpful information for primary care physicians and other caregivers interested in occupational medicine. . . . General readers; professionals."
—*Choice, Association of College & Research Libraries, May '01*

"Recommended reference source."
—*Booklist, American Library Association, Feb '01*

"Highly recommended." —*The Bookwatch, Jan '01*

Worldwide Health Sourcebook

Basic Information about Global Health Issues, Including Malnutrition, Reproductive Health, Disease Dispersion and Prevention, Emerging Diseases, Risky Health Behaviors, and the Leading Causes of Death

Along with Global Health Concerns for Children, Women, and the Elderly, Mental Health Issues, Research and Technology Advancements, and Economic, Environmental, and Political Health Implications, a Glossary, and a Resource Listing for Additional Help and Information

Edited by Joyce Brennfleck Shannon. 614 pages. 2001. 0-7808-0330-2.

"Named an Outstanding Academic Title."
—*Choice, Association of College & Research Libraries, Jan '02*

"Yet another handy but also unique compilation in the extensive Health Reference Series, this is a useful work because many of the international publications reprinted or excerpted are not readily available. Highly recommended." —*Choice, Association of College & Research Libraries, Nov '01*

"Recommended reference source."
—*Booklist, American Library Association, Oct '01*

SEE ALSO *Traveler's Health Sourcebook*

Teen Health Series
Helping Young Adults Understand, Manage, and Avoid Serious Illness

List price $65 per volume. **School and library price $58 per volume.**

Alcohol Information for Teens
Health Tips about Alcohol and Alcoholism
Including Facts about Underage Drinking, Preventing Teen Alcohol Use, Alcohol's Effects on the Brain and the Body, Alcohol Abuse Treatment, Help for Children of Alcoholics, and More

Edited by Joyce Brennfleck Shannon. 370 pages. 2005. 0-7808-0741-3.

"Boxed facts and tips add visual interest to the well-researched and clearly written text."
— *Curriculum Connection, Apr '06*

Allergy Information for Teens
Health Tips about Allergic Reactions Such as Anaphylaxis, Respiratory Problems, and Rashes
Including Facts about Identifying and Managing Allergies to Food, Pollen, Mold, Animals, Chemicals, Drugs, and Other Substances

Edited by Karen Bellenir. 410 pages. 2006. 0-7808-0799-5.

Asthma Information for Teens
Health Tips about Managing Asthma and Related Concerns
Including Facts about Asthma Causes, Triggers, Symptoms, Diagnosis, and Treatment

Edited by Karen Bellenir. 386 pages. 2005. 0-7808-0770-7.

"Highly recommended for medical libraries, public school libraries, and public libraries."
— *American Reference Books Annual, 2006*

"It is so clearly written and well organized that even hesitant readers will be able to find the facts they need, whether for reports or personal information. . . . A succinct but complete resource."
— *School Library Journal, Sep '05*

Cancer Information for Teens
Health Tips about Cancer Awareness, Prevention, Diagnosis, and Treatment
Including Facts about Frequently Occurring Cancers, Cancer Risk Factors, and Coping Strategies for Teens Fighting Cancer or Dealing with Cancer in Friends or Family Members

Edited by Wilma R. Caldwell. 428 pages. 2004. 0-7808-0678-6.

"Recommended for school libraries, or consumer libraries that see a lot of use by teens."
— *E-Streams, May 2005*

"A valuable educational tool."
— *American Reference Books Annual, 2005*

"Young adults and their parents alike will find this new addition to the *Teen Health Series* an important reference to cancer in teens."
— *Children's Bookwatch, Feb '05*

Complementary and Alternative Medicine Information for Teens
Health Tips about Non-Traditional and Non-Western Medical Practices
Including Information about Acupuncture, Chiropractic Medicine, Dietary and Herbal Supplements, Hypnosis, Massage Therapy, Prayer and Spirituality, Reflexology, Yoga, and More

Edited by Sandra Augustyn Lawton. 405 pages. 2006. 0-7808-0966-1.

Diabetes Information for Teens
Health Tips about Managing Diabetes and Preventing Related Complications
Including Information about Insulin, Glucose Control, Healthy Eating, Physical Activity, and Learning to Live with Diabetes

Edited by Sandra Augustyn Lawton. 410 pages. 2006. 0-7808-0811-8.

Diet Information for Teens, 2nd Edition
Health Tips about Diet and Nutrition
Including Facts about Dietary Guidelines, Food Groups, Nutrients, Healthy Meals, Snacks, Weight Control, Medical Concerns Related to Diet, and More

Edited by Karen Bellenir. 432 pages. 2006. 0-7808-0820-7.

"Full of helpful insights and facts throughout the book. . . . An excellent resource to be placed in public libraries or even in personal collections."
— *American Reference Books Annual, 2002*

"Recommended for middle and high school libraries and media centers as well as academic libraries that educate future teachers of teenagers. It is also a suitable addition to health science libraries that serve patrons who are interested in teen health promotion and education."
— *E-Streams, Oct '01*

"This comprehensive book would be beneficial to collections that need information about nutrition, dietary guidelines, meal planning, and weight control. . . . This reference is so easy to use that its purchase is recommended."
— *The Book Report, Sep-Oct '01*

"This book is written in an easy to understand format describing issues that many teens face every day, and then provides thoughtful explanations so that teens can make informed decisions. This is an interesting book that provides important facts and information for today's teens."
— *Doody's Health Sciences Book Review Journal, Jul-Aug '01*

"A comprehensive compendium of diet and nutrition. The information is presented in a straightforward, plain-spoken manner. This title will be useful to those working on reports on a variety of topics, as well as to general readers concerned about their dietary health."
— *School Library Journal, Jun '01*

Drug Information for Teens, 2nd Edition

Health Tips about the Physical and Mental Effects of Substance Abuse

Including Information about Marijuana, Inhalants, Club Drugs, Stimulants, Hallucinogens, Opiates, Prescription and Over-the-Counter Drugs, Herbal Products, Tobacco, Alcohol, and More

Edited by Sandra Augustyn Lawton. 468 pages. 2006. 0-7808-0862-2.

"A clearly written resource for general readers and researchers alike."
— *School Library Journal*

"This book is well-balanced. . . . a must for public and school libraries."
— *VOYA: Voice of Youth Advocates, Dec '03*

"The chapters are quick to make a connection to their teenage reading audience. The prose is straightforward and the book lends itself to spot reading. It should be useful both for practical information and for research, and it is suitable for public and school libraries."
— *American Reference Books Annual, 2003*

"Recommended reference source."
— *Booklist, American Library Association, Feb '03*

"This is an excellent resource for teens and their parents. Education about drugs and substances is key to discouraging teen drug abuse and this book provides this much needed information in a way that is interesting and factual."
— *Doody's Review Service, Dec '02*

Eating Disorders Information for Teens

Health Tips about Anorexia, Bulimia, Binge Eating, and Other Eating Disorders

Including Information on the Causes, Prevention, and Treatment of Eating Disorders, and Such Other Issues as Maintaining Healthy Eating and Exercise Habits

Edited by Sandra Augustyn Lawton. 337 pages. 2005. 0-7808-0783-9.

"An excellent resource for teens and those who work with them."
— *VOYA: Voice of Youth Advocates, Apr '06*

"A welcome addition to high school and undergraduate libraries." — *American Reference Books Annual, 2006*

"This book covers the topic in a lucid manner but delves deeper into every aspect of an eating disorder. A solid addition for any nonfiction or reference collection."
— *School Library Journal, Dec '05*

Fitness Information for Teens

Health Tips about Exercise, Physical Well-Being, and Health Maintenance

Including Facts about Aerobic and Anaerobic Conditioning, Stretching, Body Shape and Body Image, Sports Training, Nutrition, and Activities for Non-Athletes

Edited by Karen Bellenir. 425 pages. 2004. 0-7808-0679-4.

"Another excellent offering from Omnigraphics in their *Teen Health Series*. . . . This book will be a great addition to any public, junior high, senior high, or secondary school library."
— *American Reference Books Annual, 2005*

Learning Disabilities Information for Teens

Health Tips about Academic Skills Disorders and Other Disabilities That Affect Learning

Including Information about Common Signs of Learning Disabilities, School Issues, Learning to Live with a Learning Disability, and Other Related Issues

Edited by Sandra Augustyn Lawton. 337 pages. 2005. 0-7808-0796-0.

"This book provides a wealth of information for any reader interested in the signs, causes, and consequences of learning disabilities, as well as related legal rights and educational interventions. . . . Public and academic libraries should want this title for both students and general readers."
— *American Reference Books Annual, 2006*

Mental Health Information for Teens, 2nd Edition

Health Tips about Mental Wellness and Mental Illness

Including Facts about Mental and Emotional Health, Depression and Other Mood Disorders, Anxiety Disorders, Behavior Disorders, Self-Injury, Psychosis, Schizophrenia, and More

Edited by Karen Bellenir. 400 pages. 2006. 0-7808-0863-0.

"In both language and approach, this user-friendly entry in the *Teen Health Series* is on target for teens needing information on mental health concerns."
— *Booklist, American Library Association, Jan '02*

"Readers will find the material accessible and informative, with the shaded notes, facts, and embedded glossary insets adding appropriately to the already interesting and succinct presentation."
— *School Library Journal, Jan '02*

"This title is highly recommended for any library that serves adolescents and parents/caregivers of adolescents." — *E-Streams, Jan '02*

"Recommended for high school libraries and young adult collections in public libraries. Both health professionals and teenagers will find this book useful."
— *American Reference Books Annual, 2002*

"This is a nice book written to enlighten the society, primarily teenagers, about common teen mental health issues. It is highly recommended to teachers and parents as well as adolescents."
— *Doody's Review Service, Dec '01*

Sexual Health Information for Teens

Health Tips about Sexual Development, Human Reproduction, and Sexually Transmitted Diseases

Including Facts about Puberty, Reproductive Health, Chlamydia, Human Papillomavirus, Pelvic Inflammatory Disease, Herpes, AIDS, Contraception, Pregnancy, and More

Edited by Deborah A. Stanley. 391 pages. 2003. 0-7808-0445-7.

"This work should be included in all high school libraries and many larger public libraries. . . . highly recommended."
— *American Reference Books Annual, 2004*

"Sexual Health approaches its subject with appropriate seriousness and offers easily accessible advice and information." — *School Library Journal, Feb '04*

Skin Health Information for Teens

Health Tips about Dermatological Concerns and Skin Cancer Risks

Including Facts about Acne, Warts, Hives, and Other Conditions and Lifestyle Choices, Such as Tanning, Tattooing, and Piercing, That Affect the Skin, Nails, Scalp, and Hair

Edited by Robert Aquinas McNally. 429 pages. 2003. 0-7808-0446-5.

"This volume, as with others in the series, will be a useful addition to school and public library collections." — *American Reference Books Annual, 2004*

"There is no doubt that this reference tool is valuable."
— *VOYA: Voice of Youth Advocates, Feb '04*

"This volume serves as a one-stop source and should be a necessity for any health collection."
— *Library Media Connection*

Sports Injuries Information for Teens

Health Tips about Sports Injuries and Injury Protection

Including Facts about Specific Injuries, Emergency Treatment, Rehabilitation, Sports Safety, Competition Stress, Fitness, Sports Nutrition, Steroid Risks, and More

Edited by Joyce Brennfleck Shannon. 405 pages. 2003. 0-7808-0447-3.

"This work will be useful in the young adult collections of public libraries as well as high school libraries."
— *American Reference Books Annual, 2004*

Suicide Information for Teens

Health Tips about Suicide Causes and Prevention

Including Facts about Depression, Risk Factors, Getting Help, Survivor Support, and More

Edited by Joyce Brennfleck Shannon. 368 pages. 2005. 0-7808-0737-5.

Tobacco Information for Teens

Health Tips about the Hazards of Using Cigarettes, Smokeless Tobacco, and Other Nicotine Products

Including Facts about Nicotine Addiction, Immediate and Long-Term Health Effects of Tobacco Use, Related Cancers, Smoking Cessation, Tobacco Use Prevention, and Tobacco Use Statistics

Edited by Karen Bellenir. 430 pages. 2007. 0-7808-0976-9.

Health Reference Series

Adolescent Health Sourcebook,
2nd Edition

AIDS Sourcebook, 3rd Edition

Alcoholism Sourcebook, 2nd Edition

Allergies Sourcebook, 2nd Edition

Alzheimer's Disease Sourcebook,
3rd Edition

Arthritis Sourcebook, 2nd Edition

Asthma Sourcebook, 2nd Edition

Attention Deficit Disorder Sourcebook

Back & Neck Sourcebook, 2nd Edition

Blood & Circulatory Disorders
Sourcebook, 2nd Edition

Brain Disorders Sourcebook, 2nd Edition

Breast Cancer Sourcebook, 2nd Edition

Breastfeeding Sourcebook

Burns Sourcebook

Cancer Sourcebook, 4th Edition

Cancer Sourcebook for Women,
3rd Edition

Cardiovascular Diseases & Disorders
Sourcebook, 3rd Edition

Caregiving Sourcebook

Child Abuse Sourcebook

Childhood Diseases & Disorders
Sourcebook

Colds, Flu & Other Common Ailments
Sourcebook

Communication Disorders Sourcebook

Complementary & Alternative Medicine
Sourcebook, 3rd Edition

Congenital Disorders Sourcebook,
2nd Edition

Consumer Issues in Health Care
Sourcebook

Contagious Diseases Sourcebook

Contagious & Non-Contagious Infectious
Diseases Sourcebook

Death & Dying Sourcebook, 2nd Edition

Dental Care & Oral Health Sourcebook,
2nd Edition

Depression Sourcebook

Dermatological Disorders Sourcebook,
2nd Edition

Diabetes Sourcebook, 3rd Edition

Diet & Nutrition Sourcebook,
3rd Edition

Digestive Diseases & Disorder
Sourcebook

Disabilities Sourcebook

Domestic Violence Sourcebook,
2nd Edition

Drug Abuse Sourcebook, 2nd Edition

Ear, Nose & Throat Disorders
Sourcebook, 2nd Edition

Eating Disorders Sourcebook

Emergency Medical Services Sourcebook

Endocrine & Metabolic Disorders
Sourcebook

Environmentally Health Sourcebook,
2nd Edition

Ethnic Diseases Sourcebook

Eye Care Sourcebook, 2nd Edition

Family Planning Sourcebook

Fitness & Exercise Sourcebook,
3rd Edition

Food & Animal Borne Diseases
Sourcebook

Food Safety Sourcebook

Forensic Medicine Sourcebook

Gastrointestinal Diseases & Disorders
Sourcebook, 2nd Edition

Genetic Disorders Sourcebook,
3rd Edition

Head Trauma Sourcebook

Headache Sourcebook

Health Insurance Sourcebook

Healthy Aging Sourcebook

Healthy Children Sourcebook

Healthy Heart Sourcebook for Women

Hepatitis Sourcebook

Household Safety Sourcebook

Hypertension Sourcebook

Immune System Disorders Sourcebook,
2nd Edition